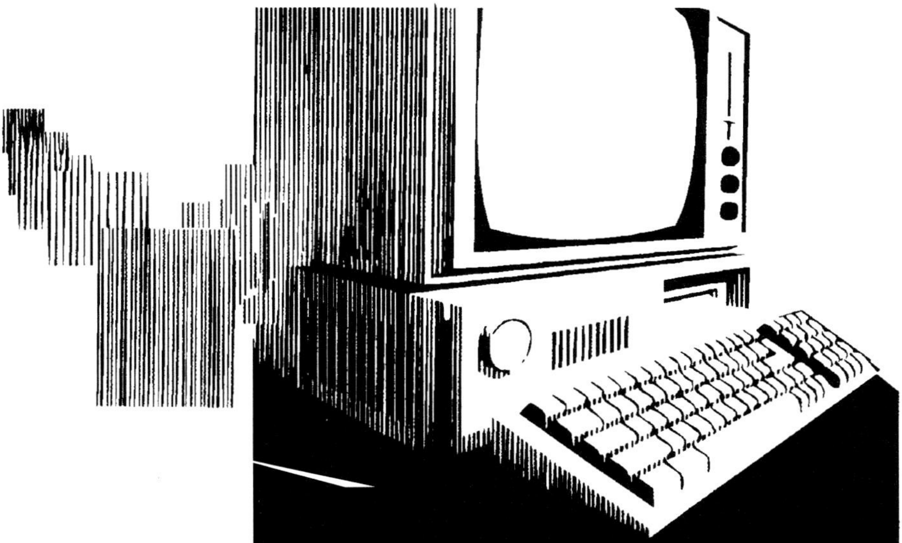

THE
13th CONFERENCE
ON
COMPUTER
APPLICATIONS
IN
RADIOLOGY

SCAR 96

SYMPOSIUM FOR COMPUTER APPLICATIONS IN RADIOLOGY

This program is jointly sponsored by the American College of Radiology and the Society for Computer Applications in Radiology (SCAR)

DENVER, COLORADO
JUNE 6–9, 1996

SCAR 96

COMPUTER APPLICATIONS TO ASSIST RADIOLOGY

Editors

Ray F. Kilcoyne, M.D., F.A.C.R.
Professor of Radiology and Orthopaedics
Vice-Chairman, Department of Radiology
University of Colorado Health Sciences Center,
Denver, Colorado

James L. Lear, M.D.
Professor of Radiology
University of Colorado Health Sciences Center,
Denver, Colorado

Alan H. Rowberg, M.D.
Associate Professor of Radiology
University of Washington,
Seattle, Washington

Published by

Symposia Foundation

A Public Non-Profit Organization Dedicated to the Health Care of the Public

Founded 1979

University of Colorado
Health Sciences Center (UCHSC)

Planning Committee

Ray F. Kilcoyne, M.D., F.A.C.R. – Chairman

Mary Ann Hamm
Jim Lear, M.D.
John Lewin, M.D.
Michael Manco-Johnson, M.D.
Morgan Nields
Ann Scherzinger, Ph.D.
Victor Spitzer, Ph.D.
Steve Swanson

RISC & SCAR Staff

Anna Marie Mason	– Executive Director
Pamela Mechler	– Senior Meeting Manager
Vickie Giannotti	– Administrative Assistant

This book produced directly from camera ready mechanicals furnished by the authors.

Symposia Foundation
P.O. Box 2107
Carlsbad, CA 92018
Telephone: (619) 632-8882

Library of Congress Catalog Card Number 90-643663
International Standard Book Number 0-88372-005-1

Printed in the United States of America

S/CAR 96 Program Committee

Program Chair

Ray F. Kilcoyne, M.D.
University of Colorado Health Sciences Center
Denver, Colorado

Organizing Committee

Michael L. Manco-Johnson, M.D.
University of Colorado Health Sciences Center
Denver, Colorado

Morgan Nields
Fischer Imaging Corporation
Denver, Colorado

Scientific Program

Alan H. Rowberg, M.D.
University of Washington
Seattle, Washington

James L. Lear, M.D.
University of Colorado Health Sciences Center
Denver, Colorado

Tutorials

Steven C. Horii, M.D.
University of Pennsylvania Medical Center
Philadelphia, Pennsylvania

Joseph N. Gitlin, D.P.H.
Johns Hopkins Hospital School of Medicine
Baltimore, Maryland

Poster Session/ Demonstrations

John M. Lewin, M.D.
University of Colorado Health Sciences Center
Denver, Colorado

Technical Exhibits

John Vanden Brink
Technology Marketing Group
Des Plaines, Illinois

John M. Boehme, Ph.D.
Bowman Gray School of Medicine
Winston-Salem, North Carolina

1996 EXHIBITORS/SPONSORS

ADAC HealthCare Information Systems

Agfa Medical, Bayer Corporation

Algotec Systems, Ltd.

CEMAX-ICON

DeJarnette Research Systems

Dictaphone Corporation

Eastman Kodak Company

EMED

Fischer Imaging Corporation

Fuji Medical Systems USA, Inc.

GE Medical Systems

Howtek, Inc.

Kurzweil Applied Intelligence, Inc.

Philips Medical Systems

Siemens Medical Systems, Inc.

Shared Medical Systems (SMS)

Sterling Diagnostic Imaging, Inc.

Storage Technology Group

TeleMedicine and TeleHealth Networks

VIDAR Systems Corporation

REVIEWERS OF PROFFERED PAPERS

Robert Allman, M.D.
Katherine Andriole, Ph.D.
David Avrin, M.D., Ph.D.
Daniel Bednarek, Ph.D.
F.H.Barneveld Binkhuysen, M.D.
John Boehme, Ph.D.
Davide Caramella, M.D.
Anna K. Chacko, M.D.
Robert Choplin, M.D.
David Clunie, M.B., B.S.
Philip Drew, Ph.D.
Bob Gaylor, M.D.
Nancy Giacobbe, M.D.
Lynwood Givens, Ph.D.
Mark Goldberg, M.D.
Ben Harmon, M.D.
Janice Honeyman, Ph.D.
Tim Hunter, M.D.
R. Gilbert Jost, M.D.
Kenidrizo Kajwawa, M.D.
Ray F. Kilcoyne M.D.
Edmond Knopp, M.D.
Elizabeth Krupinski, Ph.D.
Richard Morin, Ph.D.
Lawrence J. Moss, M.D.
Marilyn Noz, Ph.D.
Chul Paik, Ph.D.
William Pavlicek, Ph.D.
David Pickens, Ph.D.
David W. Piraino, M.D.
George Popky, M.D.
Michael Richardson, M.D.
Monica Rivera, M.D.
Eliot Siegel, M.D.
Walid Tohme, Ph.D.
Douglas Tucker, Ph.D.
Paul Weiss, M.D.
Lawrence Williams, Ph.D.
Byrn Williamson, M.D.
Robert Witt, Ph.D.
Beverly P. Wood, M.D.
Akiteru Yoshikawa, M.D.
Jeremy Young, M.D.

COOPERATING ORGANIZATIONS

Society for Computer Applications in Radiology

Radiology Information System Consortium

American College of Radiology

International Society of Optical Engineering

Society of Nuclear Medicine

NEXT MEETING

Beginning in 1996, the symposium will become an annual meeting. Mark your calendar as follows:

SCAR 97
Mayo Clinic
June 22-25, 1997
Rochester, Minnesota

Introduction

Background

The 13th Conference on Computer Applications in Radiology is one of a series of meetings which began in 1964 in cooperation with the American College of Radiology (ACR). These symposia emphasize recent developments related to medical imaging with particular attention to advances in computer technology that affect information systems, image management and communication networks.

Beginning with the 9th Conference, held in Hilton Head, South Carolina in 1988, and continuing through S/CAR 96 hosted this year by the University of Colorado Health Sciences Center in Denver, Colorado, the meeting's primary supporting organizations have been the Radiology Information System Consortium (RISC) and the Society for Computer Applications in Radiology (SCAR). RISC is an organization of university affiliated medical centers and community hospitals dedicated to stimulating the application of computer science and telecommunications technology to medical imaging. SCAR, an organization sponsored by RISC, is composed of individual and corporate members interested in the exchange of technical and scientific information related to the use of computers in radiology.

Beginning in 1996, the symposium will become an annual meeting. The next meeting, SCAR 97, will take place June 22-25, 1997, in Rochester, Minnesota hosted by the Mayo Clinic.

S/CAR Program

This year's program consists of tutorials, invited speakers, scientific presentations, technical exhibits, poster sessions and computer-based demonstrations. The meeting will be held in its entirety at the Marriott City Center Hotel in downtown Denver.

Tutorials

A series of ten tutorials in two concurrent sessions are planned for the meeting. These cover a broad range of topics related to PACS, image manipulation and standardization, and computer privacy issues. Outstanding experts in the several specialized fields related to medical imaging and informatics will present current information on the topics and participate in question and answer sessions. Among the selected subjects, the regulation of medical software by the FDA, and recent changes in telecommunication policies will highlight the early tutorials. Later sessions include strategic thinking and quality assurance in medical imaging and progress in the development of the computer-based patient record.

Current Federal Projects

The opening scientific program session will include an exploration of current federal projects related to digital imaging. Filmless teleradiology will be an important part of the medical practice of the future. Government programs in military medical facilities that are based on technological advances in computers and telecommunications will be presented. Several programs supported by the National Cancer Institute to determine the utility of computer-assisted radiology will be described and a preliminary assessment will be discussed. This session will conclude with a discussion of the transfer of defense, intelligence, and space technologies to health care.

Teaching Applications

While teaching applications have been of great interest since the early days of the use of computers in radiology, it has been the widespread availability of personal computers with good image display capability which has allowed a large expansion of these capabilities. In addition, the more recent development of multimedia capability has allowed 3-D displays, addition of sound and more graphics, and the use of larger datasets. The integration of these capabilities with the clinical workstation is the next logical step in this progression.

Information Management

While the RIS was the site of the first widespread use of computers in radiology, it continues to be an area of growth. Recent improvements are in the area of integration with other information management systems, and using the information in quality assurance and other areas more generalized than the patient encounter and its transactions.

PACS and Archiving

The issues surrounding image archiving continue to be central to PACS implementation, with both better methods of data compression and better data storage hardware providing more overall capability, higher levels of integration, and the possibility of cost reduction.

Digital Mammography

The use of digital imaging techniques in mammography is growing rapidly, with the development of new image receptors as well as new techniques for acquiring and processing the images. In this area of growing clinical need and public visibility, there are opportunities for innovation in digital imaging.

DICOM/RIS/HIS

The clinical availability of systems which can use DICOM is leading to new opportunities to connect more equipment, creating more interest in integrating different types of systems, and providing a higher level of functionality. Management of information is replacing communication of data.

Workstation Design

Because the radiologists' contact with the PACS is at the workstation, there is a great deal of interest in how convenient, fast and reliable the workstation is in assisting in patient care, through several interpretation and communication processes. More tools and a wider variety of capabilities may lead to more efficiency.

Expert Systems/Artificial Intelligence/Speech Recognition

Faster processing speeds are leading to the ability for more sophistication in algorithms at the lowest levels, and giving more capability to the radiologist at the highest levels. Neural network techniques can now be applied in many environments, and speech recognition is fast and accurate. The next step is determining how these capabilities can best be used and integrated into clinical practice.

Telemedicine

While the public interest in telemedicine now far exceeds teleradiology, partially because of the wider visibility of telemedicine, serious issues of evaluation must be solved. There is a great deal of interest in diagnostic accuracy of the overall process, and in using faster networks, multimedia, and videoconferencing. Reports of experiences which cover more than one year will provide insight into the eventual role of these technologies in healthcare.

PACS Integration

As PACS is integrated with the process of healthcare delivery in multiple areas outside radiology, the total system allows measurement of diagnostic impact, utilization, and effectiveness.

Image Processing

Faster processing makes more applications possible in the clinical environment, and leads to issues of evaluation. Physiological measurements are possible in several areas, and newer display techniques give expanded capability, but make more demands on the image processing algorithms. It may take a large amount of automation to make many of these processes fast enough for routine clinical use.

21st Century Telemedicine

The topics of Telemedicine, the Visible Human Project, and Virtual Reality in Medicine have all captured the imaginations of the general public, as well as healthcare practitioners. This session focuses on the present and future in these areas, and how they may impact the practice of medicine.

Alan H. Rowberg, M.D.
Associate Professor
of Radiology
University of Washington,
Seattle, WA

Ray F. Kilcoyne, M.D.
Professor of Radiology
and Orthopaedics
Vice-Chair, Department of Radiology
University of Colorado Health
Sciences Center, Denver, CO

Contents

TUTORIALS

SESSION 1
Teaching Applications

SESSION 2
Information Management

SESSION 3
PACS and Archiving

SESSION 4
Digital Mammography

SESSION 5
DICOM / HIS / RIS

SESSION 6
Workstation Design

SESSION 8
Telemedicine

SESSION 9
PACS Integration

SESSION 10
Image Processing

FOCUS SESSION
21st Century Telemedicine

POSTERS AND DEMONSTRATIONS

Tutorials

Everything You Need to Know About FDA Regulation of PACS Equipment

Loren A. Zaremba and Mary P. Anderson
Center for Devices and Radiological Health, Food and Drug Administration, Rockville, Maryland

I. Introduction

The term "picture archiving and communications systems (PACS)" is used to describe an extremely diverse array of radiology products with wide differences in their intended use and technical characteristics. Consequently, it is not suprising that, although these products have been on the market for some time, there is still some confusion amongst manufacturers and purchasers regarding when, how and why they are regulated by the Food and Drug Administration (FDA). The purpose of this tutorial is to present an overview of medical device regulation by the FDA, and how this scheme is applied to PACS. A few of the more frequently asked questions and misconceptions regarding FDA's regulation of PACS will be addressed. Also, the major safety and effectiveness issues and some possible future changes in FDA's regulatory requirements for these products will be discussed.

II. Regulation of PACS by the FDA

The FDA's Center for Devices and Radiological Health (CDRH) has the responsibility for assuring the safety, effectiveness and proper labeling of medical devices. For most new medical devices the premarket (section 510(k)) notification procedure, provides the mechanism by which they are brought to market. CDRH evaluates the notification and determines if the product is substantially equivalent to a legally marketed device. If not, the device is evaluated through a more stringent process called premarket approval, which requires evidence of safety and effectiveness.

Radiology devices such as radiographic and fluoroscopic x-ray machines, x-ray computed tomography scanners, nuclear medicine scanners, diagnostic ultrasound devices and magnetic resonance imaging systems, which are used to produce medical images, have always been considered to be Class II medical devices requiring premarket notification. Most PACS products did not exist when the radiological device classifications were first proposed in 1982. However, CDRH has been treating them as accessories to the imaging modalities with which they are used. Consequently, premarket notification has been required to bring these devices to market.

CDRH developed a guidance document for the submission of premarket notifications for PACS devices in 1991, which it updated in August 1993. This document outlines the suggested information for a premarket notification for PACS devices and related components in order to enable the evaluation of substantial equivalence. Although there are no formal classifications for PACS, product codes have been developed for recordkeeping purposes. Currently, there are five categories of PACS products; image digitizers (video frame grabbers and film scanners), communications devices (networks, gateways and interfaces), storage devices (digital memory, tape and disk), hardcopy devices (multiformat cameras and laser imagers), and image processing systems (workstations, monitors and image processing software).

III. Frequent Questions

A number of devices which are utilized in the transmission, storage or display of medical images are similar to products which are used to perform related functions for non-medical images. General purpose imaging or telecommunications products which are not promoted for use in medicine are not considered to be medical devices. Medical products have emerged which are intended to perform bookeeping functions such as patient billing. Also, there are expert systems which catalogue symptoms and diseases for reference by physicians, much like a medical textbook. These systems do not handle the medical images of individual patients, and are not considered to be radiology devices.

We have been frequently asked if standalone software products which are marketed for use on a purchaser's own personal computer are subject to regulation. A software product is not exempt from regulation simply because it consists of a set of instructions, rather than tangible hardware. If it meets the definition of a medical device it may be subject to regulation. Recently, we have been asked by companies if a premarket notification must be submitted for a system which is comprised of components for which marketing clearance has been obtained by their original manufacturers. This is not necessary since the FDA has already evaluated the components.

A number of persons appear to be under the impression that the FDA does not allow the use of lossy (irreversible) compression. This is not the case. However, we do recommend that images which have been subjected to lossy compression bear a label advising the user of this along with the approximate compression ratio.

IV. Possible Future Changes

In August of 1994 we presented a set of proposed classifications for PACS at a public meeting of the Radiology Devices Panel. We expect that this proposal will be published in the Federal Register for public comment in the very near future. We encourage all interested parties to examine and comment on this proposal.

The Internet and Advanced Telecommunications for Medical Imaging

Dr. Peter D. Bergstrom, Vice President and
Frank E. Ferrante, Senior Principal Engineer
Center for Information Systems, Mitretek Systems, Inc., McLean, Virginia

I. INTRODUCTION

Within the past five years the World Wide Web[1] has become the most explosive application on the Internet; it is second only to electronic mail. As of early this year over 50 million users existed on the Internet. Correspondingly, Web sites have grown from 100,000 in August of `95 to more than 450,000 this past month and are continuing to grow exponentially. As a result, the Internet and its Web applications, once used primarily by experienced computer scientists, engineers, and hackers, are now becoming household words.

Within the radiology community, as well as within all of the professional medical disciplines, a change in the paradigm of how medicine of the future will be practiced is foreseen as inevitable. The distributed intelligence offered by a high speed World Wide Web offering is expected to allow multi-billions of characters of information (voice, video, and high resolution imaging and data) to be processed rapidly through individual channels among a diverse set of user facilities. To accommodate the future that is foreseen, high speed, multi-media transmission systems, coupled with enhanced processing capabilities of Pentium-speed desktop computers, all at low cost to the users, are needed.

This tutorial examines the current status of the Internet and its popular application, the World Wide Web, and reviews advances in telecommunications and information processing technologies that are expected to impact both everyday medical practice as well as the specialized field of radiology and its corresponding information dissemination.

The tutorial will focus on the changes that are occurring in the Internet and how these in-turn are being viewed as positive factors related to the processing of high resolution radiological images. A brief review will be given of the Internet

---

[1] For WWW history, see http://www.w3.org/hypertext/WWW/History.html

design and of the corresponding broadband design being used by the National Science Foundation to interface their national laboratories across the nation. Terms will be defined such as Asynchronous Transfer Mode (ATM) and Synchronous Optical Network (SONET) so that open discussion and relationships of these new technologies can be discussed. Collaborative computing tools, now available to support the high resolution image transfers at giga-bit per second transmission rates offered through ATM applications, will be illustrated. Information will be provided on data requirements needed to represent a variety of commonly used medical data ranging from the basic ultrasound signaling that requires but a few thousands of characters (bytes) to mammography images which require more than 24 million characters per image to be accurately represented. A relationship between image size and transmission speed requirements will be developed.

Given the security and privacy issues being raised within the Internet users community, a discussion will be presented on the design and use of firewalls and their application relative to protecting information carried across the Internet onto new enterprise network structures (local Intranets). Encryption processes that can be applied to protect the privacy of vulnerable patient information will be reviewed and related methods of introducing digital signatures in the transmission of information will be described. The application of encryption processes and use of a legal digital signature procedures are vital to the success of using the Internet as a media for handling medical information dissemination in the near future.

Finally, highlights of on-going interactive trials using the Internet and a review of proposed broadband experiments that are in process and aimed at validating the benefits of using advances in telecommunications technology will be discussed.

Medical Image Management – The Future of PACS

Sridhar B. Seshadri
Medical Imaging Systems, Health Imaging Division, Eastman Kodak Company, Dallas, Texas

TUTORIAL OUTLINE

1. The evolution of PACS: the last 15 years and the next 5 years
    a. Change in industry focus
    b. Change in customer expectations
    c. What can we expect in the next few years ?

2. PACS: The three generations
    a. Users find images
    b. Images find devices
    c. Images and information find the user

3. Image Management and Distribution - The Future of PACS
    a. What is it ?
    b. What does it do for me, the user ?
    c. Why is it important ?
    d. Where is the technology today ?
    e. What can we expect in the next few years ?

4. Image Management and Distribution - Second Order Effects

5. Lessons learned
    a. Questions that customers should ask themselves
    b. Questions customers should ask their PACS vendor
    c. Mapping out the big picture ...
    d. Other lessons

6. Discussion

Medical Imaging and Computer-Based Patient Record: A Tutorial

W. Ed Hammond
Division of Medical Informatics, Duke University Medical Center, Durham, North Carolina

1. INTRODUCTION

The computer-based patient record plays an increasingly important role in the dissemination and management of clinical, administrative, and financial data in a highly competitive, cost-contained managed care environment. New health care models require the linking of traditionally independent and competitive sites, and the flow of health care data among these sites is essential for success. The computer-based patient record, a common data model and vocabulary, data interchange standards, and a networking framework is required to meet these requirements.

The computer-based patient record is now viewed to be a life-long collection of data associated with the patient's health. All data from all sources, for all time, of all types will be contained in the ideal record. The multi-medial repository will include text, images, pictures, scans, motion video, and sound.

This tutorial will define in some detail the content of the computer-based patient record; methods of managing content, structure and vocabulary; data presentation; data interchange standards; integration of multi-media objects; and requirements for successful human/machine integration.

II. COMPUTER-BASED PATIENT RECORD

The computer-based patient record can be viewed as a class-structured document containing a mixture of structured data, free text and non-textual objects. The classes may be defined by the categories of data required in the care of the patient. This tutorial will provide detail but generally the content categories are:

1. **Demographic data** - includes patient names, addresses and telephone numbers, identifying characteristics, household data, family data, health status and related data, confidentiality filters, employment data.
2. **Pertinent Provider data** - includes names, addresses and telephone numbers, clinical specialties, required identification numbers, roles, and patient contact data for those providers involved in the care of this patient.
3. **Reimbursement data** - includes insurance data, HMO, benefit plans, subscriber information, effective dates.

4. **Summary Problem List** - high-lighted items key in a person's health care status and care. Includes diagnoses, problems, critical events, risk factors. Management plans may be coupled to problems to insure constancy and completeness in care. Management plans also provide a method of expediting the collection of data and the ordering of studies, treatments, and consultations.
5. **Studies** - includes laboratory tests, radiology (including images), pathology, microbiology, diagnostic studies, etc. Each study object will be identified by name and code, date/time of result, result, and source (person , place, and type of data).
6. **Therapies** - includes drugs, allergies, immunization, blood products, diets, radiation therapy, speech therapy, rehabilitation therapy, etc. A record of current and past treatments is retained.
7. **Subjective and Physical Findings** - time-oriented health care objects organized around the concept of subjective, objective and plans. Each object is detailed similarly to studies objects.
8. **Encounter data** - details of each patient encounter - including inpatient, outpatient, telephone conversations, consultations, lab only visits, etc. Data includes involved providers, places, dates and times, problems dealt with, procedures done, tests ordered, therapies prescribed, supplies dispensed, health status, dispositions, referrals, authorizations, etc.
9. **Appointment data** - includes date and times, facilities and resources, support data, scheduling.
10. **Accounting data** - management of accounting associated with patient encounter . Includes record of payments, adjustments, etc.
11. **Supplemental support data** - includes lists, protocol management, indices, etc.

III. DATA DICTIONARY

1. The data dictionary is a directly accessible database which contains structure, codes and vocabulary, framework, linkages, messages - specifications for a generalized framework. The tutorial will address how the data dictionary can be used to manage and integrate images and other multi-media objects into the patient record.

IV. DATA INTERCHANGE STANDARDS

Health Level Seven (HL7) is the data interchange standard which is most widely used for the interchange of clinical data. ACR/NEMA DICOM standard is the most widely used standard for the transmission of image-type data. The tutorial will briefly discuss these two standards and give examples of their use in real systems. A brief discussion will also be included in identifying appropriate file types used to store image data (JPEG, GIF, etc..

V. VOCABULARY

The problem with a common vocabulary is that there are too many sets of vocabulary standards (ICD9-CM, CPT, Read, SNOMED, etc.) and not an adequate clinical set. The tutorial will discuss briefly the vocabulary coding problem and potential solutions.

VI. CONCLUSIONS

The tutorial will include implementation examples from a real system.. Adequate time will be available for questions and answers.

Strategic Thinking for Radiologists

Ronald B. Schilling
RBS Consulting Group, Los Altos Hills, California

The new approach to business analysis is STRATEGIC THINKING. Thinking can be considered to be the initial step of "doing the right things," followed by planning - "doing things right."

If one searches the files of the Futurists today for "Success Dynamics," one finds terms like Global Connectedness, Real Time Responsiveness, Always in the Process of Becoming - aimed at positioning for change.

The most rapid rate of change in history is upon us. It is occurring on a global basis. And, it is occurring even faster in the field of healthcare.

Tools for Strategic Thinking (TST) is an approach to providing the user with frameworks and processes for meeting the challenges created by rapid change. The focus is on effective communications and decision making by a diverse group of individuals.

TST achieves the Success Dynamics brought to us by the Futurists. It does it by raising the right questions. The user will determine the right answers. The frameworks and processes that have been developed provide for an integration of ideas among the user team members.

A series of tools are presented along with case studies demonstrating their use and effectiveness. After the user gains some facility with the tools they will naturally modify the tools to better fit their specific situations. In addition, the users will find themselves creating new tools together with members of their teams.

Several of the benefits to be derived from TST are as follows:

1. Developing a Common Framework for Solving Problems.
2. Identifying a Common Language for Addressing Problems.
3. Thinking with Simultaneous Focus and Flexibility.
4. Stimulating Creativity in Problem Resolution.
5. Communicating by Asking the Right Questions to Find the Right Answers.
6. Promoting Teamwork in Problem Solving.

The case studies presented are based (for the most part) on Radiology. A brief synopsis of several of the cases is presented below.

Vision - The "Vision" tool consists of a Purpose and a Mission. The Purpose states what an entity is trying to achieve in the future (3-5 years). The Mission includes approximately five strategic elements that enable the entity to achieve the Purpose. The case discussed is for The Radiology Vision. This was presented as works-in-progress at the 1995 RSNA in the FutuRad exhibit.

High Five - The "High Five" tool is usually used to address the needs of a customer. It asks the question, "What are the five reasons the customer will select one product or service over another?" The case discussed is for the Radiologist as customer when purchasing diagnostic imaging equipment.

Real-Win-Worth - The "Real-Win-Worth" tool is used whenever an entity is making a major decision regarding expenditure of capital and/or resources. Three basic questions are asked. Is the opportunity real? Can the entity improve its competitive position by making the expenditure? Is it worth doing financially? The case chosen is for the purchase of a PACS system.

Two-by-Two - The "Two-by-Two" tool is a square divided into four parts. For problems with two complex dimensions, this tool provides a method for breaking the problem into four simpler situations. The case selected relates to technology Assessment of PACS. This was utilized at the 1993 and 1995 CAR meetings.

The session will be highly interactive so that those attending can take away ideas and approaches that can be immediately applied.

Quality Assurance for Digital Imaging

John C. Weiser, Kenneth T. Drummond, Brian D. Evans, Dan J. Shock and Mathis P. Frick

Robert C. Byrd Health Sciences Center and West Virginia University Hospitals
Department of Radiology, West Virginia University, Morgantown, West Virginia

I. Introduction. The continuing proliferation of digital imaging networks both within and between hospitals indicates the need to consider the requirements for a comprehensive network-wide quality assurance (QA) program. The term, Quality Assurance is usually applied to the broad spectrum of management practices that are implemented to ensure that radiology examinations are appropriate, that the necessary image information is obtained, that the correct interpretation is made available in a timely fashion, and that radiation exposure, cost, and inconvenience to the patient are minimized. The subset of QA which specifically deals with tests of equipment function is called Quality Control (QC).[1] The general principles of radiology QA which apply to a conventional, film-based department must be extended to incorporate the new components and processes which make up a digital image management and communication system (IMACS). Although there is a considerable volume of information available which provides guidance for QC of individual digital imaging modalities such as CT, MRI, and DSA, [2-4] there is little information on QC requirements for the network which connects these modalities, the archive where the images are stored, the database which links these images with relevant patient and examination information, or the cathode ray tube (CRT) display workstations on which the images are displayed. Film digitizers (FD) and computed radiography (CR) are two additional imaging modalities which are prevalent in digital radiology departments, and some recommendations for QC of these devices have been published in recent years.[5,6] Recommendations for QC of the components of the IMACS, and the QA of the processes which are used in the implementation of the complete digital system into the operation of the radiology department are crucial requirements for the successful transition to filmless medical imaging.

II. Quality Assurance in an IMACS. An IMACS can be categorized into four subsystems, based on a functional classification. These subsystems are network/communications, database/storage, image output/display, and image acquisition.[7] Within each of these subsystems we can list a set of relevant components which may or may not be present, depending on the configuration of the IMACS. For example, the image output and display subsystem could include several categories of CRT display workstations, laser film imagers, low end paper print imagers, and 35mm slide printers. Conventional QC is directed at tests which are sensitive enough and frequent enough to detect slowly changing parameters which affect image image quality before the problem becomes clinically significant. One might suppose that in a digital system, there are no slowly changing parameters, and that any corruption of a digital system would be immediately evident. However, at both the input end and the output end of the imaging chain there are analog-to-digital (ADC) and digital-to-analog conversions (DAC) whose performance can slowly degrade with time. In the case of a CR reader acquiring an image do be displayed on laser printed film, there is an analog chain which includes a laser, a photomultiplier tube and an ADC in the CR reader and a DAC and a laser in the film printer. The drift of CRT monitors and degradation of the phosphors with time are also important parameters to monitor. The purely digital portions of the system, such as the archive and database also have indicators, such as error logs, which can be used to monitor system problems and correct them before they become more serious. In addition, software programs can be used to monitor network performance and utilization and provide trend analysis. The implementation of a comprehensive QA plan for a digital radiology department requires us to explore new areas of analysis and develop new skills which were not required in a conventional film-based system.

IV. References.

1. NCRP Report No. 99, Quality Assurance for Diagnostic Imaging, (National Council on Radiation Protection and Measurements, Bethesda, MD, 1988).

2. AAPM Report No. 39, Specification and Acceptance Testing of Computed Tomography Scanners, (American Institute of Physics, New York, 1993).

3. M.L. Wood and R.R. Price, "Quality Control Programs for MRI," in The Physics of Magnetic Resonance Imaging, P. Sprawls and M.J. Bronskill, eds., (AAPM Summer School, 1992).

4. AAPM Report No. 15, Performance Evaluation and Quality Assurance in Digital Subtraction Angiography, (American Institute of Physics, New York, 1985).

5. J.H. Trueblood, S.E. Burch, K. Kearfott and K.W. Brooks, "Radiographic Film Digitization," in Digital Imaging, W.R. Hendee and J.H. Trueblood, eds., (Medical Physics Publishing Corp., Madison, WI, 1993).

6. J.A. Seibert, "Photostimulable Phosphor System Acceptance Testing," in Specification, Acceptance Testing and Quality Control of Diagnostic X-ray Imaging Equipment, J.A. Seibert, G.T. Barnes and R.G. Gould, eds., (AAPM Summer School, 1991).

7. M.A. Cawthon, J.C. Weiser and D.V. Smith, "Applications of IMACS: The Military Model", in Digital Imaging, W.R. Hendee and J.H. Trueblood, eds., (Medical Physics Publishing Corp., Madison, WI, 1993).

How to Write an RFP for PACS

Michael M. Abiri, M.D., Nanda S. Kirpekar, M.S. and Ronald C. Ablow, M.D.
Beth Israel Medical Center, New York

Purpose of RFP

The purpose of a Request for Proposal (RFP) for a Picture Archiving and Communications System (PACS) is to provide a mechanism by which to do the following:

- Describe your institution to the vendors that you have selected to receive the RFP.
- Describe your Radiology Department.
- Describe the information systems in use at your institution.
- Describe the kind of PACS that you wish to install.
- Give the vendors an opportunity to describe their company and products.

The RFP and its Components

Even before you begin to work on the RFP itself, a great deal of preparation must be done. In this phase, you need to do the necessary research and coordination with other departments at your site to enable you to create a comprehensive RFP: a literature search, site visits, attendance at national radiological meetings, and consultations within (radiologists and support personnel) and outside (other physicians, MIS, Telecommunications) your department. The RFP is divided logically into several components, broadly falling into the following categories, each of which will be discussed in detail. You need to supply information about you and about the kind of PACS system you want to install, and request information about the vendor.

<u>Information about you</u>

There are several categories of information that need to be supplied:

- a general description of your facility as a whole, including future plans;
- a description of your Radiology department, including computer systems (RIS, dictation system), staffing, examination rooms, acquisition equipment you have installed/plan to install (e.g. CR), number of procedures performed annually, and any plans for future expansion.
- a description of other computer systems at your facility (HIS, ADT etc.).

<u>Information about the kind of PACS system you want to install</u>

In defining your PACS to the vendor, it is critical to describe the system in as much detail as possible. In general, every PACS has the following key components:

- image acquisition subsystem;
- image output and display subsystem: number and type (2K vs 1K) of viewing stations, number and type of printers;
- communications and network subsystem: LAN vs WAN, kind of throughputs desired, network topology (star, ring; FDDI, CDDI, ATM), and teleradiology (to physicians' offices and radiologists' homes);
- image database and storage subsystem: primary (local and distributed storage), secondary (RAID and jukebox), and tertiary storage (archival storage); and
- interfaces with: other computer systems (e.g. RIS, HIS), acquisition systems (e.g. CT, CR) and the standards on which they are based (DICOM, HL7).

The software requirements of your PACS should be described in a functional specifications document detailing the user interfaces and capabilities of the system. Among the issues that should be discussed in this section are: image acquisition (DICOM), image retrieval at various points in the system, graphical user interfaces, image output (including hardcopy), image archival and storage, interfaces, network structure (transmission speeds), and report generation capabilities.

Finally, you should discuss the kind of support services that will be required for your PACS: on-site and off-site support personnel provided by the vendor, support personnel provided by you, training and education, status meetings, acceptance testing, how program errors or bugs are identified and fixed, whether and how customizations requested by you will be incorporated into the product, how product enhancements (hardware and software) will be installed, new releases, emergency services provided by the vendor to handle critical situations, and disaster recovery.

<u>Information about the vendor (requested) and their PACS</u>

In this section, the vendors are asked to describe their company and their PACS:
- general description of the company;
- general description of the proposed application, including support services, network design, and compliance with governmental regulations;
- information about other sites with components of their PACS; and
- a detailed timetable for the implementation.

Post-RFP

Once the RFP has been sent to the various vendors, a mechanism should be put in place to respond to vendor inquiries and to evaluate vendor responses. One individual should be the point-of-contact at your facility, and the evaluation process must be clearly defined. In the first stage, it is hoped that you will be able to eliminate all but two or three vendors from consideration. Once the field has been narrowed to this point, you must allow yourself time to select one specific vendor. Once a specific vendor has been selected, contract negotiations can begin. For a moderately complex PACS project, the entire process, from the beginning of pre-RFP research through the signing of a contract with the chosen vendor, should take approximately six to nine months.. At this stage, the first phase of your PACS implementation can begin.

PLENARY SESSION

Current Federal Projects

Co-Chairs:

Anna K. Chacko
Joseph Gitlin

Deployable FIlmless Teleradiology Through a DICOM3 Interface: A Transparent Reality?

Jay F. Cook, M.D., James Breitweser, M.D., Brian Goldsmith, M.D. and Mark F. Hansen, M.D.
Tripler Army Medical Center, Honolulu, Hawaii
Charles E. Willis, Ph.D.
Department of Radiology, University of Texas Houston Health Science Center, Houston, Texas
Charles Suitor
Medical Advanced Technology Management Office, Fort Detrick, Maryland

I. INTRODUCTION

Project AKAMAI is a medical imaging project with the intent to install a telemedical network serving the federal beneficiary population in the Pacific basin. This population consists of approximately 834,000 members distributed within an area encompassing one-half of the world's surface area. Isolated population clusters and clinics are separated from the few federal hospitals by thousands of miles of blue water, time zones and the International Date Line. Radiology service needs vary, ranging from a few films per day to medical center volumes. Some facilities are staffed with organic radiology support. However, many are not, and those that are do not have subspecialty personnel on site, with the exception of Tripler Army Medical Center. One military base in Japan acquires once per week professional radiology coverage from a local source. The professional cost is averages $85 per exam. Several isolated atolls in the Pacific must fly their examinations to Honolulu. The turnaround time is approximately one week and at a cost of approximately $35 per examination. Okinawa, with organic radiology assets, has a need for subspecialty consultation and continuing medical education.

The Medical Diagnostic Imaging Support (MDIS) System provides for teleradiology links, but these are expensive and currently limited to linking with the MDIS PACS. Korea was the first full utilization of networked teleradiology. The installed MDIS system of hubs and spokes reduced report turnaround times from in excess of a week to 24 hours or less. However, the system is costly, and additionally, the communication links are nonscalable, functioning with T1 lines. The requirement for T1 precludes use of the system in most regions where this level of service is not available. While other Teleradiology systems are now available that use cheaper communication lines, until ACR-NEMA DICOM version 3.O, none were able to communicate with MDIS or any other proprietary system[1].

In August 1995, a system created from commercial off-the-shelf (COTS) components was installed in an Air Force International Standards Organization (ISO) Shelter for prototype testing as a DICOM 3.0 based Computed Radiography (CR) Teleradiology system. In October the system became fully operational as the temporary radiology service for the 15th Medical Group clinic at Hickam Air Force

Base while the permanent facility was undergoing renovation. A review of the current scientific literature was unrevealing regarding previous reports of actual diagnostic use of this standard in a CR based system, however, several sites are known to exist. We will describe the system architecture as well as the lessons learned from our experience in obtaining processed diagnostic CR images through Teleradiology.

II. MATERIALS AND METHODS

The Hickam to Tripler system was installed utilizing COTS components. The key hardware at the remote site is depicted in Figure 1. Exposures were obtained with a Continental single phase generator irradiating a photostimulable phosphor plate and processed through a Fuji AC3 CR. The CR was linked to a Dejarnette workstation through a DASM. Output to a GE Advantage Review workstation (GE ARWS) for Quality Control and local softcopy review was configured. The workstation included a 1.2 GB hard drive. The Dejarnette workstation was configured with a look up table (LUT) for conversion of the flat file. Fuji processing parameters were thus restored according to the organ code obtained in the header file.

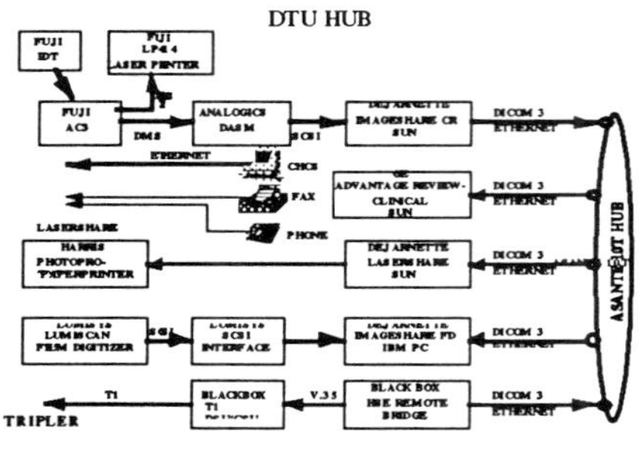

Fig. 1: The remote ISO shelter

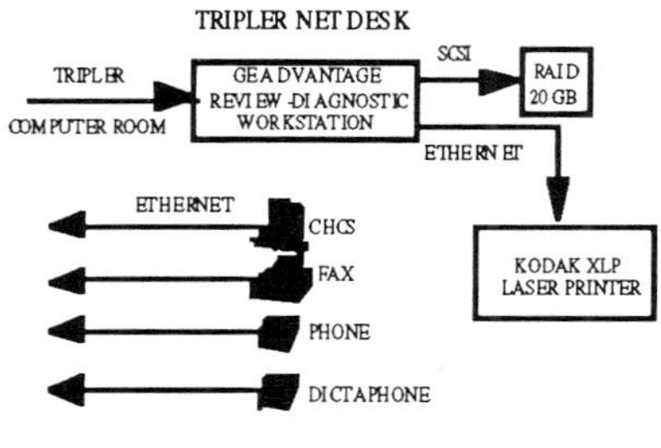

Fig. 2: The Teleradiology receive site

Additionally, output to a Fuji 414 (8 bit) laser printer for local film archive and input from a Lumisys 75 digitizer for prior examination comparison were configured. A Harris PhotoPro-2000 connected to a Dejarnette print server for trial of local dry print consultation quality images was also available.

Communication was established through a T1 line to Tripler Army Medical Center through a Black Box CSU/DSU. The receive site at Tripler was established as in Figure 2. The Black Box CSU/DSU was linked through a Dejarnette DICOM Gateway to the local area network. A two monitor GE Advantage Review Diagnostic (GE ARDS) workstation and 16 Gigabyte RAID local Archive were placed in the Department of Radiology. The workstation monitor resolution was 2300X1700 pixels. Files were transmitted using FTP and IP addressing protocols.

Notification of examination transmittal was made through facsimile transmission of the consultation request. A status window on the GE ARDS could also be accessed to identify transmission activity. Results were provided by return facsimile as well as providing a finalized report through the Composite Health Care System (CHCS) wide area network. Immediate 'wet' results were provided telephonically.

Softcopy interpretations without hardcopy overreads have continued since October 1995. Five American Board of Radiology certified radiologists have used the system during this period. An initial survey consisting of multiple statements regarding the teleradiology system based on a Likert rating scale was administered to the five participating radiologists. Responses were given by levels of agreement or disagreement, ranging from 1 as "strongly agree' to 5 as "strongly disagree." Three of the survey questions were directed toward identifying user satisfaction with the processed softcopy image appearance on the DICOM CR system. The statements concerning image acceptance were as follows:

Statement 1: You have a high degree of confidence in the image quality seen on the teleradiology workstation.

Statement 2: You prefer hardcopy to softcopy in CR generated images.

Statement 3: You prefer plain film to softcopy CR images.

A final test of the transmission of images over the internet was performed between two workstations not of the same manufacturer. Both had T1 internet access rates. Five images, each of 7.5 MB size, were transmitted intermittently during business hours PST from California to Tripler Army Medical Center in Honolulu, Hawaii.

III. RESULTS

During the initial six months of operation, 2,008 examinations, 4,186 'films', and 5,072 exposures were performed. Operations are continuing until the new facility is completed. The system has performed well, although not without problems.

Initial efforts disclosed a software error causing transmission failure in approximately one in six examinations. The affected exam could be accessed via query and retrieve; however, this action precluded simultaneous use of the viewing application. Examinations could only be retrieved serially instead of in batch mode when multiple examinations were missing. Approximately one in twenty examination files contained an incomplete set of images.

The LUT created some problems due to the field size allotted to each anatomic region. A maximum of 25 processing codes can be assigned to each anatomic region. If the region in the CR contains greater than 25, those images using an 'excess' code are automatically assigned a default algorithm for processing. This has resulted in receipt of several suboptimal or nondiagnostic images at the ARDS.

The results of the radiologist survey are found in Figure 3. All estimated they spent at least 25% more time reading softcopy than hardcopy. Results of the Internet preliminary transmission time trials are at Figure 4. Note that the transmission times did not significantly differ over the course of the day. Longer transmission times were to be expected during peak business hours for the entire United States.

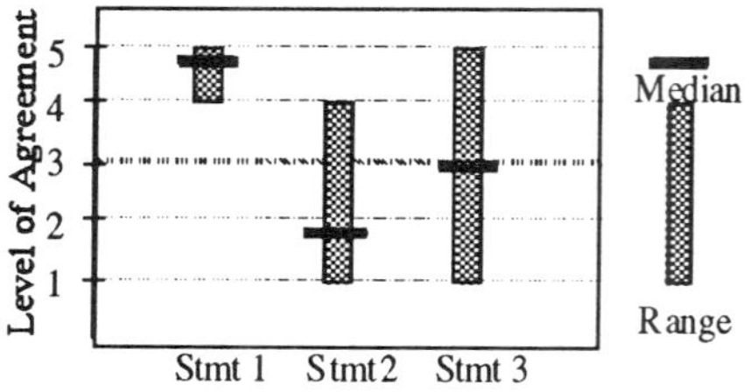

Fig. 3. Radiologist Survey

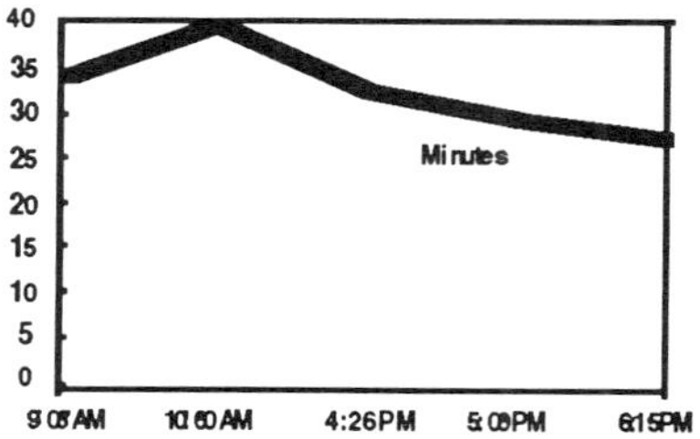

Fig. 4. Internet transmission times of 7.5 MB images through T1 access

IV. DISCUSSION

The system has operated reliably during the past six months with greater than 95% system "up-time." The original software problem of failure of examination transmittal was corrected. An occasional missing image from a file folder persists. While the direct cause has not been identified, it is felt that this is a result of operator error on the part of the technologist. Each image on the Dejarnette DICOM workstation must be individually pushed to the GE ARWS. Interruptions while performing this task probably result in the technologist not sending the entire set. An inventory of the number of images in a folder is currently passed along with the consultation request by facsimile.

The LUT has been reconfigured. Where the Dejarnette does not have sufficient space for the number of processing codes a default procedure code closely resembling that code is selected. This has been remedied in subsequent software releases not yet installed in this system.

Although overall the user survey did not contain a robust sample size, it suggests that the system produces a diagnostic quality images and that user confidence is definitely positive. The preference of four of the five surveyed for softcopy over hardcopy CR may be accounted for by the fact that the softcopy workstation display allows for better overall contrast resolution than hardcopy CR. This is due to the full use of 12 bit grayscale rather than the 10 bit available on a laser film of the CR image.

The preference of two of the radiologists for softcopy over plain film and the neutrality of the third was surprising but was felt to be related to the presentation of a processed image as well as the ability to window and level and grayscale invert. The imagery technology at the ISO Shelter consisted of a single phase generator and a table with a fixed grid. Such a system at the community clinical level would normally produce a low contrast image with generally decreased resolution due to motion unsharpness for the longer exposure times required. In addition control for exposure technique was not performed. Increased technique may account for some of the improvement.

Under the MDIS system the Fuji processing parameters are not understood by Loral PACSNET. Only the raw data is received and a flat image file produced, essentially attempting to replicate a plain film, but with a linear curve. The improvement of image quality at our institution and others revolves around adjustment of the pre and post processing algorithms. These parameters influence contrast resolution and spatial frequency. The resulting improvement in image quality by preserving the effect of the processing algorithms has changed our PACS installation plans. We are now preparing to initiate DICOM output from all CR's within the institution. This will provide improved functionality in two respects. A processed image will be available at the outset of MDIS operations. Because of DICOM standard for IP addressing, images can be made available to any workstation on the hospital wide network. This can be accomplished through establishment of an 'intranet' server. Acquisition of expensive vendor proprietary workstations can be decreased and desktop availability of CR images will be possible.

DICOM output for Teleradiology also provides a solution to Project AKAMAI's need for a variety of Teleradiology platforms. Platforms suitable for the local demand and available communications can be procured which can then communicate with the tertiary care center or any radiologist location. Again it should be noted that only two levels of Teleradiology are available under MDIS[2]. A consultation level system does not exist. A teleradiology interface to remote CT or MR also is not available under MDIS.

DICOM output also allows transmission through the internet at reasonable speeds if a large bandwidth access can be obtained. With appropriate security, large data set images can routinely be passed between institutions for after-hours second opinions. This will significantly reduce communication costs for some remote locations that have access to internet nodes, such as those US facilities in Japan. For

Tripler, establishment of after-hours staff supervision of residents, centralized teaching file libraries, and development of radiological Center's of Excellence will become a reality by networking tertiary care institutions within the Department of Defense[3,4].

V. CONCLUSIONS

The inclusion of DICOM 3.0 in an operational teleradiology system demonstrated some temporary shortcomings which are resolvable with further vendor support. Radiologist acceptance of the images generated by a single phase generator system were surprisingly high and some of the sustained confidence level may be attributable to the preservation of the ability to use processing algorithms. The benefits extend to the realization of the need to internalize DICOM standards within our PACS.

REFERENCES

1. Digital Imaging and Communications in Medicine. National Electronic Manufacturers Association. PS-xx, 199x

2. Lyche DK, deTreville RE, Norton GS and Leckie RG. MDIS Teleradiology in North America. S/CAR 1994.

3. Lyche DK, deTreville RE, Norton GS and Leckie RG. MDIS Early Experience in Wide-Area Intercontinental Teleradiology; Medical Imaging 94, SPIE 1994.

4. Cook JF, Francoise J, Leckie RG, et al. Digital Imaging Access Library; Medical Imaging 94, SPIE 1994.

Limitations of Radiology Services in a Film-based Environment

Major Morgan Williamson, M.D., Lieutenant Michael Brazaitis, M.D. and Colonel Theodore Raia, M.D.
Walter Reed Army Medical Center, Washington, D.C.
Commander Richard Bakalar
National Naval Medical Center, Bethesda, Maryland
Joan Fetter, Ph.D.
Johns Hopkins Applied Physics Laboratory, Laurel, Maryland
Major Krista McFarren, M.D. and Major Aimee Hawley, M.D.
Malcolm Grow Air Force Medical Center, Andrews AFB, Maryland
Elliott Pickar, M.S.
Veteran's Affairs Medical Center, Baltimore, Maryland
Joseph Gitlin, M.D., D.P.H.
Johns Hopkins University Medical Institutions, Baltimore, Maryland

Introduction

Soon after Roentgen discovered x-rays, the problem of radiology film accountability began. At some centers, the unread film rate, related to lost films, may reach twenty percent. Other problems exist in addition to lost films including delays in image interpretation, delays in patient diagnosis, as well as reduced physician productivity. In order to quantify these problems, we propose a method to measure film accountability in three major medical centers as they implement various measures to improve radiology services. After picture archiving and communications systems (PACS) are implemented, these variables will be restudied to support a pre and post analysis.

Philosophy/ Rationale

With the imminent dawn of PACS implementation in the nation's capitol imminent, a group of radiologists and scientists assembled in order to study the costs and benefits of PACS and telemedicine in a prospective fashion. This group, including the authors mentioned above, met on a weekly basis to discuss issues pertinent to PACS, teleradiology, and telemedicine. In the course of these meetings a strategy was developed to study of the effects of PACS on the economic costs and quality issues associated with a film-based system. Three computerized forms were developed in order to study the existing film based system and later study the filmless department.

Materials and Methods

The group developed three forms to record radiology operations at selected facilities within the greater Washington, DC. area. The first of these is the patient arrival log (Fig. 1). It contains an entry point for name, social security number, date, time, hospital information system examination number, and image tracking form number. The second form is the medical imaging examination tracking form (Fig. 2). This contains entries for patient information and examination numbers. Patient arrival times, examination start times, patient departure times, film preparation times, film hanging times, radiology reporting times, transcription time, radiologist's report verification, and report receipt time by the requesting physician are all captured. The third form is the patient film jacket file room study form (Fig. 3). It has entries for patient identification, file room search times, reason for request, and resolution of the study. All three forms contain printed instructions on the reverse.

Study Dates: 2/12/96 - 2/19/9

Form No:

MEDICAL IMAGING EXAMINATION TRACKING FORM

(1) Patient's Name (Last, First, MI)
(2) Patient's FMP/SSN

(3) Patient Type (a) O In (b) O Out
(4) Exam requested by:
(5) Patient location at time of request

(6) Exam 1 ID Number 9
(7) Exam 1 description
(8) Exam 1 code

(9) Exam 2 ID Number 9
(10) Exam 2 description
(11) Exam 2 code

(12) Exam 3 ID Number 9
(13) Exam 3 description
(14) Exam 3 code

Patient Arrival *(Study Coordinator)*	(15) Date (MMDDYY) 96	(16) Time (24 hr clock)	(17) Comments
Exam Begun *(Technologist)*	(18) Date (MMDDYY) 96	(19) Time (24 hr clock)	(20) Comments
Patient Departure *(QC Technologist)*	(21) Date (MMDDYY) 96	(22) Time (24 hr clock)	(23) Additional films? O Retakes O Additional views
Ready for Interpretation *(Clerical Support)*	(24) Date (MMDDYY) 96	(25) Time (24 hr clock)	(26) Old films available? O Yes O No If not, why not?
Staff Interpretation Begun *(Radiologist)*	(27) Date (MMDDYY) 96	(28) Time (24 hr clock)	(29) Did resident participate? O Yes O No
(30) STAT Report to Requester O Yes O No If yes, enter date and time. *(Radiologist)*	(31) Date (MMDDYY) 96	(32) Time (24 hr clock)	(33) Comments
Transcription Begun *(Study Coordinator)*	(34) Date (MMDDYY) 96	(35) Time (24 hr clock)	(36) Comments
Report Verified *(Radiologist)*	(37) Date (MMDDYY) 96	(38) Time (24 hr clock)	(39) Comments
Report Read by Requesting Physician *(Study Coordinator)*	(40) Date (MMDDYY) 96	(41) Time (24 hr clock)	(42) Comments

Tracking Form Completed *(Study Coordinator)*	(43) Date (MMDDYY) 96	(44) Time (24 hr clock)
Tracking Form Processed *(Data Processor)*	(45) Date (MMDDYY) 96	(46) Time (24 hr clock)

Exam 1 Label

Exam 2 Label

Exam 3 Label

O More than three exams (blacken circle and put additional labels on the reverse side of this page)

IMPORTANT

DO NOT REMOVE THIS FORM FROM THE RADIOLOGY DEPARTMENT

Fig. 1 Medical Imaging Examination Tracking Form

Study Dates: 2/12/96 - 2/19/9
Form No:

PATIENT FILM JACKET FILE ROOM STUDY FORM

(1) Patient's Name (Last, First, MI)

(2) Patient's FMP/SSN

Request received (Clerk) | (3) Date (MMDDYY) 9 6 | (4) Time (24 hr clock)

(5) Type of request
- O Comparison with new exam, CHCS No. ____________
- O Other clinical
- O Administrative/Legal
- O Academic
- O Other (specify) ____________________

(6) Requested by:
- O Radiologist
- O Provider (e.g. M.D., P.A.)
- O Support staff (e.g. nurse, secretary, ward clerk, student)
- O Patient
- O Clinic (specify) ____________________
- O Other (specify) ____________________

(7) Communication medium:
- O In person
- O Phone
- O FAX
- O CHCS
- O Other (specify) ____________________

Search begun (Clerk) | (8) Date (MMDDYY) 9 6 | (9) Time (24 hr clock)

Search complete (Clerk) | (10) Date (MMDDYY) 9 6 | (11) Time (24 hr clock)

(12) Resolution:

Jacket found:
- O Yes
- O No

Required film(s) found:
- O Yes
- O No
- O None specified

If 'No', why not?
- O No old films/new jacket created
- O Jacket found, specified films missing
- O Specified films signed out/unavailable
- O Other specify ____________________

(13) Comments:

Completed File Room Form secured and reviewed *(Study Coordinator)* | (14) Date (MMDDYY) 9 6 | (15) Time (24 hr clock)

File Room Form data entered in special study computer database *(Data Processor)* | (16) Date (MMDDYY) 9 6 | (17) Time (24 hr clock)

IMPORTANT
DO NOT REMOVE THIS FORM FROM THE RADIOLOGY DEPARTMENT

Fig. 2 Patient Film Jacket File Room Study Form

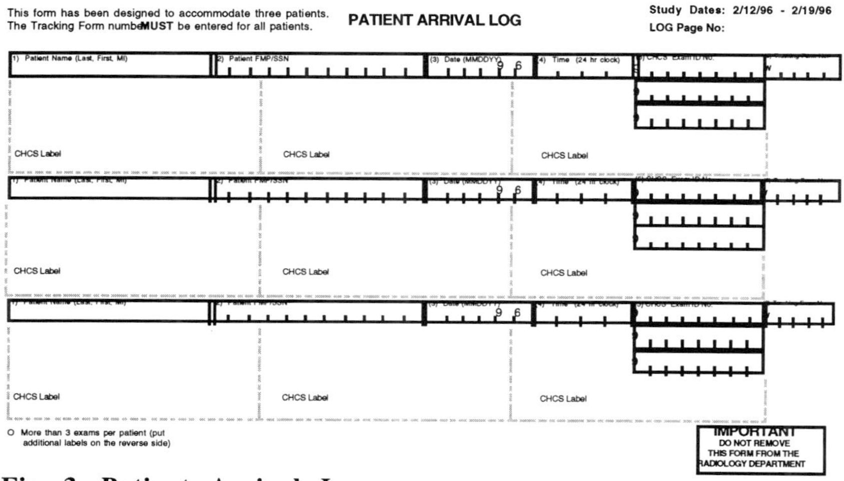
This form has been designed to accommodate three patients.
The Tracking Form numbe MUST be entered for all patients.

PATIENT ARRIVAL LOG

Study Dates: 2/12/96 - 2/19/96
LOG Page No:

1) Patient Name (Last, First, MI) | 2) Patient FMP/SSN | (3) Date (MMDDYY) 9 6 | 4) Time (24 hr clock)

CHCS Label | CHCS Label | CHCS Label

CHCS Label | CHCS Label | CHCS Label

CHCS Label | CHCS Label | CHCS Label

O More than 3 exams per patient (put additional labels on the reverse side)

IMPORTANT
DO NOT REMOVE
THIS FORM FROM THE
RADIOLOGY DEPARTMENT

Fig. 3 Patient Arrival Log

Initial versions of the forms were field tested at one of the medical centers. As a result of these dry runs, the forms were revised and the instructions were both clarified and modified. Participants on site included file room supervisors, radiologist technologist supervisors, and department chiefs. After the form was revised and finalized, instruction was given to all file clerks, patient receptionists, technologists, and radiologists.

The study was to follow all patient encounters and file room exchanges of the radiology department except angiography and nuclear medicine during a three day time period. Ample amounts of all three forms were placed at the facility prior to the start. The study began at 0001 hours on a Tuesday morning and stopped at 2400 on the following Thursday night. All members of the department were instructed to synchronize their watches with the time given by the hospital information system. Orthopedic radiology was studied the following week in a similar three day fashion.

For patients arriving in the radiology department for a routine medical imaging study, the name, social security number, and date and time of arrival were recorded on the patient arrival log by a receptionist at the entrance to the clinic. A medical image tracking form was then initiated for each patient including the name, social security number, and examination number(s) from the hospital information system (HIS). This form was attached to the examination request and placed in the queue for patient examinations. The patient then proceeded to a changing area outside an examination room. When the patient entered the room, the technologist would enter that date and time on the form. The image tracking form then moved with the exposed cassettes to the film processing area. The quality control technologist inspected the films as they came out of the processor and, if satisfactory, then dismissed the patient noting the date and time. The films were transferred with the image tracking form to the file room where a patient film jacket file room study form was initiated. This form was attached to the image tracking form after being filled out (to be covered later) by the file room personnel. The films were then taken, with the forms and any old films, to the appropriate film alternator. Once the films were placed on the alternator, the file clerk entered the date and time that the examination was ready for interpretation and whether old films were available. Next, the staff radiologist entered the date and time that interpretation began and also answers yes or no to whether there was resident participation. If a verbal report was given to the requesting physician, then the date and time of that report was recorded by the radiologist. The radiologist placed the form in a collection box by the alternator where the study coordinator later collected them. The transcription time was obtained from the HIS when the report was available. In a similar fashion, a radiologist report verification time was obtained from the HIS by the on-site study coordinator. Lastly, the HIS was queried for the date and time that the report was read by the requesting physician, and this recorded on the form by the study coordinator. The coordinator also noted form completion time and secured the completed forms for data processing.

The procedure varied somewhat for stat and portable studies. Patient arrival time was entered as the time that radiology was notified that an examination was needed on a patient (either verbally or telephonically). This information was recorded by the technologist or file clerk and one image tracking form was started. "Examination begun" time was considered to be the time that the technologist arrived with the machine for the portable exam. Patient departure was considered to be the time when the technologist had examined the films for quality control. In these cases, the films were placed on the ICU alternator next to the processor, and the technologists entered a ready for interpretation time.

For patients in remote facilities, image tracking and file room forms were created and sent with the films to the interpreting medical center. The procedure followed that for routine examinations following arrival.

The patient film jacket file room study form was initiated whenever the file room received a request for previous studies. Many of these requests came by way of the film transporter with new films and an image tracking form, as discussed above. The patient's name and social security number were entered and the date and time the request was received, as well as noting the source of the request: radiology, a patient, a practitioner, support staff, etc. A search start and completion time were entered by the file clerk. Also noted was the reason for the request, e.g. whether it was comparison with a new exam, other clinical functions such as an office visit, academic purposes, or for administrative reasons. The method of communication with the requestor was recorded, namely, person-to-person, fax, phone, or via the HIS. Finally, the resolution of the search was recorded, i.e. whether the patient jacket and required film was found and if not, the reason that they were not found. The forms were placed in a collection bin and checked by the study coordinator prior to shipment to the data collection point.

Additional information was collected from radiology department and hospital administrators. This included information on film and chemical usage and cost, number and types of examinations, number and cost of personnel in the department, space requirements, cost of file room equipment, alternators, processors, chemical disposal and their maintenance, and legal costs due to lost or unread films. This information is intended to support preliminary cost estimates.

Despite the efforts of the study coordinators, some problems were encountered. Some staff members had difficulty filling out the forms correctly despite the training provided. This was probably due to the number of items and the number of forms. On site supervision by the study team was helpful with this problem. Another problem encountered was lost forms. One week after the three day collection period, approximately five percent of the forms had not been returned.

Presumably many of these forms were associated with lost exams. Most of the information associated with the lost forms will be recaptured from the HIS. Another problem encountered was incomplete data. This was usually limited to one or two blank data fields per form, and the HIS will be queried for this information.

Perhaps the biggest problem encountered in the study was the method used to enter data on the forms. Despite instructions to use a number two pencil or black pen, writing utensils included crayons, magic markers, grease pencils, and colored inks. A related problem was poor handwriting or writing outside the spaces designed for the data. As a result most of the forms had to be entered into a database manually and not optically scanned as was originally planned. This process is still taking place at the time of writing. To accommodate for these deficiencies, data are being collected from the HIS whenever possible.

Results

Data are being entered and analyzed at the time of writing. A supplement will be provided at the conference with preliminary results. Based on our study, we expect to be able to document the time required for a medical imaging examination and report to be completed in a film-based system and the production costs for such studies. Additionally, the time required for the individual components of the radiology diagnostic cycle will be measured. Important information on the availability and the time required to locate old images also will be obtained. These data will be obtained from all three major military medical centers in the nation's capital and subsequently from comparable civilian hospitals.

Acknowledgments

Special thanks to Ms. Beverly Motley, RT., Senior Airman Sean Kirtley, and Lieutenant Phil Aldridge for their effort in coordinating the studies. Thanks also go to Ms. Bridget Gilmour for her help in data collection from the hospital information systems.

Navy Medicine Teleradiology Initiative: An Analysis of Inter-Reader Variability

CDR Maura Emerson, M.D., M.P.H. and LTC Brian Feighner, M.D., M.P.H.
Uniformed Services University of the Health Sciences, Department of Preventive Medicine and Biometrics, Bethesda, Maryland
LCDR Guillermo Olivos, M.D. and CDR David Lawrence, M.D.
Department of Radiology, National Naval Medical Center, Bethesda, Maryland
CDR Richard Bakalar, M.D.
Telemedicine Working Group, National Naval Medical Center, Bethesda, Maryland

INTRODUCTION

The US Navy has a strong interest in any technology that can expedite delivery of quality medical care to geographically remote locations. Prolonged isolation can occur during the operational deployment of US Navy ships. Should serious illness or injury occur, medical evacuation of the patient to a tertiary care center can be done. However, medical evaluation is costly and may affect the operational mission of the ship. If the use of teleradiology can increase the reliable detection of the presence or absence of clinically significant findings, shipboard medical care and the efficiency of medical evacuation can be enhanced.

The purpose of this study was to assess inter-reader variability to determine:

1. Did the use of teleradiology improve detection of the presence or absence of clinically significant findings?
2. Was teleradiology interpretation reliable in comparison to film interpretation?
3. Can the reliability of interpretation be enhanced by decreasing the number of radiologists providing interpretation of the digitized image?

METHODS

The US Navy Telemedicine Initiative, Project Challenge Athena II, was conducted during a scheduled Mediterranean deployment of an aircraft carrier, the USS George Washington (CVN 73). A commercial satellite linkage between the ship and a shore based wide area network was used to transmit digitized images to the Department of Radiology at the National Naval Medical Center (NNMC), Bethesda, Maryland. A shipboard Advanced Video Products Laser Scanner (AVP) was used to digitize images that were transmitted to NNMC on a consultative basis from May to November 1994. Analog films were interpreted by shipboard primary care providers prior to transmission. Transmitted studies were stored at NNMC where interpretation was provided by any of eight board-certified staff radiologists. Results were returned to the ship through electronic mail. The NNMC radiologists were not informed of the preliminary shipboard providers' film interpretation. At the conclusion of the ship's deployment, another board-certified staff radiologist reviewed all available analog films received from the ship and all workstation stored digitized images. The workstation monitor at NNMC provided a large matrix of 2048 x 2048 pixels with full image manipulation functions. Stored images were not annotated with the initial interpretation.

Data analysis included classification of interpretations and calculation of sensitivity (SN), specificity (SP), and kappa coefficients (k) for any of four sets of comparison groups. Interpretations were classified according to the presence or absence of clinically significant findings. A clinically significant finding was defined as one requiring either further medical treatment, additional studies, or medical follow-up. Comparison groups were matched by radiological study. Unmatched data were excluded, but reviewed for frequency of clinically significant findings.

RESULTS

During the six month deployment, 111 studies were transmitted to NNMC. Table 1 depicts the type of studies transmitted to NNMC. Missing data included 34 radiographs not sent for radiology review, 16 studies originally transmitted but not stored at the NNMC workstation, and 9 studies that lacked an initial interpretation by the shipboard provider. The frequency of clinically significant findings within these missing data, as described in Table 2, was determined through review of the original teleradiology electronic mail report returned to the ship.

Table 1
Teleradiology Studies

Study Type	Number
Chest	51
Extremity	27
Spine	11
Sinus	8
Abdominal	6
Genitourinary	6
Facial	2

Radiograph interpretation of the shipboard primary care providers was matched to that of a radiologist (N=72) with a calculated SN=69.5%, a SP=85.7%, and a k=.553 ($p<.001$). In comparison to the teleradiology interpretation during deployment (N=67), the shipboard providers had a SN=61.9%, SP=80.4%, and a k=.417 ($p<.001$). When the same radiologist interpreted matched workstation stored images as compared to the analog film (N=71), SN=79.2%, SP=87.2%, and k=.657 ($p<.001$). Comparison of initial teleradiology interpretations, provided by any of staff radiologists, with interpretation of matched radiographs of the same studies reviewed by a single, different radiologist at the conclusion of the ship's deployment (N=77) had a SN=75%, a SP=84.9%, and a k=.585 (p<.001). Table 3 summarizes these comparisons.

Table 2
Summary of Missing Data

Data Type	Number	# Findings / # Missing (%) *
Films not sent to NNMC	34	22/34 (64.7%)
No Ship Reading	9	4/9 (44.4%)
No Image Stored at NNMC	16	6/16 (37.5%)

*Clinically significant findings as determined by review of original teleradiology interpretations at NNMC

Table 3
Summary of Comparison Groups

Group *	Sensitivity[a]	Specificity[b]	kappa[c]	Total studies
1	.695	.875	.553	72
2	.619	.804	.417	67
3	.792	.872	.657	71
4	.750	.849	.585	77

*Group Definitions:
1= Interpretations of Ship providers (film) vs single radiologist (film)
2= Interpretations of Ship providers (film) vs initial teleradiology interpretation (digitized image; multiple radiologists)
3= Interpretations of single radiologist digitized image vs film
4= Initial teleradiology interpretation (digitized image; multiple radiologists) vs single radiologist (film)
[a]Sensitivity = True Positives / True Positives + False Negatives
[b]Specificity = True Negatives / True Negatives + False Positives
[c]kappa = Observed Agreement - Expected Agreement / 1 - Expected Agreement

DISCUSSION

The plain film is considered to be the gold standard in radiological interpretation, but error and variability exist (1,2). If a true gold standard truly exists, then sensitivity and specificity can be appropriately utilized to compare a new test or technology to the gold standard. If a gold standard does not exist, the kappa coefficient can provide a measure of reproducibility above that expected by mere chance. A kappa coefficient value between 0.4 and 0.75 is indicative of good reproducibility (3). All comparison groups had kappa coefficients within this range, however the shipboard providers' interpretations in comparison to the original teleradiology reading had the lowest k coefficient of all comparison sets. The lowest sensitivity values were also found when comparing the shipboard providers' interpretations to either the single radiologist's film interpretations or the teleradiology reading during deployment. These data suggest that the availability of radiology consultation during deployment did increase the detection of clinically significant findings.

When attempting to compare the reliability of teleradiology interpretation to radiograph interpretation, analysis is hampered by the consultative basis upon which digitized images were transmitted to NNMC. Because only the questionable cases were transmitted, it is possible that a significant selection bias was introduced. Ideally, all radiographic studies performed onboard ship during deployment should be transmitted. Furthermore, radiologists providing workstation interpretation should be equally trained and experienced at image manipulation at the workstation in order to standardize those effects upon inter-observer variability. Finally, in addition to standardized predeployment training, there should be randomized and equal workstation interpretations by participating radiologists. However, kappa coefficients can be used as a measure of reproducibility. A greater degree of reproducibility is an accepted indicator of reliability (4). Comparison of the matched film and digitized image interpretation by a single radiologist shows a k=.657. This implies a 65.7% agreement, above that expected by chance alone, on the presence or absence of clinically significant findings.

Comparison of the kappa coefficients obtained when a single radiologist interpreted both the digitized image and the matched films versus multiple radiologists providing the teleradiology workstation impression during deployment suggests that reliability may be enhanced by restricting the number of radiologists providing interpretation of transmitted images during deployment. As hypothesized, decreasing the number of readers did decrease the inter-reader variability as seen by the increased kappa value (k=.585 vs k=.657).

Previous field studies of teleradiology within the military setting were conducted in 1982 and 1984, but low and moderate resolution systems were used (5). Recently, the results of a prospective analysis of the diagnostic accuracy of a high resolution teleradiology system reported only 18 discrepancies out of 685 transmitted cases (sensitivity=96% and specificity=99%). As noted by the authors, the interpreter of the plain film had access to the preliminary digitized interpretation, circumstances that could introduce bias (6). The effect of performance variation between different readers was described in another study utilizing high resolution teleradiology (7). In our study, missing data may have had a significant impact upon our statistical analysis. Especially notable, 22/34 missing radiographs, excluded from analysis, had clinically significant findings on the original teleradiology interpretation during deployment. These findings would suggest that those patients may have been sent from the ship for further care. However, the lack of these data could have introduced a differential classification bias causing underestimation of sensitivity, specificity, and /or kappa coefficients.

CONCLUSION

Shipboard providers could enhance the detection of clinically significant findings through the use of radiological consultation (shipboard providers' sensitivity=69.6%). The primary care providers' radiograph interpretation as compared to teleradiology (shipboard providers' sensitivity =61.9%) also supports the clinical utility of teleradiology. Restriction of the number of radiologists providing teleradiology interpretations could decrease the inter-reader variability (k=.585 vs k=.657) and enhance the concordance between interpretation of the digitized image and the matched analog film. While missing data (64.7% of the 34 missing radiographs had clinically significant findings on initial teleradiology interpretation) may have contributed to an underestimation of sensitivity and specificity, both sensitivity and kappa coefficients were enhanced with the use of teleradiology.

REFERENCES

1. Smith, M.C. Error and Variation in Diagnostic Radiology Springfield: Charles C. Thomas Publisher; 1967.
2. Herman, P.G., Gerson, D.E., Hessel, S.G. et al. Disagreement in chest roentgen interpretations. Chest 1975; 68:278-282.
3. Landis, J.R. and Koch, GG. An application of hierarchical kappa-type statistics in the assessment of majority agreement among multiple observers. Biometrics 1977; 33:363-374.
4. Spitzer, R.L., and Fleiss, J.L. A re-analysis of the reliability of psychiatric diagnosis. Brit J Psychiat 1974; 125:341-347.
5. Gitlin, J.N. Teleradiology Radiol Clin of N America 1986; 24:55-68.
6. Goldberg, M.A., Rosenthal, D.I., Chew, F.S. et al. New high resolution teleradiology system: prospective study of diagnostic accuracy in 685 transmitted clinical cases. Radiology 1993; 429-424.
7. Yoshino, M.T., Carmody, R., Fajardo, L.L. et al. Diagnostic performance of teleradiology in cervical spine fracture detection. Invest Radiol 1992; 27:55-59.

From the *Uniformed Services University of the Health Sciences, Department of Preventive Medicine and Biometrics, Bethesda, Maryland; the +Department of

Radiology, National Naval Medical Center, Bethesda, Maryland, and #Telemedicine Working Group, National Naval Medical Center, Bethesda, Maryland.

The opinions contained herein are the private views of the authors and are not to be construed as reflecting the views of the Department of Defense or the US Navy.

PACS Training for Physicians: Experience at the Baltimore VA Medical Center

Zenon Protopapas, M.D., Eliot L. Siegel, M.D., Bruce I. Reiner, M.D. and Stephen M. Pomerantz, M.D.
Department of Radiololgy and Nuclear Medicine, Baltimore VA Medical Center, Baltimore, Maryland and Department of Diagnostic Imaging, University of Maryland Medical School, Baltimore, Maryland

Elliott Pickar, M.A.
Department of Radiololgy and Nuclear Medicine, Baltimore VA Medical Center, Baltimore, Maryland

Mike Wilson, R.T., R.D.M.S.
Loral Medical Imaging School

Frank Hooper, Sc.D.
Department of Medicine, University of Maryland Medical School, Baltimore, Maryland

In order for medical staff (attending physicians, residents, interns, and medical students) to best utilize Diagnostic Imaging services at a hospital they should be able to order studies and be able to locate studies for review from the different film libraries. Most clinicians have received some formal training on the interpretation of radiographs and many months or years of informal training on film interpretation. They were taught such "tricks" as using the bright light to bring out detail in an overexposed film, or holding the film at an angle to help determine the termination of a central line are part of the repertoire of most physicians.

Physicians practicing at the "filmless" Baltimore VA Medical Center are confronted with a hospital in which imaging studies are not stored in the film library, where there are very few film view boxes for them to review studies. Many of the "tricks" that worked when using film do not apply in a filmless hospital.

They need to be proficient in the use of the Picture Archival and Communication System (PACS) in order to be able to view radiologic images and accompanying reports. Such training is necessary to assure optimal patient care and potentially to satisfy medico-legal requirements. Providing such training is the responsibility of both the Imaging Department and the hospital. The rapid influx of housestaff and medical students each month at an academic institution poses further training challenges for the imaging department.

Training in the use of the PACS at the Baltimore VA is conducted by an on-site application specialist. We identified two goals of a PACS training program. The first is to teach physicians how to retrieve images and reports from current as well as prior studies and display them on a computer workstation. Secondly the training should include instruction on the use of the various workstation tools to enhance image interpretation. Imaging requirements and utilization by different physician groups vary, and PACS training should be tailored accordingly.

The two, one hour radiologist training sessions cover the use of the database structure in greater detail. For example, radiologists are taught to use conference folders and how to create teaching files. The use of the annotation tool allows the radiologist "draw" on the image in a manner analogous to using a wax pencil with film. The main focus of the sessions however is to equip the radiologist with the necessary expertise to use workstation tools for optimal image interpretation. They are also taught to use macros to perform certain repetitive tasks and the use of default display protocols ("intelligent" display of current and previous images on a multiple monitor workstation) to increase throughput.

PACS training is ideally performed individually or in small groups. This allows the trainer to tailor the session according to the individual's computer experience and clinical needs. Familiarity with computers and with the use of a pointing device such mouse or track ball seem to, in our experience, facilitate the training. A second advantage to training users individually is that the training can be tailored to the physician's subspecialty. We have found the PACS requirements of the various specialists and sub-specialists to be quite different. For example, an orthopedic surgeon may need to measure angles and distances, functions that are usually less critical for an internist.

Data were collected from interviews of the trainer, training log sheets, and physician surveys. While 100% of radiologists received formal training, only 22% of non-radiologists were formally trained; 32% of these physicians identified themselves as having been trained by their peers and 41% stated they were self trained.

Difficulties in the scheduling of training sessions during working hours and the widespread use of a "generic" log-on identification have contributed to the low (22%) compliance of non-radiologists with the formal training program. Although we believe that one-on-one training is most effective and can be best tailored to the needs and computer expertise of a particular physician, computer based training (both on and off-line) may provide an acceptable, and in some cases, a preferred alternative.

In conclusion, we found that a filmless hospital poses new challenges to a radiology department with regard to training physician staff. Both the radiology department and the hospital have the responsibility to provide a PACS training program in order to assure optimal use of the imaging services. Training could be provided by a combination of one to one training sessions and computer based training.

SESSION 1

Teaching Applications

Co-Chairs:

David R. Pickens
Byrn Williamson, Jr.

Images in the Electronic Medical Record

Byrn Williamson, Jr., M.D. and Nicholas Hangiandreou, Ph.D.
Mayo Clinic and Foundation, Rochester, Minnesota

INTRODUCTION

Interest in picture archiving and communication systems (PACS) is increasing dramatically in the radiologic community. The initial development of these systems naturally focused on image management within the radiology department and delivering images to dedicated viewing stations outside radiology. This "image-centric" approach is natural in view of the significant technical challenges involved in developing and implementing PACS; however, it is not suited to the needs of non-radiologists. For clinicians, images are only a small part of the information needed to care for patients. Our medical center, like many others, plans to implement an Electronic Medical Record (EMR) to replace the traditional paper-based patient chart. This EMR will contain all the pertinent clinical data for each patient including clinical notes, problem list, test results, medication records, and other data. In order to meet the needs of clinicians, PACS systems must be able to provide images in the context of an electronic medical record.

In order to determine the needs of clinicians for access to images and to determine the relationship between PACS and the EMR, questionnaires were sent to representatives of 48 clinical departments and divisions at our institution, a large medical center providing inpatient and outpatient care. Forty questionnaires were returned representing 772 clinicians.

RESULTS

Clinicians generally would prefer display of images on the EMR workstation and would be willing to accept a moderate decrease in image quality to get it. Seventy nine percent of the respondents indicated that they would prefer that images be displayed on the same workstation as the electronic medical record, while 4% preferred display on a separate workstation. Seventeen percent indicated no preference. EMR workstations eventually will be located in each examining room in our outpatient facility and each patient room in the hospitals. Thus images will be available widely if they can be displayed on EMR workstations. Conversely, placing separate image display workstations in each of these locations would be impractical. Not only is space inadequate to accommodate two separate workstations, but the current price of dedicated image display workstations is too high to allow purchase of the large number that would be required. In addition, the necessity to navigate two databases, one for EMR data and the other for images, would be an inefficient use of clinician time. We believe that radiology images and reports should be provided by a software module within the EMR.

Clinicians' requirements for image quality will vary with specialty. For many clinicians, convenient access to images will be more important than image quality unless quality is markedly degraded. In our study, 61% of respondents indicated that they would be willing to accept a moderate decrease in image quality in order to view images on the same workstation as the EMR. Sixteen percent of respondents indicated that a decrease in image quality would be unacceptable, and 22% were undecided.

Most images will be viewed as part of a review of a specific patient rather than a series of patients. This mode of access is fundamentally different from that used by radiologists who usually interpret a series of examinations. Current PACS systems are usually designed to accommodate the type of viewing used by radiologists, while the EMR needs to present all the clinical data for a single patient including x-ray reports and images. Eighty percent of respondents indicated that they would frequently view images in the context of a particular patient, and only 9% of respondents indicated that they would frequently need to review the images of a series of patients such as when making rounds on a hospital ward.

Most clinicians require access to both digital and conventional images. Approximately 30% of imaging examinations in our practice originate from digital modalities such as CT, MRI, Ultrasound, and Nuclear Medicine. One potential approach to providing images to clinicians would be to begin with these digital images, but few clinicians would be satisfied with this situation. Only 5% of the respondents indicated that more than 90% of the images they need to view are from digital modalities while 12% of respondents indicated that more than 90% of the images they need to view are conventional radiographs. The remaining respondents indicated a need to access images from digital modalities and conventional radiography. Radiology departments must migrate from analog to digital technology for projection radiography if we are to provide all the images our clinical colleagues need to view in the EMR.

The needs of a few clinicians can be satisfied by images only or by reports only, but usually both are needed. Approximately 4% of respondents indicated that their needs would be satisfied by access to images without a report more than 50% of the time. Eighteen percent reported that their needs for radiologic information would be satisfied by access to reports without images more than 50% of the time. Sixty three percent of the clinicians indicated that they require access to images and reports more than 50% of the time. Because of differences in technology and database requirements, RIS and PACS systems have generally been provided by separate vendors who provide interfaces to each other, but from the user's point of view, images, reports, and other radiologic information are all required to care for patients. Ideally, all pertinent radiologic information, including images, should be accessible in the EMR.

PACS vendors commonly provide a variety of viewing features within their workstations to facilitate interpretation and management of images. In response to our questionnaire, clinicians indicated that they would use the following features when viewing images in the EMR:

	frequently	occasionally
Images from prior examinations	36%	51%
Resolution comparable to current film	31%	59%
Simultaneous display of multiple images	27%	68%
Contrast and brightness adjustment	7%	55%
Ability to measure distance and angles	6%	24%
Ability to produce a paper copy of images	3%	46%

Many clinicians indicated that they would like access to non-radiology images in the EMR:

Endoscopic images	58%
Pathology slides	49%
Patient photographs	45%
Blood smears	34%
Electrocardiograms	17%
Echocardiograms	11%

PACS systems need not be limited to radiology images. There is little difference in the technology required for the storage, communication, and display of radiology images and other images, particularly if a color monitor is used as in most EMR workstations. On the other hand, linkage of non-radiology images to the appropriate reports in the EMR would need to be provided, either by entering these reports into the Radiology Information System or by interfaces between the EMR and the systems containing the appropriate reports.

CONCLUSION

Electronic medical record technology will be deployed widely in the coming years. Images will comprise a significant component of the electronic medical record. A number of issues must be addressed as radiologic information and images are integrated into the EMR, because the needs of clinicians are different from those of radiologists. The radiologic community should begin to address these issues rather than deferring them to EMR vendors.

Creating a Database-Driven, Interactive Radiology Teaching File for Distance Learning

Michael W. Freckleton and Ralph B. Evans
Wilford Hall Air Force Medical Center, San Antonio, Texas
Mark T. Schnur
Medical Advanced Technology Management Office, Frederick, Maryland

Overview: Radiology texts and radiology case teaching files have been the traditional mainstay of non-mentored radiology learning. Although these teaching methodologies have served us well, new technologies now present the possibility of new teaching paradigms that may be more effective in teaching the intricacies of an ever-expanding subject.

Radiology texts present information in a linear fashion, where one idea follows the next in step-wise fashion. This type of learning is often insensitive to the specific learning requirements of the student, and may be presented at a level of knowledge either above or below what the student may actually possess. Text-based education is also passive, not requiring the student to actually *use* any of the information he/she has just learned. Although "information points" (which we define as facts or data included in any teaching modality) are presented to the student, there are no "decision points" to help reinforce the information. We define "decision points" as moments in the learning processes where ideas are reinforced by requiring decisions to be made based on information recently learned.

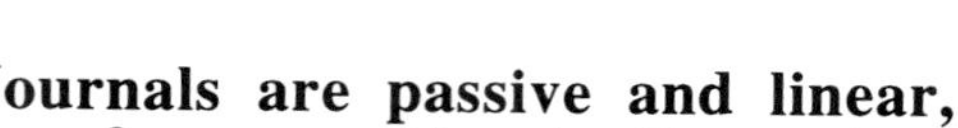

Books/Journals are passive and linear, flowing from one idea to the next.

Radiology teaching files present a slightly more dynamic approach to learning, and may be considered a two-dimensional learning technique. Although the format of the teaching files is standardized, some room remains for the student to seek additional images and to formulate a differential diagnosis. Teaching files may thus include "decision points", but to a limited degree.

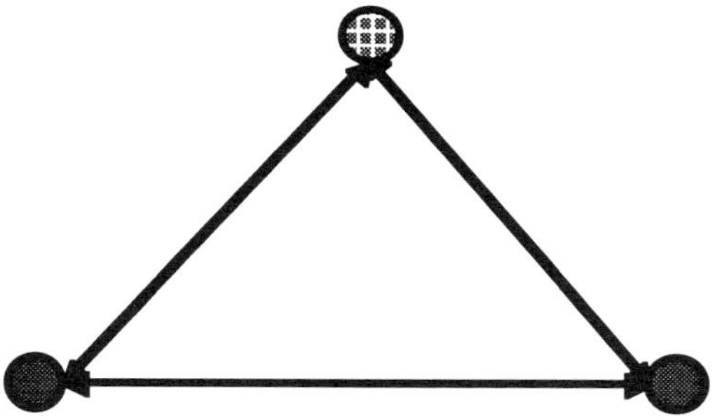

Teaching Files, Either Hard Copy or Electronic, tend to be two dimensional, with some minimal capacity for decision making.

Key:  **=Information Point** (A fact or piece of data included in any teaching modality)

 = **Decision Point** (Moments in the learning processes where ideas are reinforced by requiring decisions to be made based on facts recently learned.)

Undoubtedly, the most effective radiology learning takes place during mentored teaching, where the student sits with an instructor and discusses topics or cases in a truly interactive fashion. During mentored teaching, the educator is able to assess the learning level of the student, and then present or reinforce new information as the student's needs dictate. Questions asked by the teacher become decision points for the student, reinforcing the information being discussed. Although ideal, time constraints on student and teacher make such optimal encounters less frequent than may be desired.

Object: Our goal was to create an interactive teaching file which would closely imitate advantages of mentored teaching. Where textual learning is passive and linear, we wanted to establish a new active teaching paradigm, allowing students to browse through a *volume* of information, selecting areas appropriate to their present knowledge base. By evaluating student responses to questions posed, the next information point could be presented either to reiterate a fact that had been missed, or to go on to the next logical area.

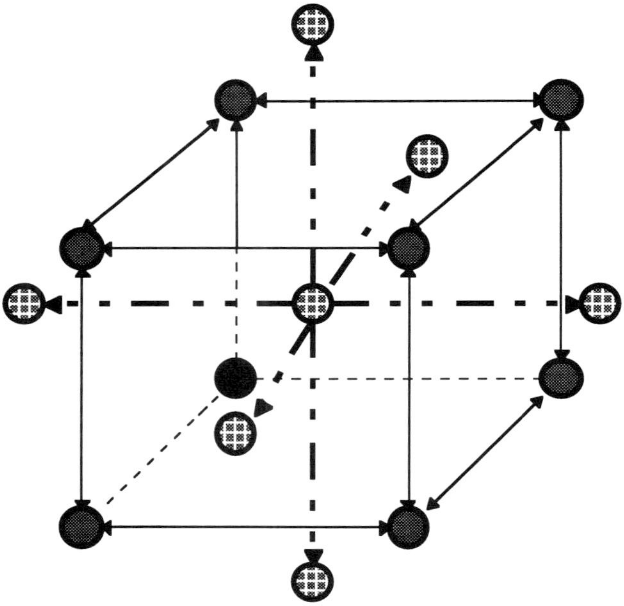

A database-driven teaching paradigm allows information to be treated as a volume through which students may browse according to their present knowledge base. Information points within the volume of knowledge are reinforced by decision points.

An additional goal was to provide Internet access to our interactive teaching resource, recognizing that a repository of information is only valuable when it can be tapped. By providing access to **Radiology Central Resource (RCR)** through the Internet, we could thus serve educational needs of radiologists, clinicians, and patients in all regions of the world where there is connectivity to the Internet. Our intent has also been to copy sections of **RCR** onto CD-ROM for stand-alone, computer-based radiology teaching.

Other goals of **RCR** have been to provide medical information relevant to military and humanitarian concerns over the Internet, especially as they apply to radiology. An entire sub-section of **RCR** is devoted to medical concerns relative to U.S. military physicians deployed overseas, addressing issues such as bomb/blast injuries, tropical radiology, etc. We also hope to be a central focus for radiology research, including diagnostic imaging, PACS, teleradiology, radiologic physics, etc.

Methods:

In its electronic teaching files, **RCR** uses standard, oral case-presentation format to present interesting or useful cases. After the student has selected a category, either pre-referenced or randomized cases are presented with only the patient age and gender as supporting information. The student is expected to view the initial image(s), identify appropriate abnormalities, and create a differential diagnosis. A list of options on the initial screen will allow the student to select information, either as history, additional images, or description of findings, that will allow the differential diagnosis to be narrowed. This additional data should allow the student to arrive at the best choice of diagnoses.

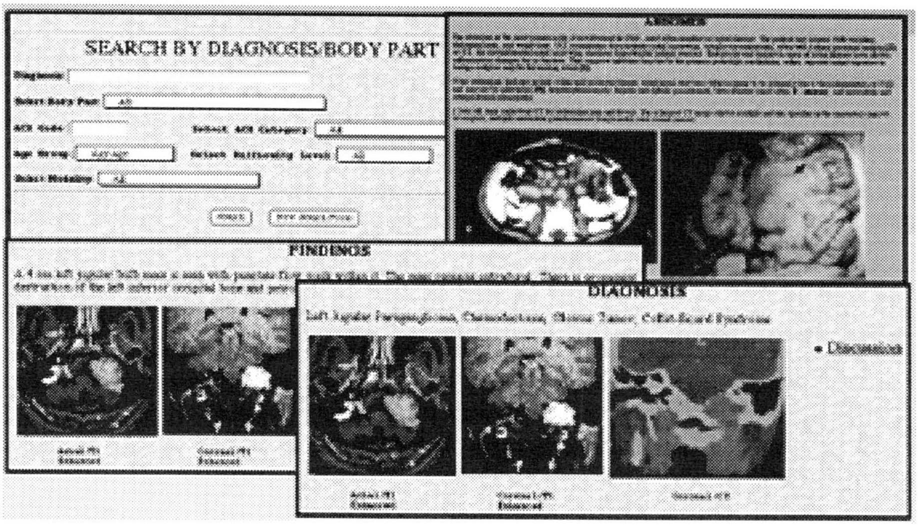

A montage of images showing a case search screen, images, findings and diagnosis.

By allowing a student to choose what information is presented, an electronic, database-driven teaching file permits various case presentation formats. More junior residents may take the cases in a linear fashion, one-by-one as they might be found in a book or standard teaching file. Residents preparing for board exams may choose to take cases completely randomly, or randomly, but within pre-defined categories. For example, the student may wish to view random cases, but only in pediatric bone. The case files may also be used as a reference source, searching on specific disease entities. Alternatively, many research applications are available through the search mechanism. For example, one may search on a specific diagnosis or ACR category, but request to see only cases where a particular imaging modality or age group have been included.

RCR not only maintains a file of interesting cases, but entire conferences, papers, posters, etc., may be found in electronic format. As with all other information within the teaching file, the information contained within these presentations is easily searchable within the database. In addition, all information within the teaching file is cross-indexed via hypertext links. Users may begin searching for an example of a particular pathology, and then find themselves linked to an entire conference on a related topic, or may be referred to research projects currently underway within a related area. We are also currently developing interactive teaching modules in several areas of diagnostic radiology which will provide the "information point/ decision point" matrix for enhanced learning.

Software components:

- The ***RCR*** Home Page is written in HTML for use with generic web browsers.

- Server Software = WEBSTAR 1.2.4 (Starnine Technologies, INC., Berkeley, CA).

- Although standard HTML format allows multiple browsers, we have used Netscape 2.0 as our preferred browser.

- Database = Filemaker Pro 3.0v2 (Claris Corporation, Santa Clara, CA).

- Search Script = WEB FM (Web Broadcasting Co., Palo Alto, CA).

- The data entry form for **RCR**'s database, and script modifications linking HTML text to the database were created by Michael Freckleton, MD, and Ralph Evans, RT.

- Graphic Manipulations are performed by Adobe Photoshop 3.0 (Adobe, Mountain View, CA).

- Graphic Conversions are performed by Graphics Converter 2.3 (Lemke Software, Germany).

HTML text is edited with HTML Editor 1.0 (Shareware, Canada).

Hardware Components:

- **RCR** is presently served from a Macintosh Power PC Workgroup Server 6150/66, with access within Wilford Hall Medical Center via a local Ethernet connection. Our teaching files are also served from the Medical Advanced Technology Management Office (MATMO; Ft. Detrick, MD) server at the Internet address http://www.matmo.army.mil.

- Films are digitized via a Lumiscan 200 film digitizer (Lumisys, Inc.), although we will shortly be publishing images obtained digitally from our Medical Diagnostic Imaging Support PACS system (Loral Medical Imaging Systems, San Jose, CA).

Conclusion:

It would appear that part of the strength of computer-based learning is its ability to approximate mentored teaching. This is facilitated by linking a large archive of images and textual information to a database, adding maximum flexibility to how information is presented. Where such learning falls short of teaching at the view-box, it is accentuated by convenience and linking information from multiple sources.

Radiology Central Resources proposes to provide access to an information/decision matrix of Radiology data for computer-based education in civilian, military and humanitarian applications. As with all teaching files, we view our efforts as a process rather than a product. Having developed a relational platform for display of cases, future efforts will focus on adding content within the teaching files through a broad, multi-institutional consortium including military and university teaching programs.

The Production of Multimedia Educational Tools with HyperText Markup Language

Richard H. Wiggins, III

Department of Radiology, University of Mississippi Medical Center, Jackson, Mississippi

I. INTRODUCTION

The ability to create effective multimedia educational tools has been severely hindered by the requirement of programming knowledge. In order to connect text with graphics or sound in an adequate graphical interface, a broad foundation of programming experience has previously been needed, as well as access to multiple operating systems.

Web browsers (clients), which are software programs normally used to view documents on the World Wide Web (WWW), can be used locally with HyperText Markup Language (HTML) documents for quick access to interactive teaching files and materials. The WWW has been described as a wide area hypermedia information retrieval initiative [1]. This retrieval system can, however, be used on a single computer, directed at the hard drive or compact disc, read-only memory (CD-ROM) media, without actually connecting to the Internet.

The plethora of hardcopy teaching materials at academic institutions can form the infrastructure for relatively quick production of excellent digital teaching materials. Text can easily be digitally scanned using a flat bed scanner and optical character recognition (OCR) software. Extensive development time is not needed for the simple translation of text into HTML. Current technology provides relatively inexpensive and easy to use image manipulation hardware and software. Modern Picture Archival and Communication Systems (PACS), flat bed scanners and 35mm slide scanners allow for quick digitization of teaching file images for association with HTML text documents. The use of cross platform HTML files with Web browsers avoids the extensive programming and long man hours that has hindered the creation of quality multimedia educational tools [2].

II. BACKGROUND

The *Introduction to Radiology* (Radiology M-IV) [3] course for fourth year medical students consists of a 100 page spiral handout and over 300 hard copy radiologic films. This was somewhat limiting, since there was only one copy of the films, and the films could only be viewed in the radiology department. It has been difficult for a student to check out many films to bring home for study outside the department, and the films are best viewed in an optimal environment with a view box. Clearly, the bulk of this material limits its use by students. Although the material is of excellent content, a firm course requirement or a motivated student is required to complete the course.

III. MATERIALS AND METHODS

The *Introduction to Radiology* HTML CD-ROM project was created using relatively common hardware and software. The images were obtained by digitally scanning the hard copy films or transferring the digital images directly from the PACS at the University of Mississippi Medical Center (UMC), Department of Radiology. The images were then edited as needed with Adobe Photoshop™ (Adobe Systems, Incorporated, Mountain View, CA) imaging software. Text was scanned digitally on a flat bed scanner with OCR software, Omnipage Professional (Caere Corporation, Los Gatos, CA), and was then edited for HTML using ClarisWorks™ (Claris Corporation, Santa Clara, CA) for word processing.

The image and text manipulation was performed on a relatively low-end (Performa 636CD, 66/33 MHz, 68LC040 CPU) Macintosh platform computer (Apple Computer, Cupertino, CA). The Macintosh platform was chosen for its ease of use with multimedia production and image processing [4-6]. The images were then linked with the text appropriately, and the files (text and graphics) were then pressed onto a CD-ROM with a CD-ROM recorder, Phillips LMS CDD 522 (Phillips Key Modules, San Jose, CA), and designed Macintosh CD-ROM recording software, CD-It-All (Phillips Media Optimage, West Des Moines, IA). Any computer with CD-ROM capability and a Web browser can view the files on the CD-ROM.

IV. TECHNOLOGY

CD-ROM Versus Laser Disc

Recently there has been an exponential growth in medical interactive educational material. The most common of which includes both laser disc and CD-ROM media. Although laser discs have been popular recently, many instructors are recognizing the limitation of this media; a laser disc player can be a costly investment for home use. The bar-code book with laser disc has been compared to a computer-driven laser disc program, and students usually prefer the computer driven media [7].

With the explosion of home computer use many educators are now recognizing the ability of CD-ROM media to bypass these limitations. Computers sales are exceeding the sale of televisions today, and most of these home computers have CD-ROM and modem capabilities, or external CD-ROM drives and modems can be added at relatively little cost. A laser disc player may not be used at home for purposes other than presenting the teaching material and movies; however, for approximately the cost of a computer compatible laser disc player and connections, the home computer is a wealth of innovative technology from word processing to creating projects, to the great number of available distractions. A similar project, created on CD-ROM, would be easily transported and easily used at work or home for further study.

CD-ROM media has now overcome the limitation of prior multimedia programs with an increased removable data source (650 megabytes) in a type of media with a large installed user base. CD-ROM media also has a relatively low distribution cost compared with hard copy film and other media, allowing CD-ROM technology to surpass prior laser disc advantages [8,9].

WWW

The WWW began in 1989 when a consortium lead by the French National Institute for Research in Computer Science and Control (also known as CERN) proposed a set of protocols for the exchange of information between computers. This group now exists as the W3 Consortium which is a collection of organizations which set Internet standards for protocols and the transmission of information between computers [10]. Concurrent with the growth of the WWW, there has been an explosion in home computer use. There are now over 9 million host computers forming the backbone of the Internet, and estimates place as many users as hosts actively using the WWW [11]. At the current rate of growth, it is now estimated that by the year 2003, every inhabitant of our planet will have at least access to the Internet [12]. The basic requirements to "surf the net" include a modem, connection to a server, and a Web browser. Computers with Internet connections will require Web browsers to allow them to view the multimedia rich WWW, which now exists primarily in HTML format.

HTML

HTML is a markup language, not a programming language. It consists of a set of tags or elements, which define text, graphics, audio, and video and their relationships [Figure 1]. HTML files exist independent of operating systems, hardware and platforms. This neutrality makes HTML very useful and powerful for multimedia productions, especially in fields similar to teleradiology where networks with multiple different platforms may be connected. Different Web browsers may display a file with the same unaltered content but in slight variations, based partially on preferences set by the user and partially on the browsers interpretation of the HTML formatting commands of that individual document [Figure 2].

```
<HTML>
<HEAD><TITLE>Introduction to Radiology</TITLE>
<CENTER><H1>Introduction to Radiology</H1></CENTER><HR></HEAD>
<BODY><A HREF="intro.html">Introduction</A><HR>
<CENTER><H2>Welcome to <B>Radiology!</B></H2></CENTER>
</BODY><I>Version 1</I>
</HTML>
```

Figure 1. HTML text document with formatting elements

Introduction to Radiology

Introduction

Welcome to **Radiology!**

Version 1

Figure 2. The interpretation of the HTML text and elements by a Web browser. The word "Introduction" would be a different color than the other text, chosen by the user, and linked to the file named "intro.html".

Since many homes in the United States will have home computers with CD-ROM drives and Web browsers of some type on their computer, the ability to create multimedia educational tools in HTML on CD-ROMs, will allow prepared information to be viewed by all of these computers, independent of platform and operating system. Therefore, HTML CD-ROMs can be created with essentially no programming experience in a fraction of the time, since different versions would not have to be created for each platform (Macintosh, Windows-based PC or UNIX).

These same files could also be placed on a server connected to the Internet, and the documents could then be accessed through the WWW. Each document on the WWW has a Uniform Resource Locator (URL), which is equivalent to the street address of a house. The Web browser can be directed to a URL on a CD-ROM as easily as a URL on the WWW, with faster access time.

V. FUTURE WORK

Using HTML, effective multimedia teaching tools can be created without the extensive knowledge and "man-years" previously needed. Initial preliminary testing with UMC medical students and radiology residents demonstrates a preference for this type of education on CD-ROM media over laser disc bar-code, laser disc-computer workstations, and even hard copy films with workbooks. The reasons for this include ease of use, cost and availability.

A prospective, controlled crossover experiment is now being designed at UMC with pre- and post-testing to compare CD-ROM media with hard copy text and films, as well as laser disc with bar-coded books. Initial results demonstrate a preference for CD-ROM technology. The results from this and other comparisons will be forthcoming in the near future, however, the author expects CD-ROM technology to be clearly favored over other types of media.

VI. CONCLUSIONS

Recent advances in the technology of hardware and software with a reduction in cost have made multimedia productions easier to develop with less investment in time and money. This, combined with the cross platform capabilities, makes HTML CD-ROM productions an attractive alternative for multimedia teaching applications, meeting criteria previously described for such computer assisted instruction [9]. Extensive collections of hard copy teaching cases can quickly and easily be developed into effective HTML CD-ROM teaching modules.

VII. REFERENCES

1. Hughes K. Entering the world-wide web: a guide to cyberspace. http://epics.aps.anl.gov/demo/guide/www.guide.html.
2. Binet EF, Trueblood JH, Macura KJ, et al. Computer-based radiology information system: from floppy disc to CD-ROM. Radiographics 1995; 15:1203-1214.
3. Raila FA, M4 Radiology Study Manual. Unpublished research and teaching notes. Last updated June 2, 1992.
4. Macura KJ, Macura RT, Morstad BD. Digital case library: a resource for teaching, learning, and diagnosis support in radiology. Radiographics 1995; 15:155-164.
5. Berlangieri SU, Schifter T, Hoffman JM, et al. An interactive, computer-based atlas of neurologic positron emission tomographic studies for use in teaching. AJR 1993; 160:1295-1298.
6. Richardson ML, Gillespy T, III. An inexpensive computer-based digital imaging teaching file. AJR 1993; 160:1299-1301.
7. Chew FS, Lanier L. Learning radiology from interactive videodiscs: bar-code book versus computer-assisted instruction. Acad Radiol 1995; 2:1016-1020.
8. Chew FS. Interactive videodisc for teaching radiology. AJR 1994; 162:987-991.

9. D'Alessandro MP, Galvin JR, Erkonen WE, et al. An approach to the creation of multimedia textbooks for radiology instruction. AJR 1993; 161:187-191.
10. Metcalfe ES, Frisse ME, Hassan SW, et al. Academic networks: mosaic and world wide web. Acad Med 1994; 69:270-273.
11. Lottor MK, Network Wizard's Internet Domain Survey. http://www.nw.com/zone/WWW/report.html.
12. Savola T, Westenbroek A, Heck J. Special Edition Using HTML. Indianapolis, IN: Que Corporation, 1995: 17.

VII. ACKNOWLEDGEMENT

The author wishes to thank Dr. Frank A. Raila, UMC Department of Radiology, Associate Professor of Radiology, for the chance to turn his years of hard work into another form and entrusting his hard copy materials for this use.

Integration of a Digital Teaching File at the Diagnostic Workstation

David E. Avrin, M.D., Ph.D., Katherine P. Andriole, Ph.D. and Ronald L. Arenson, M.D.

Laboratory for Radiological Informatics
Department of Radiology, University of California at San Francisco

I. INTRODUCTION

One of the many motivations for establishing picture archiving and communication systems (PACS) in an academic environment is the potential to migrate digital image and related data from the clinical to the educational environment. Our departmental vision of the future is one of seamless digital integration from imaging modality to PACS, through the diagnostic workstation, to the academic network and faculty/resident desktop.

Dissemination of PACS technology has provided the impetus for developing computer-based teaching file archives and databases (1-5). Two basic approaches have been described: (a) migrating image and associated data from the clinical archive to a "high-interest" case file (HICF) archive; and (b) identifying clinical cases by some manual method as "high-interest" for later access and retrieval (6). Some mini-PACS also have the ability to tag cases and images within the clinical archive for academic interest.

In a large-scale clinical PACS environment, the first approach has significant advantages, but creates technical difficulties in the convenient migration of image and associated data from the clinical to the high-interest archive. One of the difficulties is related to the optimum time and environment for selection of these cases, and initiation of migration. We believe that selection and migration is best initiated and performed at the time of diagnostic interpretation, at the digital workstation. Software development to support this activity is the specific topic addressed in this paper.

We have previously reported on a high-interest archive maintained in the Macintosh environment with the 4D object-oriented database (6-8). Macintosh is the preferred environment for our faculty because of its highly intuitive graphical user interface (GUI). Our PACS, however, is Sun/UNIX-based, integrated with a Sybase database (9). Tools developed at the University of California at San Francisco (UCSF) for selecting case and image data stored in the clinical PACS from the departmental Macintoshes for population of the HICF have been previously demonstrated and described (6-8). This client-server software suite, the Radiology Workshop, permits limited controlled access to the clinical archive from Macintosh PC's on the academic/departmental network. Image data is passed as either raw 16 bit or windowed and leveled PICT formatted data. The Workshop, which can be used to populate the HICF through cut and paste operations, has had limited use since performance is slow.

An alternative approach is direct export of image data to the HICF, selected at the time of diagnostic interpretation. The objective of this project is to demonstrate workstation tools that select ACR-NEMA images, convert them to PICT format, packaged with relevant demographic and descriptive information, and export them to a folder swept by the 4D HICF application. This direct export feature is implemented on a prototype Macintosh-based diagnostic workstation for CT and MR, interfaced to the clinical PACS network, and running 4D client (10,11). The improved functionality of this approach will be demonstrated.

This paper specifically addresses the software design and inter-operability issues involved in affecting image data transfer directly from diagnostic interpretation to the HICF.

II. MATERIALS AND METHODS

At UCSF, the clinical PACS, developed in house (9), receives input from 5 MR units, 5 CT units, 3 CR devices, an US minipacs and scanned film. Digital image data is passed through the PACS Controller, and is stored initially on magnetic hard disks, and long term on a magneto-optical disk (MOD) jukebox.

The prototype Macintosh/DOME three monitor 1K diagnostic workstation provides a well-understood development platform for this project. All software is written with Think C and Macintosh Toolbox (12,13), and the DOME (14) support library. This workstation is on the PACS network Ethernet, and has a TCP/IP link to the PACS controller, as shown in Figure 1. It can receive all CT and MR studies pushed to it by the UNIX PACS controller. In addition, the workstation has the 4D HICF application running as a standalone module, but can also be running as client with a second separate network connection to the departmental/academic network (refer to Figure 1).

When a case is selected from the local workstation archive (disk) for interpretive viewing, it is loaded in full spatial and density resolution to the DOME offscreen memory (11). An "image selection" function has been developed to associate the image data in memory with the selected image on screen. On activation of the "Export to HICF" command from

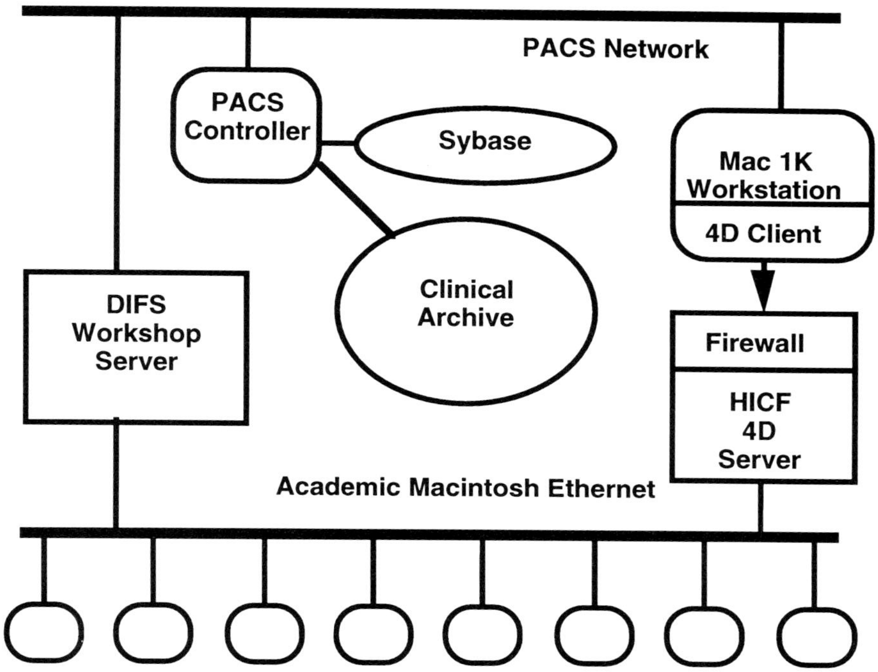

Figure 1. Workstation Bridging Clinical PACS and Academic Networks

a pop-up menu, twelve to eight bit window and level are performed using the existing tools to copy the selected image data to Macintosh memory. The image data is then packaged as a Color QuickDraw "PICT" format pixel map (15), and exported to an HICF "sweep" folder. Relevant history, radiographic findings, and teaching file coding is performed at the time of export. This case data is then incorporated into the 4D HICF application for teaching file creation.

III. RESULTS

The presentation will demonstrate the software functionality described above in which a digitally acquired imaging study is processed through the Sun-based UCSF PACS and distributed to the Macintosh-based workstation. At the time of simulated readout at the Mac display station, specific key images are selected as appropriate for teaching. Relevant clinical data is entered at the time of HICF image tagging. Both text and image data are exported to an HICF "sweep" folder from which the 4D database application seamlessly retrieves the new teaching file case.

IV. DISCUSSION

Cross-platform interoperability and interprogram image data transfer remain a challenge at this time, especially when interfaces to commercial packages are attempted. The existence of standards like "PICT" are generally helpful. However, "PICT" is a complex standard, and its intricacy can make export implementation difficult. It does facilitate compatibility with Macintosh desktop publishing applications.

This project was accomplished using the specific workstation developed on the Macintosh platform at the UCSF Laboratory for Radiological Informatics. Ideally, these software components could be packaged and ported to other commercial workstation platforms. However, end-users are infrequently allowed access to commercial workstation source code for installation of modules such as these. Further, this type of functionality does not appear to be a high-priority for most commercial workstation vendors.

This proof-of-concept demonstration addressing cross-platform interoperability and integration of digital teaching file creation at the diagnostic workstation needs to be evaluated in a working clinical environment. We feel that the ideal time to identify cases including images of high educational or research content is at the time of interpretation. The software applications developed and presented here accomplish these goals.

ACKNOWLEDGMENTS

Mohan Ramaswamy, M.D., generously provided some of the source code for implementing the PICT format conversion. The assistance of Wyatt M. Tellis with coding of the 4D database is greatly appreciated.

REFERENCES

1. Arenson RL. Teaching with computers. *Radiol Clin NA* 1986;24:97-103.
2. Arenson RL, Greenes RA, Swett HA, Allman RM. Digital radiology learning library (DRILL): A standardized teaching platform. *SCAR* 1990:674-680.
3. Apicella PL, Blaine GJ, Jost RG. A prototype of a high-resolution computerized radiology teaching file. *Journal of Digital Imaging*, 1991;4:43-50.
4. Richardson ML, Gillespy T 3rd. An inexpensive computer-based digital imaging teaching file. *AJR* 1993;160:1299-1301.
5. Richardson ML, Rowberg AH, Gillespy T 3rd, Frank MS. An on-line digital Internet radiology teaching file server. *AJR* 1994;162:1239-1242.
6. Avrin DE, Andriole KP, Ramaswamy M, et al. The digital academic radiology department: automation and enrichment of teaching and research. *SCAR*94:631-633.
7. Avrin DE, Andriole KP, Ramaswamy MR, Huang HK, Arenson RL, Tellis WM. Issues in converting conventional teaching and research files in a digital academic department. *RSNA* 1994, Chicago.
8. Ramaswamy MR, Wong AWK, Lee JK, Huang HK. Accessing picture archiving and communication system text and image information through personal computers. *AJR* 1994;163:1229-1243.
9. Huang HK, Arenson RL, Lou SL et al. Second generation PACS (abst). *Radiology* 1993;189:410.
10. Avrin DE, Lou A, Andriole KP, Ramaswamy M, Arenson RL. Cost effective many-monitor workstation. *European Congress of Radiology*, Vienna Sept., 1993.
11. Ramaswamy MR, Avrin DE, Andriole KP, Wong AWK, Bazzill TM, Arenson RL. Use of personal computer technology in supporting a radiological review workstation. *SPIE Medical Imaging Proceedings*, 1994.
12. THINK C is a trademark and product of Symantec Corp.
13. Macintosh Toolbox is a trademark and product of Apple Computer Corp.
14. Dome Hydra imaging board is a product of Dome imaging systems, Waltham, MA, USA.
15. Gillespy III T, Rowberg AH. Radiological images on personal computers: introduction and fundamental principles of digital images. *Journal of Digital Imaging* 1993; 6:81-87.

Generation of 3D Anatomical Atlases Using the Visible Human

Thomas Schiemann, Jochen Nuthmann, Ulf Tiede and Karl Heinz Höhne
Institute of Mathematics and Computer Science in Medicine
University Hospital, Hamburg, Germany

Abstract In principle the Visible Human data sets are an ideal basis for building electronic atlases. While it is easy to construct such atlases by just offering the possibility of browsing through the 2D slices, the construction of realistic 3D models is a huge project. As one rather easy way to establish three-dimensionality, we have registered the Visible Human data to the already existing 3D atlas VOXEL-MAN/brain. This procedure enables lookup of anatomical detail in an atlas based on radiological images. Concerning the segmentation problem, which is the prerequisite for a real 3D atlas, we have developed an interactive classification method, which delivers realistic perspective views of the Visible Human.

Introduction

In our previous work we have developed a framework for generating volume based 3D interactive atlases. These atlases are based on a two layer model [6]: Images volumes, usually obtained from radiology, and congruent label volumes for different domains of knowledge like morphology or physiology form the spatial part of the model. It is linked to a semantic network containing descriptive knowledge about the objects. For extraction of the model's contents there is a large set of visualization, exploration, and simulation tools.

With this framework the VOXEL-MAN atlases of brain and skull have been completed [1] and atlases of other parts of the body are under development [3]. Their pictorial basis are radiologic cross-sectional images. While this has the advantage that anatomy can be linked nicely to radiological imaging, anatomical detail is subject to improvement. The high resolution data sets of the Visible Human project [7] are therefore an ideal basis for this purpose.

Typically the Visible Human images are presented in stacks of orthogonal slices, which can be browsed through. Compared to such simple systems, creation of a real 3D model requires detailed segmentation, which is a huge project due to the vast amount of data and anatomical detail. In our first approach we overcome this problem by registration of the Visible Human with the existing volume based atlas VOXEL-MAN/brain. This procedure introduces anatomical detail from the Visible Human into the radiological environment of VOXEL-MAN/brain, and on the other hand the detailed labelling of VOXEL-MAN can be correlated with the Visible Human.

While this procedure gives a new dimension of functionality to the existing atlas, 3D display of the Visible Human is not possible in this way. Thus we have done first steps in segmentation of some portions of the huge data set, which can thus be visualized in high quality with greatly improved realism. This procedure will be described in the second part.

Registration of the Visible Human to VOXEL-MAN

Registration of the anatomical Visible Human images to the radiological images of the VOXEL-MAN atlases is established by a linear mapping function, which is specified in an interactive environment [5]. The specification uses two different steps of interaction:

1. A set of landmarks (points and planes) is specified for a coarse mapping. For registration of the head region we use the bicommisurial coordinate system of Talairach For other body regions this can be generalized to any pair of characteristic points on an orthogonal plane.

2. For a refined registration, surface representations of structures from VOXEL-MAN are first transformed according to the specified landmarks, and can then interactively be registered on the Visible Human images in any linear manner (rotation, translation, scaling): Wire frames can be modified on perspective images and contours are manipulated on slices.

Due to the linear mapping function and the fact, that two different individuals have to be registered, this procedure cannot create a registration with a precision in the order of a few voxels. Nevertheless the procedure results in highly correlated image volumes, enabling a combination of the advantages, which each of them has: The VOXEL-MAN volume has been segmented in great detail offering information about morphology, blood supply, and function, while the anatomical images of the Visible Human present anatomical realism, which cannot be obtained from radiological procedures. Thus arbitrary slices of each of the volumes can be viewed side by side with one of them showing anatomical realism and the other one giving knowledge from the volume model (Fig. 1). In addition the Visible Human slices can also be shown in the 3D context of the perspective images.

Segmentation for high quality rendering

High quality rendering of volume data requires supersampling of the data volume on basis of an analytical description of the segmentation result. In case of scalar image volumes this is a labelled volume in combination with threshold ranges for every object. In case of the anatomical images of the Visible Human the threshold range has to be generalized to a region in RGB feature space. In order to keep computing times during rendering as low as possible, the selected description should be easy to formalize. We have thus decided to classify the regions by ellipsoids.

The segmentation is adapted from an interactive method, which has proven to be successful for many purposes with scalar images like CT or MRI [2, 4]. The procedure is based on thresholding followed by binary mathematical morphology and connected component labelling. While the latter two steps remain unchanged for color images, the thresholding step is generalized to specification of an ellipsoid in RGB-space:

1. The users outlines a (usually small) region of the object, which shall be segmented. This results in a set of RGB-triples $(RGB)_i$.

2. The median rgb-triple μ_{RGB} and the median μ_d of all distances $d(\mu_{RGB} - (RGB)_i)$ are computed.

3. For determination of the ellipsoid only those triples are further regarded, which are closer to μ_{RGB} than an interactively specified multiple of the median μ_d: The center is taken from the median of the considered sample set, the axes directions are computed from covariance analysis and their length is determined such, that all considered triples are inside the ellipsoid.

Instead of this basic ellipsoidal specification, the segmentation step could also be performed with much more sophisticated classification algorithms. However, these do usually not result in easy to formalize descriptions, which we need during ray-casting.

The proposed segmentation procedure is successful for all major constituents of the body like brain or abdominal organs. For a detailed subdivision of these structures, e.g. into gyri of the brain, manual segmentation is still needed due to a lack of image properties for this purpose.

Figures 2 and 3 show renderings of structures of the upper abdomen, which have all been segmented with the described semi-automatic procedure. The bone has been segmented from the CT images, which come along with the anatomical images and which have undergone further registration [5]. Except for bone and vascular structures, all organs are visualized according to their colors in the anatomical images. Bone colors are weighted with an artificial color in order to enhance bone appearance. Arteries and veins are visualized in pure artificial colors (red/blue) as usual on anatomical images. Further 3D images of the head are shown in [8].

Conclusions

We have proposed two different approaches for use of the Visible Human images for electronic anatomy atlases. The registration of the Visible Human with VOXEL-MAN/brain offers a new dimension for interpretation of anatomy obtained from radiology. This functionality is ready for use without limitations. In our second approach the described first steps in segmentation for high resolution volume rendering show, that the Visible Human data set represents a new quality of anatomical imaging, when used in a state-of-the-art visualization system. Nevertheless, a huge amount of work still has to be done for detailed segmentation. But unlike clinical imaging, which requires new segmentation for every case, segmentation of the Visible Human has to be done only once. If this work is completed, the results will surely have great impact on many applications of visualization such as education and simulation.

Acknowledgements

We are grateful to all members of our department, who have supported this work. Special thanks to Rainer Schubert for anatomical and Uwe Pichlmeier for statistical support.

References

[1] Höhne, K. H. (Ed.): *VOXEL-MAN, Part 1: Brain and Skull, Version 1.0.* Springer-Verlag Electronic Media, Heidelberg, 1995. (ISBN 3-540-14517-6).

[2] Höhne, K. H., Hanson, W. A.: Interactive 3D-segmentation of MRI and CT volumes using morphological operations. *J. Comput. Assist. Tomogr. 16*, 2 (1992), 285–294.

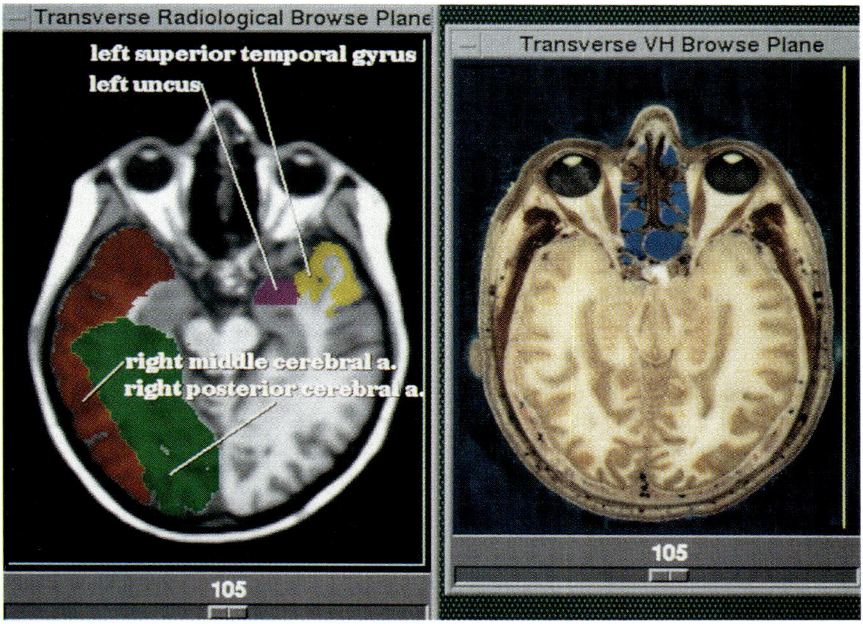

Figure 1: Correlation of slices from the Visible Human and VOXEL-MAN/brain after registration has been performed: The VOXEL-MAN slice (left) shows semantic regions of the volume model (morphological objects on the right and blood supply areas on the left). The Visible Human slice adds pictorial anatomical detail to the context.

[3] Höhne, K. H., Pflesser, B., Pommert, A., Riemer, M., Schiemann, T., Schubert, R., Tiede, U.: A new representation of knowledge concerning human anatomy and function. *Nature Med. 1*, 6 (1995), 506–511.

[4] Schiemann, T., Bomans, M., Tiede, U., Höhne, K. H.: Interactive 3D-segmentation. In Robb, R. A. (Ed.): *Visualization in Biomedical Computing II, Proc. SPIE 1808.* Chapel Hill, NC, 1992, 376–383.

[5] Schiemann, T., Höhne, K. H., Koch, C., Pommert, A., Riemer, M., Schubert, R., Tiede, U.: Interpretation of tomographic images using automatic atlas lookup. In Robb, R. A. (Ed.): *Visualization in Biomedical Computing 1994, Proc. SPIE 2359.* Rochester, MN, 1994, 457–465.

[6] Schubert, R., Höhne, K. H., Pommert, A., Riemer, M., Schiemann, T., Tiede, U.: Spatial knowledge representation for visualization of human anatomy and function. In Barrett, H. H., Gmitro, A. F. (Eds.): *Information Processing in Medical Imaging, Proc. IPMI '93*, Lecture Notes in Computer Science 687, Springer-Verlag, Berlin, 1993, 168–181.

[7] Spitzer, V. M., Whitlock, D. G.: High resolution electronic imaging of the human body. *J. Biol. Photogr. 60*, 4 (1992), 167–172.

[8] Tiede, U., Schiemann, T., Höhne, K. H.: Visualizing the Visible Human. *IEEE Comput. Graphics Appl. 16*, 1 (1996), 7–9.

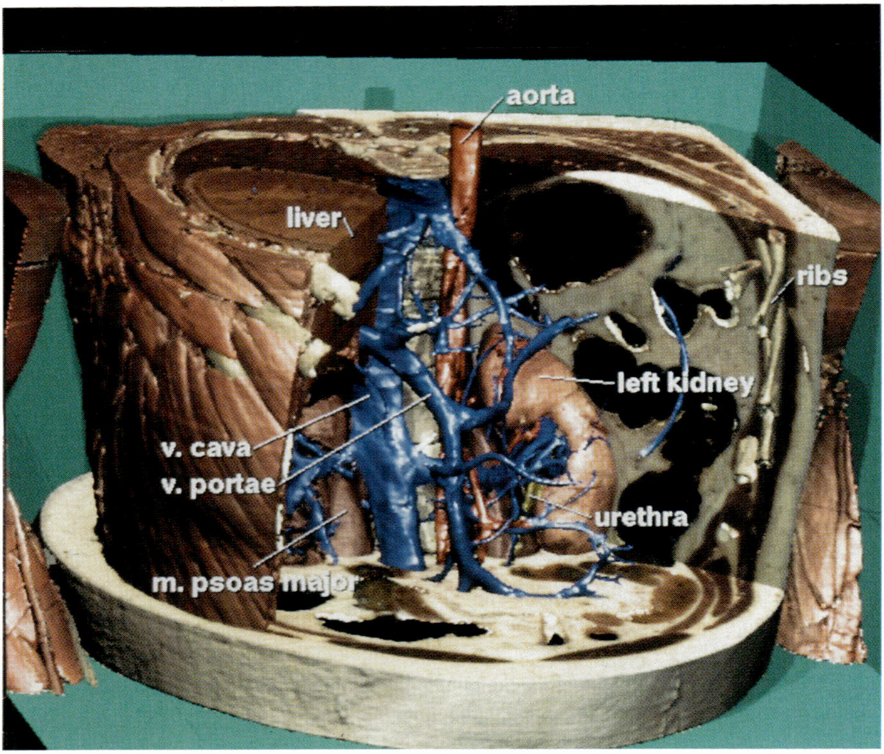

Figure 2: Frontal view of the left kidney: Several cut planes are specified in order to unveil the left kidney and the major vascular structures. Ribs, blood vessels and some muscles are excluded from cutting. The cut planes show the colors of the anatomical volume

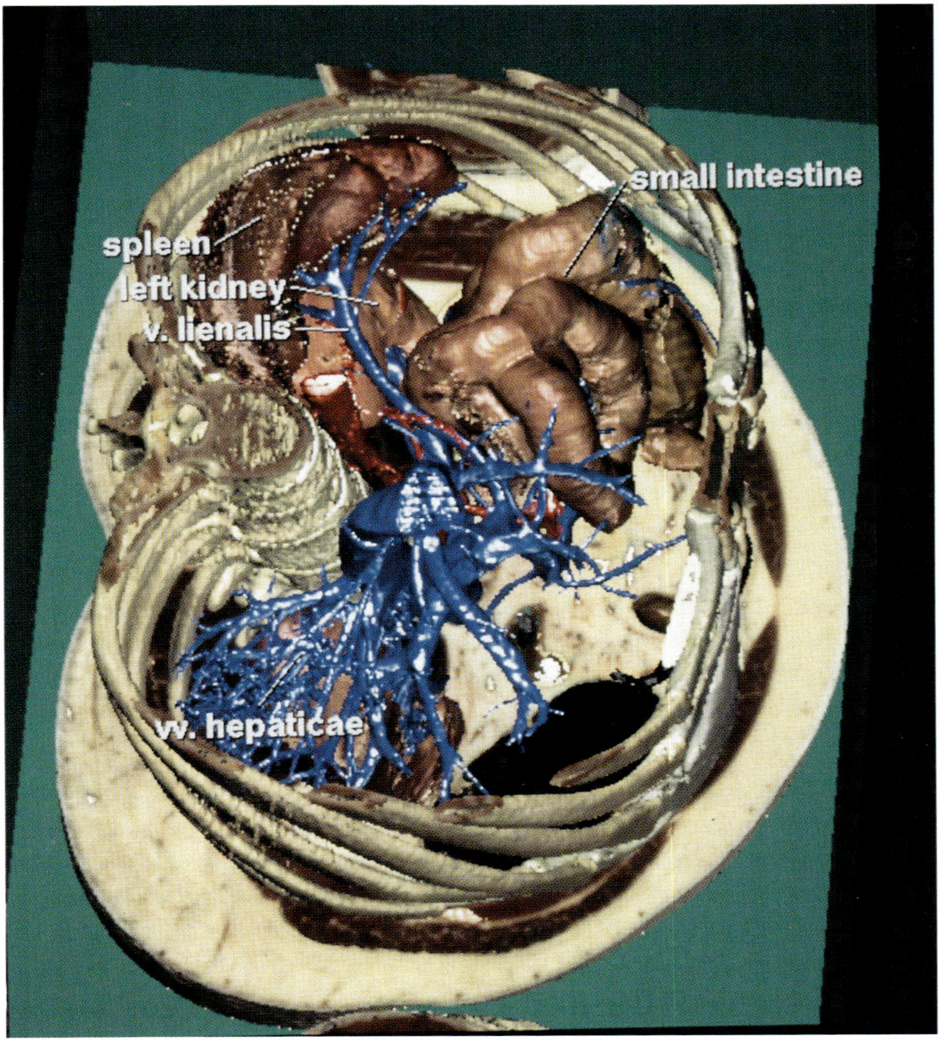

Figure 3: Cranio-caudal view of the spleen, small intestine and the hepatic veins surrounded by the rib cage.

Computer Applications in Radiology Resident Training: Evidence Based Radiology

Barbara M. Jaeger, M.D., Barbara H. Miller, M.D. and Robert M. Allman, M.D.
University of Maryland Medical Center, Department of Radiology, Baltimore, Maryland

The newest breakthrough in clinical medicine today is not a drug nor vaccine. It is a way of answering clinical problems by utilizing current research findings in real time for clinical decisions. Known as evidence based medicine, its use is rapidly spreading.

Evidence based medicine is a term coined in the 1980's at McMaster Medical School in Canada. It defines a clinical learning strategy wherein the clinician identifies questions relative to patient care and consults the literature to obtain relevant data. [1] This practice allows clinicians to update their knowledge to solve medical dilemmas in a rapidly changing field of biomedical knowledge, instead of relying on anecdotal clinical experience.

The radiologist's counterpart of clinically oriented evidence-based medicine is the radiology consultation performed at the view box for referring physicians or for the benefit of residents in training. In the course of this radiological consultation, the faculty is often called upon to furnish information on the incidence of disease, probability (specificity and sensitivity) and other statistics. Anecdotal knowledge (gamuts, pearls, mnemonics etc.) has formed the traditional basis for this transfer of knowledge. Often, the resident supplements anecdotal information from the faculty with "facts" from texts such as AFIP workbooks, Gamuts in Radiology, The Massachusetts General Primer of Diagnostic Imaging, Radiology Review Manual etc. Theories of evidence based medicine can be applied in the field of radiology, to enhance the interpretative accuracy of film reading and to form a foundation for thorough and meaningful radiologic consultation.

Requirements of evidence based radiology:[2,3]

1. Clearly define the problem.
2. Identify the information required to resolve the problem and answer the question.
3. Conduct an efficient search of the literature.
4. Critically appraise the evidence for its validity and usefulness.
5. Implement useful findings in to radiologic practice.

If radiologists are to be comfortable with evidence based radiology, the required skills should be developed during residency. Therefore, evidence based radiology has another valuable attribute in that it mimics problem based learning (PBL), a most widely discussed development in medical education today.

Over 100 years ago medical educator William Welch, realized that "the time has gone by when one mind can encompass all which has ascertained in the medical sciences".[4] In 1992, the AAMC ACME-TRI report entitled ' Educating Medical Students: Assessing Change In Medical Education' addressed the need for doctors of the 21st century to develop skills to stay current with the changes in medical practice. (Students) must be prepared to go on learning through their professional lives.[5] This philosophy holds true for graduate medical education as well. The days of formal didactic lecture oriented medical education are giving way to innovations in curricula which stress self directed learning and problem solving. "The starting point for PBL is a problem, a query or a puzzle that the learner wishes to solve."[6] Faculty serve as facilitators, providing a framework for the medical student to work on problems for himself.

Advocates of PBL believe that with self directed learning, knowledge is remembered and applied more easily when new concepts are implemented immediately. The General Professional Education of the Physician and College Preparation for Medicine Report calls upon medical education to prepare future physicians to "learn throughout their professional lives rather than master current information and techniques." It states that " lifelong learning requires active, independent, self-directed learning and the ability to identify, formulate and solve problems; to grasp and use basic concepts and principles; and to gather and assess data rigorously and critically."[7]

Likewise, for evidence based radiology, we begin with a clear definition of the problem. This may be a question of pathological mechanism, natural history of a disease, or of an epidemiologic nature. The resident is challenged to identify the necessary information to resolve the clinical question, as well as consider the appropriate resource for locating this information. "[Residents] are able to learn medicine in a way that develops their problem solving abilities, thereby making them effective, self-directed learners."[8]

Teaching evidence based radiology in residency training, faculty would serve as facilitators, rather than as lecturers or fact providers. In this manner, faculty shape the mind of the resident, bestowing upon them their cumulative experience and clinical acumen. Their personal approach to resolving questions is drawn upon in discussions that "move the resident from passive learner to active learner."[9]

Thus evidence based radiology is the application of real-time literature searching in teaching and in the practice of the art of radiological consultation. This term is an extension of clinically oriented evidence-based medicine and defines the growing practice in radiology residency training of obtaining current statistics of incidence of disease by age, race, gender, etc. and probability data, sensitivity and specificity, etc. from on-line literature databases such as Medline.

Resident training for efficient meaningful film reading and for literature searching requires a computerized work station at the site of film interpretation. With the computerized work station, practitioners of evidence based radiology have a rapid means of acquiring the necessary data for problem based resident training, and provision of the radiological consultation. Critical appraisal takes place at the work station, when the validity of research can be challenged by the team as literature comes on-line. It is at this 'teachable' moment that residents and attendings choose whether to incorporate new data into their radiology practice. In this way, the radiologist of the future may continue to be an effective contributor to patient management, and the health care team.

Scenario:

The Jr. resident is presented with a chest Xray in which there is a 5cm. solitary pulmonary nodule. The attending queries as to what it may be. Eagerly the resident states primary carcinoma, without knowing patient history, demographics or prevalence. The attending guides the resident through the process by asking what information is necessary to fully evaluate this case. Using On-line Medical records the resident determines that the patient is a 28 year old female, non-smoking. He now lowers his index for suspicion for primary carcinoma. Further investigation reveals that the patient is HIV+, homeless, with a cough. Through the PACS system old films are retrieved revealing that this nodule has appeared over a rather small period of time. Although the differential for solitary nodule is well known, a quick literature search cross-referencing HIV,and solitary pulmonary nodules reveals two pertinent articles; one on nocardiosis and one on PCP, expanding the standard differential with current research statistics, e.g. 'in 150 cases of PCP, two patients (1.3%) presented as solitary nodules".[10] Without leaving the work-station, the resident has performed his own investigation into the patients history, and into the disease he has focused his concern on. His literature search quickly provided him with statistics regarding incidence and prevalence of his suspect findings, as well as radiographic descriptions of the appearance. By thinking through the process and putting the pieces together himself, the resident takes ownership of the case, much in the way that clinical residents learn by treating individual patients.

Evidence based radiology satisfies only one of the fundamentals of the radiological consultation described in depth by legendary as well as contemporary radiologists. One early description occurred at the inception of the Registry of Radiological Pathology at the AFIP when the teaching methods of Colonel William Leroy Thompson were introduced. The following is Colonel Thompson's portrayal of the scientific criteria by which to analysis radiographic films 1) An orderly study of the evidence shown by the film with a listing of the morphological criteria;

2) Consideration of corroborative evidence might be obtained by radiographic studies of other portions of the body; 3) Considerations of the implications of such factors as age, sex, nationality and race of the patient in relation to the general incidence of the suspected condition; 4) Review of the clinical history, the physical findings and the laboratory data. [11]

In todays cost-consciousness atmosphere, Col. Thompson's criteria are no less applicable. In fact, they should be heeded more stringently than ever. Adherence to these concepts with appropriate modification for todays health care environment, provides a cost effective framework for providing radiologic consultation services to referring physicians and their patients.

With a premium on judicial use of health care dollars, the addition of standards for use of radiologic services becomes the final requirement of the radiologic consult. The ACR appropriateness criteria for imaging and treatment decisions considers the indication, benefit and cost of each imaging study and rates them for suitability for a given clinical condition. These criteria are to aid radiologists and referring physicians in choosing the proper imaging studies for a given clinical scenario, providing efficient use of resources, resulting in fewer unnecessary studies and saving patients time, money and needless exposure to radiation.

Often when the radiologist reviews images, there is insufficient clinical and demographic data to help narrow the diagnostic possibilities. The cumbersome nature of obtaining this information leads many in the interest of time to provide overwhelming and inappropriate differentials with caveat "clinical correlation suggested." This disclaimer does not do justice to the patient nor does it enhance the image of the radiologist in the eyes of the clinician. Such ambivalent reporting has contributed to the current movement by some clinicians to want to be paid for reading their own films. If radiologists wish to remain consultants, they must integrate radiographic observations with a decision-making scheme incorporating current knowledge of appropriate clinical information and epidemiological statistics.

Applying todays standards, the radiologic consultation should include: Morphological analysis, Corroborative Imaging Procedures, Probability and Statistics, Clinical information, Appropriateness.

The work station as the foundation for the radiologic consultation.

Finding and incorporating relevant data from computer sources (including literature) into clinical interpretations of radiographs is the foundation of evidence-based radiology. It's use can statistically support a diagnosis and produce a reasonable differential list. The ideal work station for the radiologist should include more than just film reading; there must be access to old studies, clinical, pathological and epidemiologic data. In addition to a PACS system for accessing current and previous radiographic studies and their reports, the work station of the future will contain a state of the art computer allowing one to rapidly switch from On-line medical records to Laboratory and Surgical-Pathology records, ACR Standards and Appropriateness Criteria, Medline and literature databases. With these databases readily available, information can readily be incorporated into the radiologic consultation.

Morphologic Analysis and Corroborative Imaging Procedures:

Correlation of new studies with old examinations, or other modalities is often limited to what is available in the patient's film folder when that folder is available. With todays rapidly advancing technology, current as well as prior radiographs and reports are immediately available via PACS system. Images can be darkened or lightened, as well as magnified to maximize the information obtained.

Incidence and probability statistics:

Previously, a search of the literature to evaluate clinical research or answer a clinical question required a trip to the library, and perhaps hours to root out a relevant article. It was inconvenient and time consuming. Development of peripheral brains or pocket references were the key to survival and learning, but not always very practical. Many residents choose to carry reference texts to read-out. While this facilitates rapid verification of information, carrying your library with you is cumbersome and not a very practical proposition. With the advent of electronic data bases, access can be available at the site of film interpretation. Information is always up to date and correct, not always the case with reference texts.

Clinical Information:

Clinical information usually comes from a request form, often giving the patient history as only "pre-op" or "pain". In order to be effective as a consultant, the radiologist must know any relevant patient history. Ordinarily, obtaining the patients medical history and records requires a trip to medical records, often finding the chart to be not in file. Contacting the referring physician can take hours awaiting a return call, particularly if they are in clinic or the Operating Room. With work station access to On-line medical records a patients medical history may be accessed to facilitate interpretations and/or provide concordance with previous studies. Additionally, through the use of the Internet, information related to radiographs and/or hospitalizations at other institutions could be obtained in seconds. Similarly, surgical and pathological information may be obtained to correlate findings and learn from them.

Appropriateness:

As clinical physicians choose studies they want, they may select a non-diagnostic or totally inappropriate study based on their training or comfort level with the study. The ACR Appropriateness criteria must be made available to referring physicians quickly and efficiently. With a CD-ROM system at the radiologists fingertips, any request for a study can immediately be followed with feedback on appropriateness, along with recommendations for the proper course of diagnostic imaging.

Use of readily available information in decision support and problem solving prevents errors in diagnoses secondary to inaccurate assumptions. Accurate diagnosis enhances patient care, and may reduce costs and unnecessary procedures. Additionally, the radiologic consultation gains favor in the eyes of the clinician, and the services of the radiologist become a necessary component of good patient care.

In training of residents:

The benefits to residents, attendings and patients through the use of evidence based radiology include the following: 1. Enables attendings as well as residents to upgrade their knowledge routinely. 2. Enables residents to make a useful contribution to the team. [12] 3. Improves confidence in diagnostic decision making by reinforcing correct information. 4. Indications for study, patient history, laboratory findings, and surg-path correlation's can be obtained, improving patient care and communication with the care team.

Conclusion:

Evidence based radiology is a new approach to film interpretation that provides for meaningful radiologic consultation through the use of computers to access patient history and demographic data as well as to perform rapid searches of the literature to answer a clinical question with contemporaneous research findings. The knowledge and skills required to practice evidence based radiology should be taught at the resident level, in order to assure that comfort with the skills necessary for lifelong learning is developed. In turn, performing evidence based radiology during resident read-out, allows residents to participate in the learning process, making a useful contribution to the team. By having the resident perform his own data search, self directed, active learning takes place, fostering lifelong learning skills for critical review of the literature and problem solving. In times of rapidly changing breakthroughs in medicine, residents are learning a skill that will enable them to remain current in their knowledge base throughout their careers.

References:

1. Rosenberg, W. and Anna Donald. Evidence-Based Medicine: An approach to clinical problem-solving. BMJ 1995; 321:1122-6.
2. Ibid.
3. McCulluch,Christopher, DDS, PhD. Can Evidence Based Dental Care Assure Quality? Journal of Dental Education. vol.58#8, 1994.
4. Ende,Jack and Elaine Atkins. Conceptualizing curriculum for Graduate Medical Education. Academic Medicine. Volume 67 #8 Aug. 1992 pp528-534.
5. Association of American Medical Colleges (1992) ACME-TRI Report on Educating Medical Students: Assessing Change in Medical Education - The Road to Implementation Association of American Medical Colleges, Washington D.C.
6. Bligh,John Problem-Based Learning in Medicine: An Introduction. Postgraduate Medicine 1995, 71:323-326.
7. Schilling, K. et al. Integration of Information-seeking Skills and Activities into a Problem-based Curriculum. Bull. Med. Library Ass. 83(2) Aoril 1995 pp.176-183.
8. Eldredge, Jonathan D. A Problem Based Learning Curriculum in Transition: The Emerging Role of the Library. Bulliten Medical Library Association 81(3) July 1993. 310-315.
9. Ende, J and E Atkins. Conceptualizing Curriculum for Graduate Medical Education. Academic Medicine Vol 67 #8 August 1992 p.532.
10. Barrio, J.L. et al Pneumocystis Carinii Pneumonia presenting as cavitating and noncavitating solitary pulmonary nodules in patients with the acquired immunodeficiency syndrome. Am Review of Resp Disease 134(5):1094-6 1986 Nov.
11. Allman, Robert M. Educational Concepts of the Radiologic Pathology Branch, AFIP. Digest. Nov.1970;volume XXI Number XI:11-14.
12. Rosenberg, W and Anna Donald. Evidence-Based Medicine. An Approach to Clinical Problem Solving. BMJ 1995;310:1122-6

The Development of a Computer-Based Teaching Library On Imaging Chest Disease

Debra S. Dyer, M.D., Valerie A.E. Hale, M.D., John M. Lewin, M.D., Denise C. Garcia, R.T., Vic Spitzer, Ph.D., Helen Pelster, B.A. and John Newell, M.D.

University of Colorado Health Sciences Center, Denver, Colorado

I. INTRODUCTION

Thoracic radiology is a rapidly growing area of diagnostic radiology. While clinicians and radiologists have previously relied upon the chest radiograph, a number of imaging modalities including conventional computed tomography (CT), high-resolution CT (HRCT), and magnetic resonance imaging now aid tremendously in the diagnosis of pulmonary diseases. Although this considerable growth in diagnostic capability has occurred, the ability to distribute and transmit this information to health care professionals has been limited. An innovative educational tool is needed that could be continuously updated and universally accessible. One such tool, The Virtual Hospital, has been developed by the University of Iowa[1]. This successful program contains a digital medical library stored on computers that can be accessed in distant locations via the Internet.

The ideal teaching tool for imaging lung disease should contain textual information and representative images to convey the important concepts in pulmonary medical imaging. We have developed a computer-based teaching file, modeled after The Virtual Hospital, but dedicated to imaging chest diseases. The teaching file was designed to teach thoracic radiology to radiology residents and fellows, but is also a valuable reference for practicing radiologists, pulmonary physicians, primary care providers, other residents and medical students. Via the Internet, it is accessible to health care providers in distant cities, small towns, and rural areas.

II. PROGRAM DESIGN

Our computer-based teaching file was developed through a Bridge to the Future Innovation Education Grant from the University of Colorado Health Sciences Center (UCHSC). Teaching file cases were selected from a large pool of interesting and unique cases of pulmonary disease from the National Jewish Center for Immunology and Respiratory Medicine and UCHSC. Each case includes digitized chest radiographs and CT/HRCT images. (See Figures A and B.)

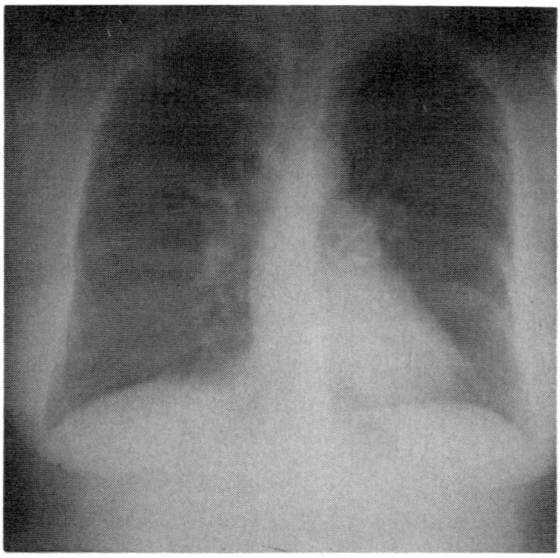

Figure A

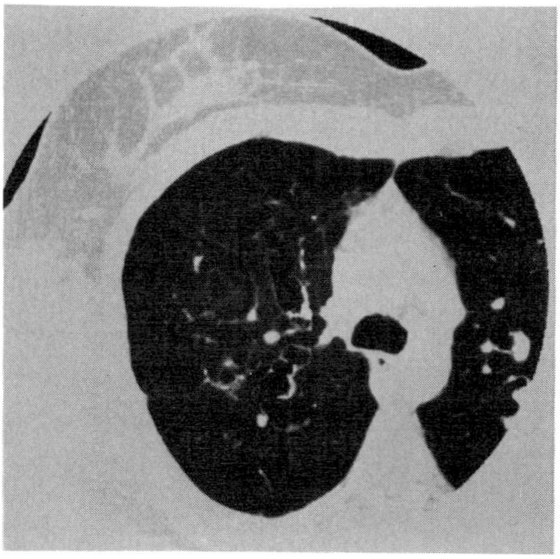

Figure B

Figures A and B illustrate a case of Allergic Bronchopulmonary Aspergillosis reproduced from our teaching file.

The file is still under construction. Our goal is to have 65 cases of usual and unusual chest diseases entered into the teaching file cases. The cases will be distributed as follows:

1. approximately 20 cases of typical manifestations of common lung diseases (examples are tuberculosis, lung cancer, lobar collapse)
2. approximately 20 cases of atypical manifestations of common lung diseases (examples are atypical lobar collapse, atypical tuberculosis)
3. approximately 25 cases of manifestations of uncommon lung diseases such as lymphangiomyomatosis, pulmonary histiocytosis X, idiopathic pulmonary fibrosis

Initially six cases were developed and evaluated to delineate the optimum format for case presentation and image acquisition. Evaluators included radiology residents/fellows, practicing radiologists, pulmonary physicians, and medical students.

III. METHODS

The project was developed using the computer facilities in the Center for Human Simulation at UCHSC. Chest radiographs were digitized using a CCD camera. CT images were loaded onto a Silicon Graphics workstation in direct digital format after being transferred from optical disk onto 4 mm Digital Audio

Tape (DAT). Chest radiographs were digitized at a resolution giving 512 pixels across either a 14" or 17" wide film. CT images were all 512 x 512 pixels. The images were compressed into JPEG and GIF image formats using San Diego Supercomputer Image Tools software (San Diego Supercomputer Center). A compression parameter of 75 on a scale of 1-100 (100 gives the least compression) was used for the JPEG compression. The JPEG compression gave much smaller data sets. On average the GIF images were 160 kbytes versus 24 kbytes for JPEG. CT images resulted in smaller data sets than chest radiographs using both methods.

The text for the cases was written by a combination of our thoracic radiology faculty members, thoracic radiology fellow and residents rotating on the chest service. The text and images from the six cases were put in a known-case format using Hypertext Mark-up Language. The teaching file was then placed on the Internet using the server at UCHSC. Our Internet address is "http://www.uchsc.edu/uh/radiology/".

IV. RESULTS

Our computer-based teaching library on imaging chest disease has been in use for nine months. The teaching file has been very popular with our residents who have enjoyed developing cases and reviewing the cases developed by others. The teaching file format provided an excellent opportunity for resident-faculty interaction and allowed the resident to do in-depth study on a topic of his/her choice.

An initial task was to determine the best image format. Our radiologists unanimously agreed that the GIF format was preferable in that it offered better spatial resolution and less visible "dither" than the JPEG images. This effect was most noticeable on computers that were not capable of displaying a full 256 gray level.

Once our initial six cases were developed, a thorough evaluation was performed. Cases were scored for presentation and content and on the quality of the images. Evaluators also rated the teaching file for its accessibility and its potential usefulness in their practice.

The pilot project was evaluated by several individuals: one fourth-year medical student, one pulmonologist, one academic radiologist, one private practice radiologist and three radiology residents. Interestingly, only three individuals described themselves as being familiar with the Internet. Most (5) felt the findings by CXR and CT were easy to identify and felt that image quality was acceptable. However, one radiologist did not think the plain film findings were readily evident and one radiologist had difficulty because of technical limitations.

Two formats for visualizing the images were used: 1) Style A, where images are "called up" by highlighted text, and 2) Style B, where images are displayed in line with the text. All evaluators with the exception of one radiologist preferred Style B. The lone dissenting radiologist did not have a preference for either Style A or Style B.

Virtually all (7) evaluators found the text easy to understand, appropriate in length and correlated well with the images. One (a radiologist) suggested an outline format as an alternative. Many commented that annotating the images with arrows and text would be beneficial.

All strongly agreed that a teaching tool such as this would be helpful to their understanding of thoracic radiology and would refer to it again. Improved plain film resolution and shorter image transmission time would enhance its use.

V. CONCLUSION

The teaching opportunities using computers are boundless. Our development of a computer based teaching file on imaging chest diseases was rewarding and represents an exciting and useful application of computer technology to the field of radiology.

REFERENCES

1. Galvin JR, D'Allesandro MP, Erkonen WE, Knutson TA and Lacey DL. The Virtual Hospital: A New Paradigm for Electronic Publishing in Radiology. Proceedings of Computer Applications to Assist Radiology, Winston-Salem, North Carolina, 1994, pp. 640-645.

SESSION 2

Information Management

Co-Chairs:

Roger A. Bauman
Philip G. Drew

Custom Presentation of Medical Imaging Management Statistics Retrieved from the HIS/RIS: Use of Commercially Available Personal Computer Software

Charles A. Nortmann and Margaret J. Farrell
Primary Children's Medical Center, Salt Lake City, Utah

I. INTRODUCTION

Decisions must be made by Medical Imaging managers. Manually collected data may assist and improve the confidence in these decisions, but the mechanism for collection makes their use limited. The gathering of data and production of information through the department computer information system streamlines and increases the accuracy of this information. Some information systems produce reports that are not easily modified by the end user. Requests for modification or additional software can be prohibitively expensive or not available. Personal computers and local area networks (LANs) are readily available in most Medical Imaging departments. Timely access to procedural data assists in the evaluation of processes in this era of health care restructuring. We report our experience with data extracted from a commercial software system and reports generated with personal computer mainstream applications.

II. OVERVIEW

A commercial RIS was used to collect data (HELP,3M). The system runs on a minicomputer (TANDEM). A program supplied by the vendor is used to extract relevant fields. On a daily basis, the previous day's data is transferred in a tab separated format to the hospital LAN. The files from the individual dates are imported to a personal computer database application (Paradox, Borland). The database application is used to create custom reports, or alternatively, data can be exported to a spreadsheet application (Excel, Microsoft) for additional processing and display.

III. DATA IMPORT

Forty fields from the RIS were selected for inclusion in the database. The most useful are listed in Table 1. Several fields not listed are used for indexing and future expansion. Each record represents a single patient study, so that multiple exams performed on one patient generate separate records. The

Account#	Pt.Name	ReferringMD	ReportingMD
BirthDate	SSN	Comment	MR Number
OrderLoc	AdmitDx	OrderTime	RequestTime
ConfirmTime	CPT	ExamDescrp	ExamReason
RadiologyNo	Gender	ExamModality	Transport
PatientType	DictatedTime	TranscribedTime	SignedTime
ChargeCode	ConfirmTech0	ConfirmTech1	ConfirmTech2
ConfirmTech3	CorrectTime	CorrectedBy	TranscribedBy

TABLE 1

exam is scheduled, completed, dictated, and signed through the RIS. Department personnel must electronically complete and sign the study before a record is available for transfer. The stripping utility is activated during evening processing and creates a tab separated file on the minicomputer. A second utility copies the daily file to the LAN. An average day generates a file 16 KB in size with a range of 2 to 25 KB. The age of the tab separated files is monitored, and any over 30 days old are deleted by the copying utility. The tab separated data is imported to an unkeyed database table.

Maintenance of the table should be performed by non-programmers so it is desirable that the data import be accomplished by a "one button" function. This requirement presented the first obstacle. The database application import function for tab separated files does not support user selection of field types. This required the creation of an import module that would perform the table manipulations necessary for a successful import. The import program is written in the database application language (ObjectPAL) and it performs several tasks. The date of the last file to be imported is stored so that the import program will calculate the name of the next file to be imported. If necessary, the user may import several successive days. The tab file is imported and a database file for that day is created.

Any field on the RIS that stores a time is in the form of a Julian date. This is output in the daily tab file in the form mm/dd/yyyy.hh:mm:ss. The time is in 24 hour format. The first import results in a field of the correct format, but with a string field type. The correct field type is created by copying the data to an intermediate table with a structure similar to the original, but with the "timestamp" field correctly defined. A peculiarity of the database software resulted in the storage of incorrect times. Any time between 12:00 and 13:00 hours was transferred as 00:00 to 01:00 hours. A loop function scans all time/date fields prior to import and appends the characters "PM" to any times between 12:00 and 13:00 and the import proceeds correctly.

Data in the master table is stored by year. Studies with completion times of January 1 to December 31 are stored in one annual table.

IV. DATA EXTRACTION

Data retrieval is accomplished using the tools supplied as an integral part of the database program. Queries are created at any one of three levels of abstraction. The first two require a relatively sophisticated, knowledgeable user. It is possible to write queries in Structured Query Language (SQL) , a standard, relatively low level database query language, but the process is simplified by a function called Query By Example (QBE). The QBE function lets the user select the fields to be displayed, permits a range of values to be entered, and allows inclusion of unique or non-unique values. The QBE image is translated to SQL for processing. It is this function that makes the use of commercial PC database software attractive. The table to be queried may reside locally or on an enterprise wide server, and all users may extract information without need of programming knowledge. This method is used if the information needed is for one time use. Reports that need to be generated on a regular basis should be set up for use at the third abstraction level.

The third level is the most attractive for general use. The ObjectPAL language can be used to create query and report generation modules that proceed with a minimum of operator interaction. The users at this level are knowledgeable in that they have been instructed in the use of the application, and its related modules.

V. EXAMPLE OPERATIONS REPORTS

The management decision making process is supported by the information system. Basic department functions that need to be monitored include volume of exams, turnaround time, and employee productivity. These reports are generated using ObjectPAL methods.

EXAM VOLUME:

The number of examinations for a given date range, and a given time range can be created. Also, the volume of studies during a day, for a fixed time interval, may be reported. The time interval between points, in minutes, is chosen by the user. Any number of minutes evenly divisible into 24 hours may be selected.

TURNAROUND TIME:

The time between completion of the examination and the final electronic signature can be calculated. The results can be collated by exam, modality, or radiologist.

EMPLOYEE PRODUCTIVITY:

The technologists performing the examinations have their identification numbers included in the database at the time the exam is completed. The number of examinations performed by each technologist can be calculated. A table can be created containing a weighting factor, such as an RVU for each exam and a workload statistic, by technologist, can be generated.

ICD-9 CODING:

Insurance claims may be processed more efficiently if the clinical reason for the procedure is encoded in the ICD-9 format. Monthly reports reflecting the percentage of examinations containing codes are generated. The spreadsheet application is used to create a month to month process monitoring chart so that the effect of interventions, i.e. additional employee education, may be followed.

VI. RESEARCH SUPPORT APPLICATIONS

The collection of data for research applications can be simplified. Additional information on selected patients can be collected in a table. This information is then linked to the main database to combine age, gender, modality, or examination information with the research fields. This reduces the time and tedium for the data collection staff.

VII. FUTURE DIRECTION

An enterprise-wide database is being created (Oracle). This large scale system will receive information from the minicomputer as changes are made in each record. This eliminates the need for a daily download of the tab separated files.

VIII. SUMMARY

It is possible to use general purpose, commercially available personal computer software to extract management information from the hospital radiology information system. The flexibility in the presentation of the data supports department management decisions. Rapid access to information allows these decisions to be made in a timely manner.

Acknowledgment:

The authors wish to recognize the support of Bill Boam for authoring the TAB file creation tool.

A Computer System for Improving the Score on the NCQA Health Care Report Card

Mahfuz Ahmed, M.D., Ph.D., Pankaj J. Mowji, M.D., Curtis Anderson, R.T. and Charles Stuewe, B.S.
Kaiser Permanente Medical Center, Anaheim, California

Carol A. Ahmed, D.O.
Kaiser Permanente Medical Center, Riverside, California

Introduction

Access to health care has become one of the most discussed topics in the United States. Most of health care is purchased by the Federal and State Governments and by employers, with few individual purchasers. These purchasers demand high quality care which is affordable. To evaluate the different health-care delivery systems in a meaningful way, certain performance measures have been developed which are called the Health Plan Employer Data and Information Set or HEDIS. These measures are in a state of evolution as employers, health plan purchasers and health plans learn which performance measures are meaningful and which are not, and how best to obtain data for those that are meaningful. At this time the performance measures are: quality of care, member access and satisfaction, enrollment and utilization, and financial stability. By examining this information in its proper context, the purchasers of health care can clearly see a health plan's strengths, and understand the health plan's performance. Health plans and purchasers can use the HEDIS data to set and track progress towards mutually agreed-upon goals.

"Quality of care", goes beyond prescribing effective medical treatments for problems as they arise. Many physicians and other health care providers feel that the purchasers should receive superior care at an excellent value, which means avoiding many serious health problems, and detecting others at their earliest, most treatable stages. The purchasers need help from the providers to learn ways of staying healthy and disease free as long as possible. The providers, therefore, influenced the National Committee for Quality Assurance (NCQA) to work with HEDIS to develop quality of care indicators which are effective in the prevention and early detection of disease. The indicators are: childhood immunization, cholesterol screening, prenatal care, cervical cancer screening, breast cancer screening, and diabetic retinal examination. Some are low-cost, high-payoff, such as childhood immunization, cholesterol screening, and diabetic retinal examination; others are higher cost but vital in the fight against disease, such as mammograms and pap smears. These performance indicators are measurable and have the potential for improving the delivery of care. They are being used to track and report the performance of health care delivery systems including Health Maintenance Organizations (HMO's). In this competitive age, a health plan can be financially doomed by a low score. Information technology can help achieve a high score by providing baseline data on the health status of members, monitoring the indicators mentioned above, and automating clinical processes.

We describe a computer program, developed for a HMO serving 192,000 members, which monitors the NCQA indicators on every patient, and which alerts the physician or other health care provider when one or more of the indicators are not met. This is achieved via a "preventative health screen" which can be pulled up on a monitor whenever the patients medical record number is entered into the computer in connection with any type of interaction. It then allows the physician or other health care provider to take the appropriate action to satisfy the indicator. The system is generic, and can function as an integral and critical part of any quality of care and service improvement program while achieving reduction in cost.

Computer System

The system has been described previously(1)(2), but it has been upgraded and a new application, the "preventative health screen" has been added. The system is designed as an automated electronic medical record, in a managed care setting, for inpatients and out patients, with the ability to track any type of data. The hardware at this time consists of Data General Minicomputer Distributed Processing System consisting of twenty-one(21) DG S-280 minicomputers, 800 terminals, 150 printers and sixteen(16) Gigabytes of main storage. Further upgrades and additional applications are planned. The system operates on the RDOS/CHAMPS operating system, with application written in hybrid "Basic/Assembly" language with random access file structure.

The member base in the service area is 192,000. These members are seen in a 243 bed hospital with a medical office and seven other outlying clinics which is supported by 392 physicians and over 50 non physician practitioners consisting of physician assistants and nurse practitioners. The patient's electronic medical record can be accessed at any of these facilities.

Monitoring the NCQA indicators

The NCQA indicators described above are shown in Table 1 along with other indicators felt to be beneficial to the patient. When a patient checks in at any reception station, at the medical center or at any of the outlying clinics, the receptionist swipes his/her health plan card through a card reader and the quality of care indicators on the "preventative health screen" shown in Figure 1 is pulled up on the monitor. This screen is unique for each patient, and is generated in conjunction with a table of medical problems and risk factors (shown in Figure 2) entered for each patient. The intervals for screening and intervention change automatically according to predetermined guidelines as the risk factors and problem list change for a particular patient. This screen is available for the physician to view and take appropriate action at any computer terminal. In those locations where a computer terminal has not as yet been installed in the physician's office, the information on the screen is printed on a sheet of paper which goes with the patient's chart to the physician. If the patient is not in compliance with a particular screening procedure, such as for example, "mammography screening", the physician or his/her designee can request this test on the computer screen, and an order is automatically generated in the laboratory for the patient to go immediately and have the test performed. If the patient refuses an indicator such as for example "pneumococcus vaccination", this is entered into the computer as "refused" and tracked. If certain information is missing , e.g. "safe sex education" the physician or his/her designee is prompted by the computer to get the information. In those cases where the patient is in

Table 1

Preventative Health Screen

KPMC, O.C. **MEMBER PREVENTATIVE SCREEN SYSTEM**

Patient: Jane Doe **DOB:** 04/15/35 **Age:** 60 **SEX:** F **Pers Phys:** A. Jones MD.

Overdue!!	Mammography	X	Last: 03/02/95	*Overdue 31 days
Overdue!!	Tet-Diphtheria	I	Last: 03/15/84	*Overdue 24 months
No info on	Safe sex education	S	Please Inquire	
No info on	Clamydia	S	Please Inquire	
No info on	Syphilis Test	S	Please Inquire	
Compliant	BP Monitoring	S	Last: 03/28/96	Next due 23 months
Compliant	Diabetic retinal exam	S	Last: 03/28/96	Next due 11 months
Compliant	Breast self exam educ	S	Last: 03/29/96	
Compliant	Cholesterol	L	Last: 03/20/96	Next due 59 months
Compliant	Influenza	I	Last: 10/9/95	Next due 6 months
Compliant	PAP Smear	L	Last: 06/01/93	Next due 1 months**
Compliant	Weight recording	S	Last: 03/28/96	Next due 23 months
Refused	Pneumococcus	I	Last asked: 03/15/96	

To order, use letter code [ ](I,L,P,R,S,X) and CHAMPS Provider number [ ]

LEGEND: I - immunization, L - lab, P - prog note, R - risk/prob, S - service, X - xray

compliance at the time of seeing the physician, but will become non-compliant shortly thereafter, the system prompts the physician to advise the patient accordingly, and facilitates the process of becoming compliant.

The problem list shown in Table 2 allows the physician to review all the problems at a glance prior to providing treatment. The number of items which can be entered into the problem list and into the list of risk factors is virtually limitless. After extensive review of the literature and consultation with experts, guidelines have been developed by the physician group regarding the frequency of surveillance and intervention based on the patient's medical problems and risk factors. These guidelines have been incorporated into the program and the frequency of surveillance and intervention are automatically changed as problems and risk factors are added, deleted or modified. The screen shown in Table 2 allows the addition, deletion or modification. For example, to change the risk factor for breast cancer one types the letter "B" in the bracket following Code#[ ] as shown. Another screen appears, shown elsewhere in this volume[(3)], which

Table 2

Medical Problem list and Risk factors

KPMC, O.C. **MEMBER PREVENTATIVE SCREEN SYSTEM**

Patient: Jane Doe **DOB:** 04/15/35 **Age:** 60 **SEX:** F **Pers Phys:** A. Jones MD.

CD#	Type	LVL	Description	Onset	Resolve	Status	Mod
231	Prob		Warfarin-INR 2-3	12/1/95		Active	10925
125	Prob		Asthma	12/15/84		Presum	10925
248	Prob		Met - brain, liver	4/21/95		Active	10925
255	Prob		Cancer - GI	2/22/94		Active	10925
127	Prob		Cataract	4/17/92	8/15/95	Resolv	10925
247	Prob		Chemotherapy	4/30/95		Active	10925
026	Prob		DVT	11/25/95		Active	10925
005	Prob		Depression	3/21/94		Interm	77848
011	Prob		Hip Fracture	5/20/75	6/15/95	Resolv	67164
016	Risk	High	Alcohol use			Active	10925
011	Risk	Low	Breast cancer			Active	10925
096	Risk	High	Diabetes			Active	50989

Function [ ] A - Add, D - Delete, M - Modify, Type [ ] R-Risk, P-Problem Code# [B]

allows the change. The first column CD# is a cross reference to ICD-9 codes. The number under the column heading "Mod" is the identification number of the person entering the data.

Discussion

The Member Preventative Screen application was placed in service in January 1996. The quality of care indicators for the first quarter 1996, from the use of this application, has been calculated for mammography and is described elsewhere in this volume[(3)] . The results show an increase in mammography compliance of 2% over the 58% achieved in 1995. It is clear that without continuous monitoring of the indicators which can only be achieved by a computerized process, the quality of care results can be erratic, as shown in Table3. The performance for mammography and prenatal care decreased in 1995 compared to 1994, whereas the other indicators showed an increase. This is because the manual method does not allow continuous feedback for improvement when needed. The performance data for 1994 and 1995 was obtained through a manual sampling process. Table 3 shows the performance of our service area on the NCQA quality measures compared with health promotion and disease prevention targets established by the US Public Health Service (Year 2000 Goal). These goals, called Healthy People 2000, are set for the entire US population and are to be achieved by the year 2000. The system described here is an effective tool to achieve this goal.

Table 3
Performance on NCQA quality indicators

	Year 2000 Goal	94 Performance	95 Performance
Mammography	60%	62%	58%
Peds Immunization	90%	82%	85%
Prenatal Care	90%	88%	85%
Cervical CA Screen	85%	75%	83%

References

1. Ahmed M., Anderson C., and Stuewe C., "A Computer System for Requesting and Reporting Radiologic Examinations, Verifying Receipt of Reports by Referring Physicians, and Tracking Patients with Significant Abnormal Findings", in **Proceedings of the International Symposium CAR'93**, H.U. Lemke Editor, Springer-Verlag, pp. 179-184.
2. Ahmed M., Anderson C., and Stuewe C., "A Computer System for Providing Feedback to Physicians to Influence Their Ordering Practices", in **Proceedings of S/CAR 94**, J.M. Boehme Editor, Symposia Foundation, pp. 271-276.
3. Mowji P.J., Ahmed M., Anderson C., Stuewe C., and Ahmed C., "A Computer Based System for Tracking Compliance of Mammography Guidelines", in this issue.

Multivariate Techniques for Process Inspection of Quality Control in a Medical Imaging Environment

Dennis N. Stroud

Department of Radiology, Fitzsimons Army Medical Center

James R. Koehler

Department of Mathematics, University of Colorado at Denver, Colorado

I Introduction

Computerized statistical process control methods for quality monitoring have been implemented for a number of imaging sections in the radiology department at Fitzsimons Army Medical Center. These attempts range from purely experimental to an integral part of the routine daily quality control. The goal is to facilitate collection and maintenance of QC data as well as provide insight into what W. E. Deming and others have called the *"extended process"*. For this we need to analyze all sources of data from the processes being monitored. Part of this can be accomplished by analyzing a number of measured parameters or *"quality characteristics"* of a process. A complete analysis of multiple characteristics does not only reveal the behavior of the individual parameters but also their interactions. The multivariate methods described here allow this kind of analysis while at the same time providing simple control charting methods for display and interpretation of the results.

II Univariate Methods

The univariate methods found to be most useful are Shewhart control charts and Cumulative Sum or CUSUM[1,2,3,4]. Both are used to monitor a process quality characteristic in order to detect a change in the process. Familiar examples are film processor sensitometry control charts, the image quality charts used in mammography and uniformity measurements of gamma cameras. Examples of these kinds of control charts are seen in figure 1. The X-bar chart is an example of a Shewhart measurement chart for the mean, the range chart is also a Shewhart chart for controlling the variability of a process. The CUSUM is designed to detect small process deviation much sooner than Shewhart charts. A failure of the CUSUM, defined here as a deviation from the 0 line by more than plus or minus 4, indicates a shift of one standard deviation whereas X-bar chart control limits of three standard deviations are typically used. The CUSUM is the fastest way known to the authors for detecting small changes in a univariate characteristic with a small probability of false alarm.

Since all of these methods require that the data in question are normally distributed the normal probability plot is used as a qualitative means for evaluating

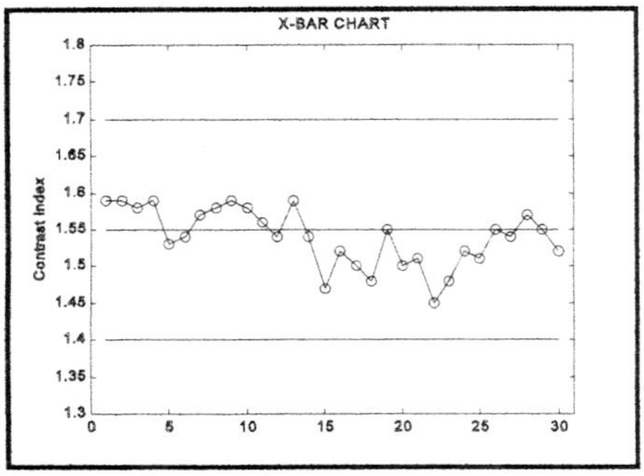

1a: X-bar chart

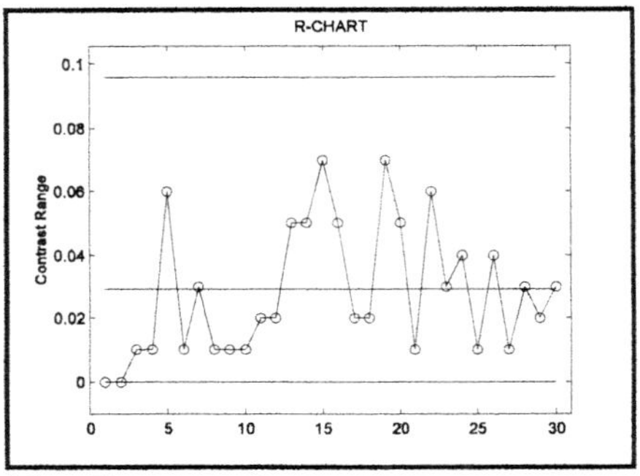

1b: Range chart

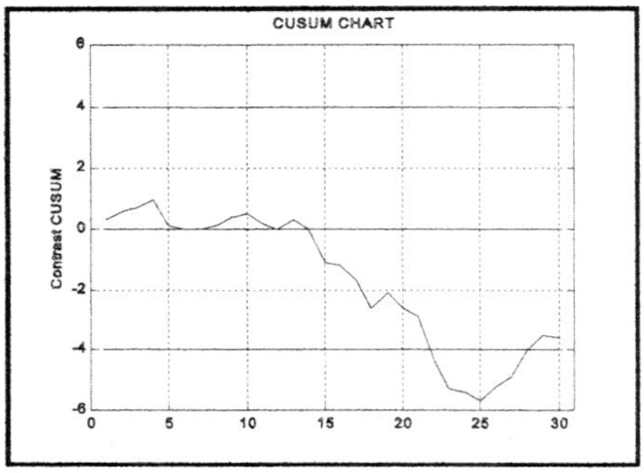

1c: CUSUM

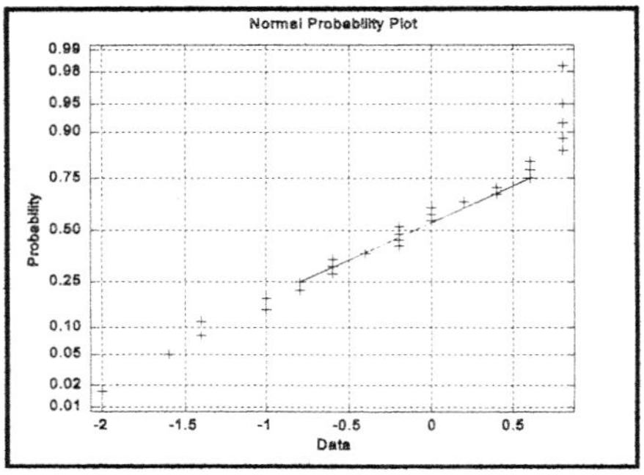

1d: Normal plot

this. The solid line represents normal (or Gaussian) data. If the points are aligned in a straight line but off the solid line then the data are normal but the mean is shifted.

III Multivariate Methods

One problem with the univariate methods is the large number charts that are needed to evaluate each characteristic. Typically, more than one characteristic is monitored. In the film processor sensitometer example, contrast and speed along with base plus fog and processor temperature are usually monitored on a daily basis. That means looking at 4 charts for every characteristic. Not only is this a lot of hard copy, it is a lot to view and interpret on a daily basis. Moreover, what is often of interest is the effect of all the characteristics together. For the film processor sensitometry example: (1) reduced contrast with the speed remaining constant and increased fog indicates possible contamination of the developer with fixer or that the fixer replenishment rate is too low. (2) If instead of the speed being constant it is increasing, the developer replenishment may be mixed improperly or underdiluted. (3) On the other hand, if the speed and contrast are both decreasing but base plus fog is constant, this could indicate overdilution of developer.

What is needed is a simple and effective means to monitor a multiplicity of process characteristics simultaneously. Multivariate techniques such as the Chi-squared (χ^2) and Hotelling's T-squared (T^2) control charts are applicable.[3,4,5] The basis for both control charts is the quadratic form of the covariance matrix with the observed deviation vector. That is, given the covariance matrix, **Σ** and the observation vectors **x** with mean **μ** the Chi-squares is defined in Equation 1.[5]

$$\begin{array}{ll} \textit{Observed values:} & X^T = (X_1, \ldots, X_i, \ldots, X_p) \\ \textit{Mean values:} & \mu^T = (\mu_1, \ldots, \mu_i, \ldots, \mu_p) \\ \textit{Covariance:} & \Sigma \textit{ with inverse } \Sigma^{-1} \\ \textit{Then:} & \chi^2 = n\,(X-\mu)^T\,\Sigma^{-1}\,(X-\mu) \end{array} \qquad \text{EQN: (1)}$$

When the covariance matrix is estimated by the sample covariance matrix **S**, the mean is estimated from a set of samples (referred to as the *training set),* and m observations determines the mean vector **X**, (each component is the mean of m values), Hotelling's T^2 method is used as defined in Equation 2.[5]

$$\begin{array}{l} \textit{Let: } \bar{\bar{X}} = (\bar{X}_1, \ldots, \bar{X}_p) \\ \textit{be the sample mean} \\ \textit{with S having inverse} = S^{-1} \\ \textit{Hotelling's } T^2 = m\,(X-\bar{\bar{X}})^T\,S^{-1}\,(X-\bar{\bar{X}}) \end{array} \qquad \text{EQN: (2)}$$

The T^2 statistic is analogous to the univariate T-test in which we test the hypothesis $\mathbf{H_0: \mu=\mu_0}$ against $\mathbf{H_1: \mu \neq \mu_0}$.[3] Consider the univariate case as an example. If sample data $X_1, X_2, \ldots, X_n$ are normally distributed with mean μ_0 and standard deviation σ, we can use the sample mean X and sample standard deviation to set a confidence interval for μ based on α , the probability of false alarm or type I error. The confidence interval $100(1-\alpha)\%$ is a random interval depending on the sample data, X and has a probability of $(1-\alpha)$ of containing μ. That means we do not reject $\mathbf{H_0}$ when μ_0 lies in the $100(1-\alpha)\%$ interval $X \pm t_{n-1}(\alpha/2)s/n^{1/2}$.

HOTELLING'S T^2 CONTROL LIMITS

For training samples, reject H_0 when:

$$T^2 > \frac{(n-1)p}{(n-p)} F_{p,n-p}(\alpha)$$

$$\text{or} \quad T^2 > \chi^2_{\alpha,p}$$

For future T^2 observations, reject H_0 when: EQN: **(3)**

$$T^2 > \frac{p(n+1)(n-1)}{(n^2-np)} F_{p,n-p}(\alpha)$$

where: n is the training sample size
α is the probability of Type I error
F is the F-distribution
with p , n-p degrees of freedom

T^2 is the generalized distance from the observed vector **X** to the mean $\boldsymbol{\mu_0}$. If the distance is "too large", the $\mathbf{H_0}$ hypothesis is rejected. We define "too large" in the manner of a control chart, with an Upper Control Limit (UCL) rather than with tables as in a univariate T-test. The control chart represents the UCL as a line above which a T^2 value is in the rejection region, the distance from the mean is too large. T^2 has a distribution related to an F-distribution with p and n-p degrees of freedom. Given random samples $\mathbf{X}_1,\mathbf{X}_2,\ldots,\mathbf{X}_n$ normally distributed p-variate data with mean $\boldsymbol{\mu}$ and covariance matrix Σ Hotelling's method tests $\mathbf{H}_0\mathbf{:}\boldsymbol{\mu}=\boldsymbol{\mu}_0$ by comparing observations with the Control Limits defined in Equation 3.[3]

The time series information for multivariate data can be preserved by plotting the T^2 values in sequence. The upper control limit (UCL) is defined in Equation 3. The "state" of the process is characterized by this value and the process is "in-control" when the values are below the UCL.

IV Hotelling's T^2 Examples

A. In figure 2 (below) a T^2 control chart is simulated based on two quality control characteristics. First, a set of 50 "training" vectors were simulated to define S, the covariance matrix. Next, 20 simulated vectors representing an "in-control" state were simulated followed by 20 more vectors in which one characteristic is shifted up the other shifted down by one standard deviation. The shifts in each characteristic do not exceed the control limits of the univariate X-bar charts but is detected by the Multivariate T^2 control chart.

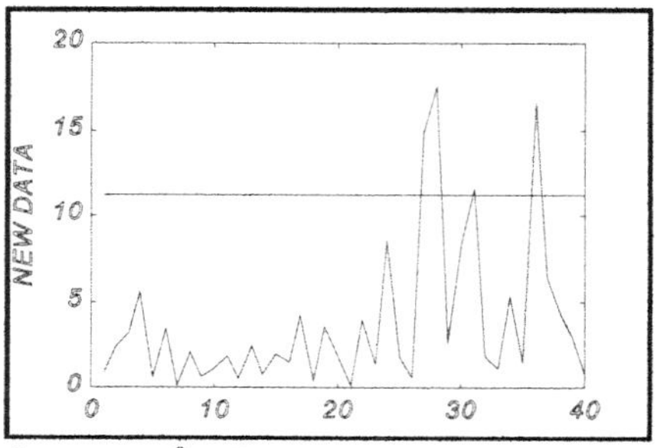

2a: A T^2 chart with values exceeding the UCL

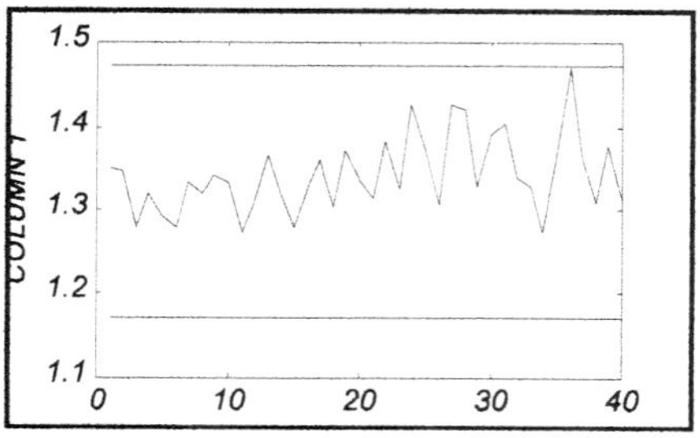

2b: Characteristic 1

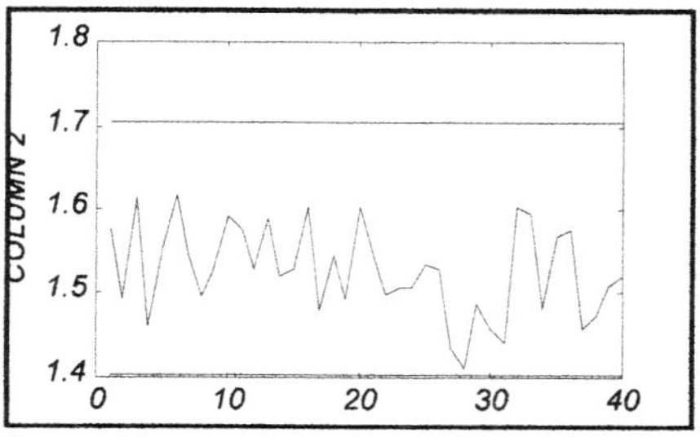

2c: Characteristic 2

The control limits for the univariate charts are based on 3 sigma, an α of 0.0027. In the Multivariate charts an α of 0.0027 and 0.0454 (3 and 2 sigma) are used to define control limits.

B. Six values are monitored on a daily basis for the film processor sensitometry in the mammography service at Fitzsimons Army Medical Center: speed, contrast, base plus fog, maximum density, average gradient and processor temperature. In figure 3, (below) a set of 40 training vectors from late 1995 through early 1996 were used to define S and to set the means of each for these six values. All six characteristics are summarized in the T^2 control chart. This example shows the processor "in-control" until the 17th value, (11 March 1996). A downward shift in the contrast index was also detected by the CUSUM univariate control charts at about the same time, (this is seen in figure 1c). The probable cause of this "out-of-control" state was contamination of developer with fixer and was remedied by cleaning the processor.

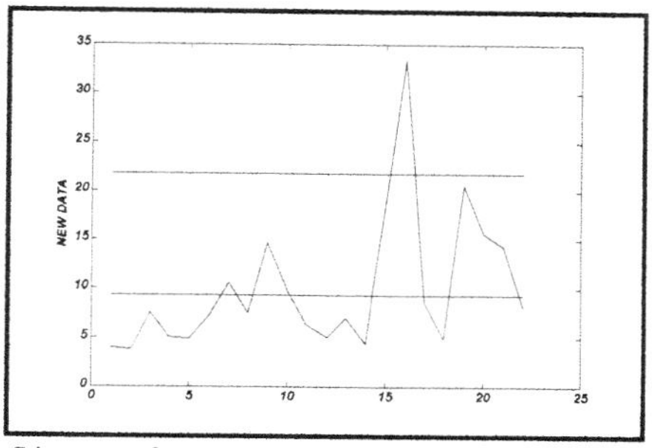

figure3: Sensitometry data from a mammographic film processor.

C. Perhaps the best use for multivariate control charts is to summarize a number of quality control parameters in a single value, T^2. Figure 4a shows the results of a T^2 control chart one month after installation of the unit in September 1992. Thirty quality control characteristics are recorded As a result of the daily calibration and QC procedure on a dual energy X-ray bone density unit at Fitzsimons. The training sample consists of 17 sample vectors using seven of the QC characteristics beginning on September 14, 1992, when the unit was installed. Twenty-two days of observed data from October and November of 1992 are shown in figure 4a. Shortly after installation, the X-ray tube failed and was replaced. The UCL was exceeded twice in October even after the faulty tube was replaced. Neither of these failures were indicated on the QC database maintained by the system but were later determined to be a misalignment of the X-ray tube and detector. After the system was determined to be "in-control" 49 training samples from the normal operation of the unit through December 1992 were used to establish the control limits. The T^2-chart figure 4b, shows "in-control" results for January through March of 1993, the UCL was never exceeded. Examination of the set of 30 univariate QC characteristics could have indicated the same results but, that kind of analysis is not typically done and is used only when a specific problem orrurs repeatedly and there is difficulty in correcting the problem.

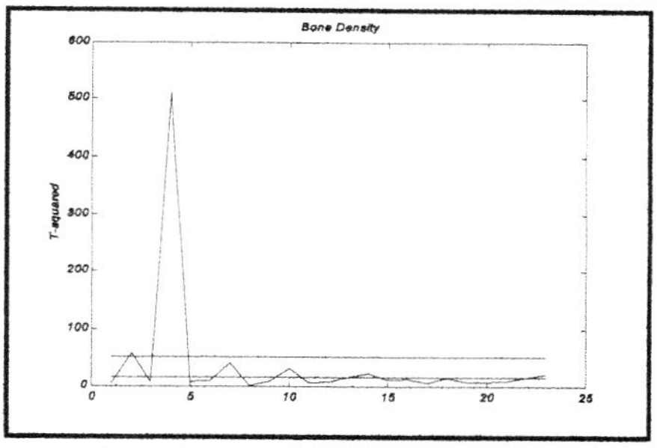

4a: "out-of-contro" bone density data from fall 1992

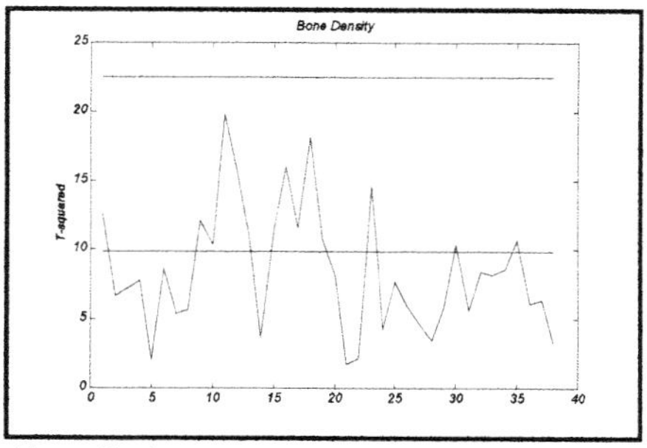

4b: " in-control" data from first quarter of 1993.

D. In nuclear medicine the quality of the gamma cameras are monitored daily by testing image uniformity. For some cameras the percentage count loss is also tested each morning. This test evaluates the "cost" (in counts) of producing a uniform image. This quantity, sometimes called *percent skim* is of value because uniform images can be produced with either high or low count loss and high or very low (even negative) count loss is an indication of some problem with the camera. Monitoring the four uniformity values separately is not always effective for detecting problems. For example, the percent skim can be very low, even a negative value and may be associated with only slightly elevated uniformity numbers that do not fail the QC criteria. Figure 5a is such an example. The third T^2 value in the chart exceeds the UCL and is a result of a skim of -0.6% with slightly elevated uniformity values of 4.54, 4.54, 3.28 and 3.01, all within tolerance. The "cause" of this state was a partial reload performed on the same day, (18 SEP 95). A full reload corrected this and the camera T^2 remained below the UCL of 26 for the remainder of the chart. Two other points on this control chart (31 and 42) correspond to possible shifts of one standard deviation in the skim values seen on the CUSUM. They are however, both within tolerance.

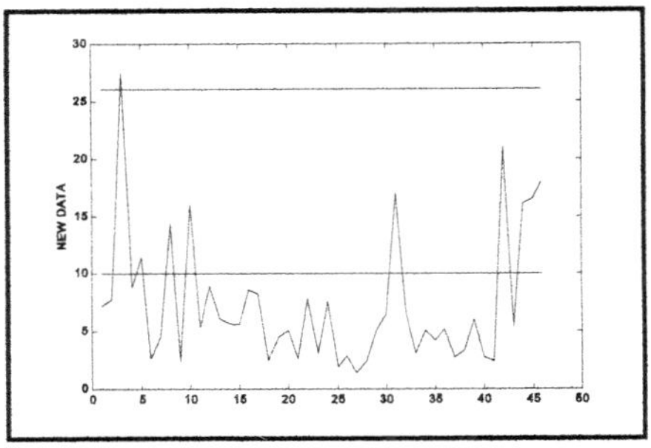

5a: camera 3

In figures 5b, T^2 values are plotted for another camera beginning at the end of August. When the weather starts to get cooler, the heat comes on in the nuclear medicine department and the cameras begin to "act up". The uniformity and skim fluctuate more than in other seasons. This requires more frequent reloads by the technologists and could possibly be corrected by improving the environmental conditions, (the air conditioners) in the Nuclear Medicine department.

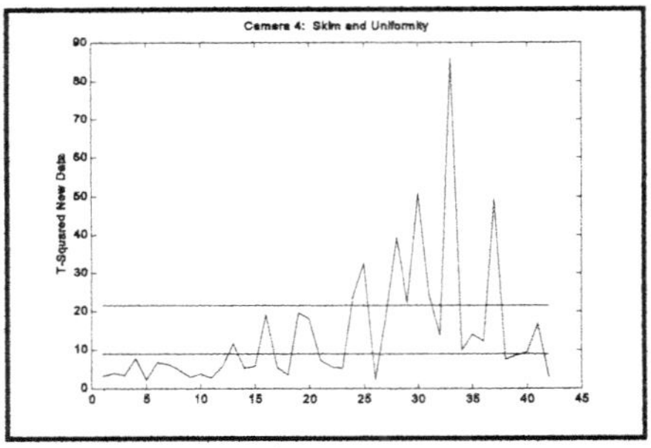

5b: camera 4

It should be noted that the choice of training samples will affect the control limits. A smaller training set will result in a higher UCL. Twenty-two vectors were used to train in figure 5a, 30 were used in figures 5b. Thus, the sensitivity of the T^2 control chart is determined by the number of training samples used.

V. Other Considerations

Two assumptions underlie the implementation of Hotelling's T^2 multivariate charts. The first, that the data are multivariate normal random variables can be tested with a normal probability plot for each characteristic. The test is not a guarantee, if however each characteristic is normal, the joint distribution is likely to be multivariate normal regardless of whether or not the variables are independent. In fact , the case where characteristics are dependent is where the most can be gained. Dependent data only changes the "shape" of the multivariate control region.

The second assumption of Hotelling's method is that the covariance matrix is nonsingular. This is often not true with multivariate QC data. Consider the base plus fog and the temperature measurements from the film processor examples above. These tend to be constant or nearly constant varying between only a few values. It can also be the case that two or more characteristics have identical data, i.e. 2 or more variables are perfectly correlated. One can drop these variables from the control charts but it may be that these are important indicators of the quality of the process. When these situations occurs, the covariance matrix is singular. To handle this case, the pseudoinverse is substituted for the inverse in equation 2, (above). The rank of **S** is used in place of p in equation 3 to compute the proper control limits and the Hotelling's method is used to monitor the other (nonsingular) components.

In order to monitor the (so called) singular characteristics, an implementation of the novelty filter was used[6]. For the training set defined by the matrix $\boldsymbol{X}$, the identity matrix $\boldsymbol{I}$ and observation vector $\boldsymbol{x}$, the novelty η is defined in equation 4. The novelty may be considered the orthogonal component of the observed vector. If one of the "singular" characteristics in the training set changes, the magnitude of η will change dramatically.

$$(I - XX^{+}) x = \eta \qquad \text{EQN: } \mathbf{(4)}$$

Figure 6a shows the T^2 chart for film processor data in which the base plus fog and temperature are constant in the training set. The remaining characteristics appear to be normally distributed and indicate a failure at the end of the chart. If this change were accompanied by changes in the constant parameters this would be seen in the novelty chart. Figure 6b in the novelty filter charted for the same period. In this case changes in the temperature and base plus fog have been modified from the real data to simulate a thermostat problem. The changes in the singular characteristics cause η to increase by many orders of magnitude.

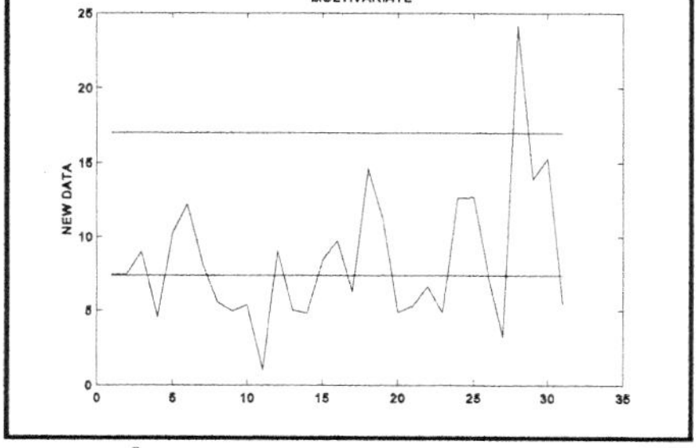

6a: T^2 chart for rank less than p

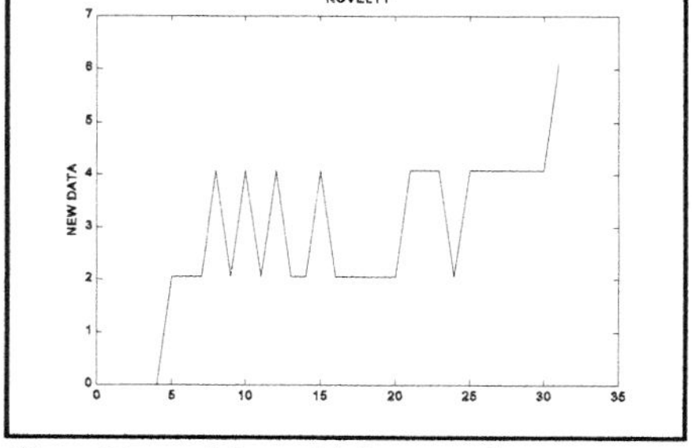

6b: Novelty filter for sensitometry data.

VI. Discussion and Conclusion

The multivariate techniques described in this paper are effective tools for monitoring multiple sources of quality control data from a process. T^2 control charts have sensitivity at least comparable to univariate charts while still having few false alarms and in many cases are better at detecting real problems in the processes being monitored becausae of natural dependencies in the data. The limitation of a singular covariance matrices may, in part be overcome with implementation of a novelty filter to monitor correlated quality control characteristics. The results of these kinds of monitoring methods can provide greater insight into process quality, are easily interpreted and may lend themselves to automated processing.

VII. References

(1) D.Stroud, J.Koehler, M.McBiles, S.Kimball and M.Toney, "A Statistical Process Control Approach to Department Quality Control and Quality Improvement", (Abstract), Med. Phys, 20, (1993).

(2) D.Stroud, J.Koehler and S.Kimball, "Computer Assisted Quality Improvement in Radiological Science", (Paper, in preparation).

(3) Thomas P. Ryan, "Statistical Methods for Quality Improvement", John Wiley and Sons, 1989.

(4) Douglas C. Montgomery, "Introduction to Statistical Quality Control, Second Edition",John Wiley and Sons, 1991.

(5) Richard A. Johnson and Dean W. Wichern, "Applied Multivariate Statistics, Third Edition", Prentice Hall, 1992.

(6) T. Kohonen, "Self-Organization and Associative Memory, Second Edition", Springer -Verlag, 1988.

An Automated System to Monitor Equipment Service and Billing Information

Kimmet B. Workman, B.S.E.E., I. Michael Harris, B.S.E.E. and Bob W. Gayler, M.D.
The Russell H. Morgan Department of Radiology and Radiological Sciences, The Johns Hopkins Hospital, Baltimore, Maryland

Our information system is the result of an evolutionary process that began in 1986. This had produced cumulative savings to the hospital approaching a million dollars by 1992 when we had a major change in imaging equipment service policy.

This new policy included an outside insurer for all service costs on covered equipment and required us to make major changes in our information system. The restrictive software used in developing the earlier system prevented modification to accomplish these changes and we decided to develop the new system in-house. It was implemented May 1, 1993

The overall design was based on input from members of the Physics and Engineering group, technologists, administrators and secretaries. Even some of the outside service engineers gave us some good ideas.

With this new design, work orders can be initiated from any networked computer in the hospital or outpatient center. Technologists from any of our divisions can initiate a work order through a computer terminal without visiting or calling our office.

This system has helped us to save over 1.2 million dollars in 2 years. All equipment service invoices were review by the assistant administrator using the information from the system to determine payment responsibility. The invoices were then routed to our insurer or accounting, depending on this determination. Payments routed to our insurer were over 1.2 million dollars greater than our premiums.

Every imaging system in our department is assigned a unique identifier, which is kept in the file SYS_ID.DBF. For the purpose of our work orders that system can consist of one or more independent subsystems. As an example, if we refer to a biplane angiography system, there may be two independent x-ray systems, a patient monitoring system, and an injector. All of these are independent systems in their own right, but together they comprise the system that the department views as a revenue generating entity. When any of the subsystems in the system fail to work correctly, the department loses revenue That makes it a system.

Since not all of the subsystems that comprise the system are necessarily bought on the same capital equipment purchase order, we need to keep them separate.

Each month the database automatically creates seven new files to hold work order information for that month. The first file is the main work order file. This file contains the information about the work order itself. Two files are created to handle in-house service information, two for outside service information, one for in-house parts used, one for outside parts used and one for in-house labor hours. Each file is named using its month, year and purpose.

WO09_95.DBF	**Work orders for Sept, 1995**
WOI09_95.DBF	**In-house service information**
WOI09_95.DBT	**Text file for in-house service**
WOO09_95.DBF	**Outside service information**
WOO09_95.DBT	**Text file for outside service**
PUI09_95.DBF	**Parts used for in-house service**
PUO09_95.DBF	**Parts used for outside service**
TIM09_95.DBF	**In-house labor hours**

This operation is automatic and transparent to the user, unless the user is the first to initiate a work order for the month. Then a message appears on the screen stating that the files are being created.

The information about the companies that provide outside service is kept in the file COMPANY.DBF which contains information about different office and contact numbers. Information regarding outside service engineers is kept in file OUTSIDE.DBF. There are two file to hold information about inside personnel. TECHS.DBF for our service personnel and RADTECHS.DBF for our radiological technologists.

In the past we have handled outside service in many different ways. At first hospital personnel brought the paper work left by the outside service personnel to the Physics and Engineering office where the information was entered into the work order database. Starting February 1, 1993 we required the outside service personnel to return the paper work to our office so we could see that it was properly completed

All of these methods required a great deal of time and effort on the part of our office staff, in-house service engineers and outside service engineers. In many cases, paper work was delayed and in others it wasn't return at all. There have been many instances where we would receive an invoice with no other documentation; When this happened, our staff had to find the information necessary to justify payment.

We have recently implemented a new set of programs that will help remove these problems.

These new programs will allow the members of outside service organizations that we deal with to enter their own service information. These people have access to computers on our departmental network and will enter their service information from the area where they performed the service. In this way, the information will be available to us over the network on the day service was performed.

The outside service engineers appreciate this newest change. They don't have to return the paper work to our office every time they service our equipment. They can mail it to us on a weekly basis.

This provides both groups with required information in a timely way. We get the data and they get the convenience. We know what work was performed on our equipment and the service personnel don't have drag all of their tools to our office and out of the institution.

This system has proven both convenient and cost effective. It has allowed us to comply with state regulatory requirements, JCAHO certification requirements and all official requests requiring written documentation.

Diagrams A and B below show the relations of the data tables that hold the information for in-house and outside work order information.

Table 1 shows despite the fact that the size of our department and the outside service rates have almost doubled in the last ten years, the percent of the value of out asset base spent for maintenance has been very stable.

Data Tables for In-house Work Order Information

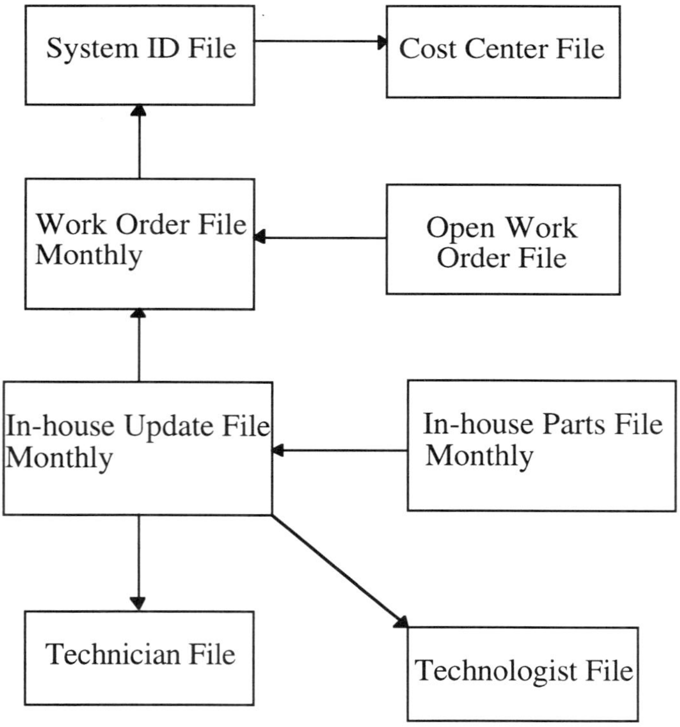

Diagram A.

Data Tables for Outside Work Order Information

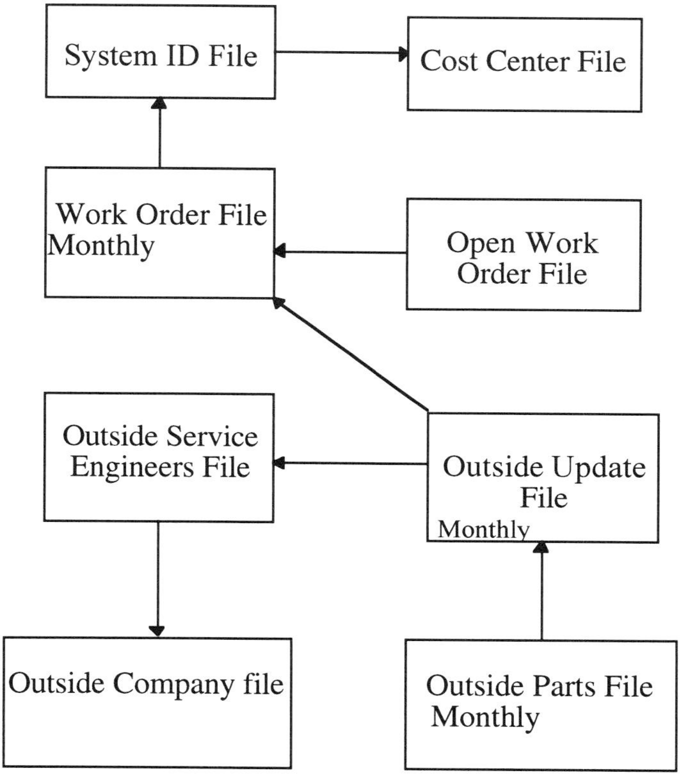

Diagram B.

Estimates of Capital Equipment Value, Maintenance Costs Percentage of Value for Maintenance Costs and Average outside Service Rates.

	1985	1991	1995
Asset Base (Purchase Value)	$26,000,000	$34,000,000	$47,000,000
Repair Cost	$1,900,000	$2,600.000	$3,500,000
Percent of Base	7.5%	7.6%	7.5%
Average Outside Service Rates. ($/Hour)	83	129	164

Between 1986 and 1991 we added two MR's and closed out our CT contracts.

Between 1991 and 1995 we expanded our Cath lab and opened our outpatient center. From 1992 to 1995 we had an insurance policy on many of our systems.

Table 1.

Academic Radiologists and Computers: Use and Attitudes

Randy D. Cork, M.D. and Charles P. Friedman, Ph.D.
Duke-UNC Medical Informatics Program, University of North Carolina, Chapel Hill, North Carolina

William M. Detmer, M.D.
Section on Medical Informatics, Stanford University, Stanford, California

Introduction

Potential benefits of computer use in medical care are well recognized [1]; however, these benefits cannot be realized unless computers are used by physicians and other health care professionals. One significant factor in the use of computers by physicians is their attitudes toward computers and medical computing [2,3,4]. A number of surveys of physicians' attitudes toward computers have been published over the last thirty years [5]; however, none specifically report on the attitudes of radiologists. In this paper we analyze the responses of academic radiologists compared to other academic physicians with regard to computer use and attitudes towards computers in medicine.

Methods

The Computers in Medical Care Survey is a questionnaire derived from an instrument originally developed by Teach and Shortliffe in 1981 [6]. It consists of eighty-nine questions in four sections measuring demographics, computer use and experience, computer knowledge, and attitudes toward computers in medicine. Psychometric properties of the instrument have been described elsewhere [5].

Demographic questions and measures of computer use and experience (Table 1, Table 2) are self-explanatory and are detailed in the Results. Four multi-item scales are also included which measure:

1. **Computer use (Table 3):** "To what extent do you personally use a computer for each of the following professional tasks?", with allowable responses of: "1. Never perform this task; 2. Perform this task but never use a computer; 3. Sometimes use a computer; 4. Often use a computer; 5. Always use a computer";
2. **Self-reported computer knowledge (Table 4):** "Below are a set of paired terms that relate to computers in medicine. Please score your knowledge of the distinction between the terms in each pair.", with allowable responses of: "1. I don't understand the distinction at all; 2. I have a general appreciation of the distinction but couldn't define it; 3. I can define the distinction precisely";
3. **Demands upon computer based systems (Table 5, Table 6):** "If you were considering the use of a computer-based system in medical care, how necessary would the following capabilities be?", with allowable responses of: "1. Vitally necessary: Any system I would use must have this capability. I would not use a system that lacked it; 2. Generally necessary: I would be much more likely to use a system having this capability, but I might use a system that lacked it; 3. Somewhat necessary: I would be somewhat more likely to use a system because it had this capability; 4. Not necessary: My decision to use a system would be unaffected by

4. the presence of this capability; 5. Unable to respond: The meaning or implication of this capability are not clear to me";
5. **Expectations of the effects of computers upon health care (Table 7):** "Given below are some effects that computers may have on medicine and health care. For each, indicate whether you believe the effect will be beneficial or detrimental using the scale below.", with allowable responses of: "1. Highly detrimental; 2. Detrimental on the whole; 3. Neither detrimental nor beneficial; 4. Beneficial on the whole; 5. Highly beneficial".

The survey was provided to full-time physician faculty in the departments of radiology, radiation oncology, internal medicine, and surgery at Stanford University, the University of North Carolina at Chapel Hill, the University of California at San Francisco, Northwestern University, and the University of Illinois at Chicago during 1993 and 1994. The institutional response rate ranged from forty-five to seventy-five percent, with 771 responses received. This is the largest survey of physicians' attitudes towards computers ever conducted.

Responses of respondents completing less than a threshold number of items were excluded on a scale by scale basis. Average scale scores were calculated (excluding missing values) as the average of the responses of the items comprising the scale. Using the respondent's self-designation of medical specialty, responses of the radiologists (N = 84) and non-radiologists (N = 687) were grouped and analyzed separately using SYSTAT for Windows version 5.05 (SYSTAT, Inc., Evanston, IL).

The distributions of most of the responses were nonparametric; therefore, the Mann-Whitney test was used unless otherwise indicated to test the null hypothesis that the responses of radiologists and non-radiologists are identical. A significance level (alpha) of 0.01 was used because of the multiple comparisons made.

Results

Demographics: The radiologists and non-radiologists did not differ significantly in mean age (46.8 vs. 44.7 years, p = 0.36), gender (75 vs. 82 percent male, chi square p = 0.11), or institutional affiliation (chi square p = 0.56).

Professional Time (Table 1): Numbers represent the respondents' self-reported distribution of time performing the listed professional tasks as a percentage of total professional time.

Table 1: Percentage Distribution of Professional Time

Percentage of Professional Time Spent in:	Radiologist Mean	Radiologist SD	Other Mean	Other SD	p
Clinical Care & Teaching	65.0	21.9	47.1	24.9	< 0.01
Didactic Teaching	9.6	8.6	8.9	9.1	0.44
Research	13.0	13.6	28.4	25.0	< 0.01
Administrative & Other	12.4	17.5	15.6	16.7	< 0.01
Total	100.0		100.0		

Computer Utilization, Training, and Sophistication (Table 2): "Computer Time" represents the number of "hands-on hours" spent each week using a computer. "Average Training Score" is the average of seven different types of computer training, each scored as zero (completed) or one (not completed). "Computer Sophistication" is a self-rating with responses ranging from one ("Very unsophisticated") to five ("Very sophisticated"). The second and third sets of items represent the percentage of respondents using that particular platform or computer type-location combination, respectively. Percentages sum to greater than one hundred because one physician may use several computers.

Table 2: Computer Utilization, Training, and Sophistication

Item	Radiologist Mean	Radiologist SD	Other Mean	Other SD	p
Computer Time	6.17	6.25	9.89	9.10	< 0.01
Average Training Score	1.06	0.70	1.17	0.81	0.35
Computer Sophistication	2.58	1.06	2.85	1.10	0.03
Percentage using:					
Macintosh	58.3		54.6		0.52*
PC compatible	29.8		47.2		< 0.01*
Terminal	36.9		30.6		0.24*
Workstation	9.5		5.8		0.19*
Other platform	2.4		1.2		0.35*
Percentage using:					
Desktop at work	65.5		82.5		< 0.01*
Desktop at home	65.5		69.9		0.41*
Laptop	34.5		35.8		0.96*
Other	13.1		10.2		0.41*

*Chi square

Computer Use (Table 3): Items are listed in descending order by non-radiologist mean response, with higher values indicating more frequent use

Table 3: Attitudes toward Computer Use

Use	Radiologist Mean	Radiologist SD	Other Mean	Other SD	p
Writing	4.06	1.13	4.42	1.06	< 0.01
Searching the medical literature	3.72	1.32	4.31	1.07	< 0.01
Preparing presentation slides or overheads	3.95	1.22	4.22	1.18	0.03
Performing statistical analysis on clinical or research data	2.88	1.43	3.78	1.52	< 0.01
Accessing clinical data	3.59	1.32	3.36	1.16	0.06
Communicating with colleagues	2.63	1.02	2.78	1.06	0.17
Teaching students and residents	2.44	0.96	2.67	0.98	0.04
Obtaining advice on a specific patient's diagnosis or therapy	1.86	0.92	2.19	0.91	< 0.01
Documenting patient information	1.77	1.02	2.01	0.92	< 0.01
Scheduling patient appointments	1.37	0.76	1.86	1.24	< 0.01
Use Scale Average	2.83	0.63	3.16	0.62	<0.01*

* Student's t-test

Computer Knowledge (Table 4): Items are listed in descending order by radiologist mean response, with higher values indicating more confident knowledge.

Table 4: Computer Knowledge

Item	Radiologist Mean	Radiologist SD	Other Mean	Other SD	p
Hardware - Software	2.88	0.33	2.85	0.38	0.65
Floppy disk - Hard disk	2.84	0.37	2.84	0.42	0.72
Digital - Analog	2.69	0.52	2.24	0.82	< 0.01
Mainframe computer - Personal computer	2.60	0.58	2.73	0.51	0.03
Sensitivity - Positive predictive value	2.47	0.70	2.36	0.77	0.24
Data in memory - Data on disk	2.41	0.63	2.57	0.62	0.01
Images - Graphics	2.41	0.66	2.19	0.69	< 0.01
Electronic mail - Electronic bulletin board	2.13	0.68	2.30	0.73	0.02
Database - Knowledge base	1.98	0.77	2.02	0.76	0.65
Full-text DB - Bibliographic DB	1.86	0.86	2.12	0.83	< 0.01
Field - Record	1.70	0.87	1.96	0.85	< 0.01
Client - Server	1.66	0.83	1.91	0.80	< 0.01
Free text - Coded data	1.63	0.74	1.92	0.80	< 0.01
Relational database - Flat-file database	1.48	0.77	1.62	0.79	0.09
Interpreter - Compiler	1.45	0.72	1.53	0.75	0.30
Entities - Relationships	1.45	0.69	1.44	0.69	0.94
ICD9-CM - SNOMED	1.19	0.45	1.35	0.59	0.02
Forward chaining - Backward chaining	1.12	0.37	1.16	0.44	0.49
Knowledge Scale Average	2.00	0.41	2.06	0.44	0.20*

* Student's t-test

Demands Upon Computers (Table 5,Table 6): Responses of "5. Unable to respond" were eliminated. Factor analysis revealed two factors in the original single scale: demand for usability and demand for sophisticated functionality [5]. The items loading upon these factors are listed in separate tables, each sorted in ascending order by radiologist mean response, with lower values indicating greater demand for the feature.

Table 5: Demand for Computer Usability

Feature	Radiologist Mean	Radiologist SD	Other Mean	Other SD	p
The system is always functioning. There is never any "down-time".	1.63	0.67	1.84	0.83	0.08
I can access the system at any place in the clinical setting.	1.89	0.79	1.72	0.76	0.07
The system always displays X-rays and other images in less than 30 seconds.	2.02	0.91	2.47	0.89	< 0. 01
The system always responds to my queries in less that five seconds.	2.16	0.88	2.27	0.90	0.42
I can enter information in my own words and not need to know any special codes.	2.23	0.99	2.15	0.87	0.72
I can learn to use the system in less than two hours.	2.42	1.01	2.29	0.93	0.29
The system can be implemented with no changes to existing clinical routines.	3.14	0.88	3.20	0.87	0.55
I can interact with the computer without using a keyboard.	3.18	0.89	3.43	0.86	0.01

Usability Subscale Average	2.33	0.48	2.42	0.49	0.13*

* Student's t-test

Table 6: Demand for Sophisticated Functionality

Feature	Radiologist Mean	Radiologist SD	Other Mean	Other SD	p
The system has been demonstrated in research studies to make diagnoses at least as accurate as human consultants.	1.84	0.98	2.08	0.99	0.04
The system has been demonstrated in research studies to provide treatment recommendations at least as accurate as human consultants.	1.84	0.95	2.04	0.97	0.09
Users can browse the information in a system as well as asking it to provide advice about care of specific patients.	2.03	0.74	2.08	0.79	0.72
The system can clearly explain the rational for advice it gives on the care of patients.	2.12	0.84	1.99	0.86	0.19
When a system provides medical advice on the care of specific patients, it can quantify the level of certainty inherent in its recommendations.	2.17	0.82	2.16	0.89	0.92
When a system provides medical advice on the care of specific patients, it always provides multiple alternative recommendations.	2.33	0.82	2.32	0.90	0.91
The system takes a patient's own preference into account when giving advice to clinicians.	2.80	0.87	2.76	0.96	0.73
Sophisticated Functionality Subscale Average	2.18	0.61	2.20	0.63	0.73*

* Student's t-test

Expectations of Computers (Table 7): Original responses (range of one to five) were recoded over the range of negative two to positive two; therefore, responses greater than zero indicate expectation of benefit, responses near zero indicate uncertainty, and responses less than zero indicate expectation of detriment. Items are listed in descending order by radiologist mean response.

Table 7: Expectations of Computers

Expectation	Radiologist Mean	Radiologist SD	Other Mean	Other SD	p
Clinicians' access to up-to-date knowledge	1.49	0.52	1.47	0.57	0.94
Continuing medical education	1.12	0.66	1.19	0.57	0.47
Access to health care in remote or rural areas	1.06	0.72	0.94	0.67	0.13
Quality of health care	0.86	0.63	0.92	0.60	0.41
Costs of health care	0.85	0.78	0.87	0.73	0.97
Interactions within the health care team	0.79	0.76	0.70	0.80	0.38
Generalists' ability to manage more complex problems	0.68	0.65	0.69	0.69	0.75

Enjoyment of the practice of medicine	0.56	0.74	0.58	0.77	0.86
Patients' satisfaction with the quality of care they receive	0.34	0.62	0.34	0.67	0.93
Status of medicine as a profession	0.26	0.84	0.26	0.69	0.85
Management of medical/ethical dilemmas	0.24	0.64	0.13	0.63	0.17
Clinician autonomy	0.17	0.82	0.18	0.80	0.99
The self-image of clinicians	0.10	0.63	0.19	0.63	0.28
Role of government in health care	-0.06	1.03	-0.14	0.93	0.69
The rapport between clinicians and patients	-0.10	0.65	-0.10	0.69	0.76
Humaneness of the practice of medicine	-0.28	0.71	-0.17	0.68	0.33
Personal and professional privacy	-0.31	0.78	-0.26	0.78	0.55
Expectations Scale Average	0.42	0.41	0.43	0.41	0.86*

* Student's t-test

Correlations between Variables (Table 8): Pearson correlation coefficients between pertinent variables (names abbreviated) for all respondents are provided. Age was significantly negatively correlated with time spent in research, computer sophistication, computer time, desktop use, and the computer use scale average but was not correlated with remaining variables. Percentage of time spent in administrative and other duties correlated positively with age and computer training and negatively with time spent in clinical duties and research but did not correlate significantly with other variables. Average computer training was significantly positively correlated with computer sophistication, computer time, desktop computer use at work, and the averages of the use, knowledge, and expectation scales. Neither of the average scores for either demand subscale correlated significantly with any of the variables in the table.

Table 8: Pearson Correlation Coefficients

	Clinical Time	Research Time	Sophistication	Computer Time	PC Use	Desktop at Work	Use Scale	Knowledge Scale	Expectation Scale
Clinical Time	1	-0.71*	-0.20*	-0.38*	-0.11	-0.18*	-0.14*	-0.23*	-0.03
Research Time		1	+0.20*	+0.41*	+0.16*	+0.19*	+0.18*	-0.20*	-0.01
Sophistication			1	+0.51*	+0.18*	+0.37*	+0.47*	+0.66*	+0.24*
Computer Time				1	+0.16*	+0.35*	+0.39*	+0.43*	+0.14*
PC Use					1	+0.25*	-0.01	+0.22*	-0.05
Desktop at Work						1	+0.30	+0.31*	+0.15*
Use Scale							1	+0.43*	+0.19*
Knowledge Scale								1	+0.20*
Expectation Scale									1

$^*p < 0.001$

Discussion

Both duration ("hands-on" hours per week) and frequency (percent using a desktop computer at work) of computer use by academic radiologists are significantly less than other academic physicians (Table 2). This is not explained by age, average computer training, or computer sophistication as these variables do not differ significantly between the two groups. As computer use is negatively correlated with clinical time and positively correlated with research time, we consider differences in computer use best explained by radiologists' significantly greater ratio of clinical to research time. We believe lower computer use represents lesser use of available resources (specifically IBM-compatible personal computers) rather than a lack of available computing resources because of the ubiquitous presence of computers in the academic environment, the differences in allocation of professional time between the groups, and the similar use of other computing platforms and computers at home. Radiologists used workstations twice as frequently as other physicians; however, the difference is not statistically significant. This lack of significant difference may reflect infrequent use of PACS/teleradiology workstations by these radiologists at the time of the survey and also the inclusion of workstation users (e.g., radiation oncologists) in the non-radiologist group.

Interesting differences in specific computer uses are present in Table 3. Uses associated with academic duties (e.g., writing, presentations, statistical analysis) are performed more frequently than more clinical (e.g., documenting patient information, obtaining diagnostic or therapeutic advice) tasks. This is likely due to both the academic orientation of the physicians surveyed and the much greater familiarity and availability of software associated with general applications (word processing, presentation graphics) as opposed to clinical (electronic medical record, expert systems) applications. Consistent with radiologists' lesser use of computers overall and their lesser time spent in research, their use of computers for most "academic" purposes is significantly lower than non-radiologists. Although radiologists spent a greater percentage of their time in clinical care, their use of the computer for clinical purposes is also less than their colleagues for all tasks except "Accessing clinical data". We surmise this is due to the nature of radiologists' work, with less need to perform tasks associated with direct patient care but greater need to access information by computer given the frequent lack of other avenues (e.g., patient chart, direct contact with referring physician) of obtaining it.

While computer knowledge correlates with variables in which radiologists and non-radiologists significantly differed (clinical time, research time, and measures of computer use) overall self-assessment of computer knowledge did not differ between the groups (Table 4). With the exception of "Digital-Analog", no significant differences between the groups are seen in the first five items nor the last five items listed in descending order by radiologist mean. We believe the initial items are "easy" enough for all physicians to understand and the latter items "difficult" enough for few physicians to understand. Considering the middle eight items which may be more discriminant of general computer knowledge, radiologists scored lower than their clinical colleagues. Only for items relating to their specialty training in imaging (Digital - Analog, Images - Graphics) do radiologists display significantly greater confidence in their knowledge than other physicians.

The two groups' demands upon computers did not differ significantly for either factor constituting the Computer Demand Scales (Table 5, Table 6). Compared to other academic physicians, radiologists placed significantly greater emphasis upon rapid display of x-rays and other images and the ability to interact with the computer without using a keyboard. This does not seem surprising given the necessity of rapid image display for adequate productivity in image interpretation and the experience of radiologists using pointing devices rather than keyboards to access images in digital workstations. Both groups placed a greater value upon usability than sophisticated functionality although the difference is not statistically significant.

Although expectations of the effects of computers upon medical care significantly correlate with measures of computer use which differ significantly between radiologists and non-radiologists, the two groups did not differ in their expectations, either overall or for specific items. Overall, expectations of the effects of computers on health care are positive, especially for access to up-to-date knowledge, access to health care in remote areas, and continuing medical education; however, deleterious effects of computers upon the role of government in health care, clinician-patient rapport, humaneness of medical practice, and privacy are expected.

In summary, academic radiologists, although similar in age, computer training, and self-rated computer sophistication, significantly lag behind non-radiologists in computer use and computer knowledge but differ little in their demands upon computer systems and their expectations of the effects of computers upon health care. This lag is largely explained by greater professional time spent in clinical activities as opposed to research. Radiologists must continue to provide excellent clinical care; however, they must also become more knowledgeable of medical computing and increase their use of computers in the professional setting if they are to survive in a future increasingly based upon digital technology [7,8] and computers.

References

1. Remmlinger E., Grossman M. Physician utilization of information systems: bridging the gap between expectations and reality. Proceedings of the 1992 Annual HIMSS Conference. Healthcare Information and Management Systems Society, American Hospital Association, 1991: 119-23.
2. Kjerulff KH, Salloway JC, Counte MA. The impact of computer systems in a medical environment. Computerized Medical Imaging and Graphics. 13. 1989:137-43.
3. Young DW. What makes doctors use computers?: discussion paper. Journal of the Royal Society of Medicine . 77. 1984:663-7.
4. Anderson JG, Jay SJ, Schweer HM, Anderson MM. Physician utilization of computers in medical practice: policy implications based on a structural model. Social Science and Medicine . 23. 1986:259-67.
5. Cork RD, Detmer WM, Friedman CP . Physicians' attitudes toward computers: Measurement study and validation of four attitude scales. In publication.
6. Teach RL, Shortliffe EH. An analysis of physician attitudes regarding computer-based clinical consultation systems. Computers and Biomedical Research . 14. 1981:542-8.
7. Staab, EV, Stewart DA. FutuRAD 2: Work in progress. RadioGraphics. 14. 1994:1187-1190.
8. Staab, EV, Stewart DA. FutuRAD: Work in progress. Radiology. 190. 1994:43A-49A

Integrated Mission-Critical Radiology Departmental Computing on a Shoestring Budget: The Bellevue Experience

Jeffrey V. Chapnick, M.D., Tamar E. Waldhauser, L.L.B. and Albert F. Keegan, M.D.
NYU-Bellevue Hospital Center, New York, New York

The core problems which afflict public hospitals and their Radiology departments in the 1990's include ever-increasing service demands and regulatory burdens coupled with rapidly-shrinking levels of funding and personnel. In order to maintain operational excellence and continue to fulfill Bellevue's historic mission as the nation's oldest public hospital, our department of Radiology has had to make innovative and integrative use of a number of different types of information systems.

The tasks which we face include the following: the intake and scheduling of large numbers of ambulatory, emergency and in-patients with only a modicum of available clerical personnel; the tracking of exam data by an overburdened technical staff; achieving timely and accurate transcription of the complex reports generated by our large rotating pools of attending subspecialist radiologists, residents and fellows despite a dearth of trained typists; rapid dissemination of these results to a large, heterogeneous group of referrers; accurate capture of vital quality assurance and regulatory compliance data with very little staff which can be dedicated to those purposes.

In order to effectively accomplish these tasks, we utilize a number of different information systems, employing them in innovative ways to meet our needs. We have customized and streamlined the use of our Radiology Information System to allow for its straightforward, efficient use by broadbanded personnel with highly variable levels of skill and training. All of our personnel can and do perform all types of system tasks on a daily basis. With regard to report generation, we utilize a multi-pronged approach: some of our reports are generated on a voice-recognition system which provides both immediate hard copy and immediate uploading of report data to the RIS for electronic archival and promulgation. Another group of our reports is dictated into a digital storage system, which allows for immediate telephone access to the report in the radiologist's own voice. These reports then get typed by on-site and remote off-site typists. Still other reports are entered directly into the RIS by the radiologist, using bar codes. Our RIS is itself interfaced to a facility-wide Clinical Inquiry System, which allows for even more effective report promulgation. With regard to image storage and teleradiology, we utilize such systems both on an intra- and interhospital basis. Capture of data for quality assurance and regulatory compliance purposes is also accomplished on a broadbanded basis (as we have essentially no staff which can be so dedicated).

SESSION 3

PACS and Archiving

Co-Chairs:

David E. Avrin
Fred Goeringer

A New Spline Wavelet Based Medical Image Compression Algorithm

John D. Hazle, Stephen K. Thompson and Don F. Schomer
The University of Texas M.D. Anderson Cancer Center, Department of Diagnostic Radiology, Houston, Texas

Álmos A. Elekes
Houston Advanced Research Center, Houston, Texas

Steve J. Liu and Charles K. Chui
Texas A&M University, College Station, Texas

John Huffman
Silicon Graphics, Inc., Mountain View, California

I. Introduction

The spatial resolving requirements of radiological imaging result in digital image file sizes of 8 MB for current 2k x 2k computed radiography formats, but are being driven to 40 MB for individual full-frame 4k x 5k mammographic image formats. Estimates of data generation for a typical academic radiology department suggest that tens of terabytes (10^6 MB) may be generated annually. Additionally, outside images must be available in the digital archive for diagnostic correlation. The cumulative archive data is then "accessed" for use several times including hard copy output, differential diagnosis and consultation. Multiple accesses result in a communication amplification factor that is likely to be greater than ten. This magnitude of information access puts significant demands on image archive and communication systems (PACS). One solution to reduce the demands of this avalanche of data on PACS is to use data compression technology.

Mathematically lossless compression algorithms seldom exceed compression ratios of about 3:1. The advent of wavelet theory in the late 1980's has produced a new class of image compression algorithms. Appropriate choice of wavelet basis filters, combined with careful quantization or thresholding and matched lossless encoding schemes may lead to compression ratios exceeding 50:1 with no significant perceptual degradation of the diagnostic information. This would significantly increase archive depth and expand communication bandwidth.

A new algorithm has been developed for medical image compression based on spline wavelets (Chui 1992, Chui 1996) with optimized quantization and lossless encoding (Said & Pearlman 1993). This algorithm was submitted to the ACR/NEMA Working Group IV (WG-IV) to be considered as a lossy compression standard for the DICOM image format standard by our group in late 1995. The algorithm wavelet basis function achieves near optimal time-frequency energy compaction: less than 1% from the theoretical limit imposed by the Uncertainty Principle. Additionally, the side-lobe/main-lobe ratio is very small (below -40 dB).

The resulting algorithm was tested on a suite of images, provided by WG-IV. In this article we overview the algorithm and provide a summary of quantitative performance measures from a test suite of radiologic images.

II. Methodology

II.1. Spline modeling

The first step in our approach is modeling of the image data. Because the integral wavelet transform (IWT) is defined only for analog (continuos-time) signals with finite energy, the digitized signals must first be mapped into the continuous-time domain in order for the IWT be meaningful. This is achieved through appropriate modeling of the image. The IWT possesses the "perfect reconstruction" property: if no processing is applied to the transformed signals the inverse transform exactly reproduces the input signal.

II.2. Wavelet transformation

The aim of wavelet space representation is to convert the spatial image into a “spectral image” with good energy compaction. Wavelet representations are determined by the choice of wavelet basis functions. Although wavelet theory was formalized only about a decade ago (Daubechies 1988) these transforms are excellent for image compression. The Chui-Wang (1990) wavelets on which this work is based can be formulated explicitly in the time or spatial domains. Other wavelets must be computed either iteratively or by taking the inverse Fourier transform of certain infinite products.

We chose cubic spline wavelets because they are symmetric, semi-orthogonal and compactly supported (Chui 1996). The Wavelet Research Laboratory at Texas A&M University has been working with these types of wavelets for several years and their properties are well understood.

II.3. Quantization

The wavelet transform coefficients are quantized by mapping them to a smaller range of values based on analysis of their statistical characteristics. This removes information that, if done properly, is not perceived by the viewer. The quantized coefficients are compactly represented with binary codewords. Unlike blocked frequency-based compression methods such as JPEG and lapped orthogonal transforms, the output of the wavelet transform can be statistically modeled in the general case. This allows the design of a quantizer which minimizes distortion for a target compression rate. Although a vector code book could be designed that would outperform a general uniform scalar quantizer, the computational overhead for designing the code book is prohibitive and a static code book performs poorly. The use of a scalar quantizer in conjunction with an entropy coder was considered a better solution.

II.4. Lossless encoding

The lossless encoder achieves compression by efficiently representing the quantized wavelet coefficients according to their statistical characteristics. It is based on the work of Said and Pearlman (1993). Our tree parsing structure is similar to the one described in that paper, but different methods for updating the list of insignificant sets and for storing the coefficients were implemented. The coder was also designed to take more care in determining the presence of descendants in sub-trees, leading to a more efficient algorithm. The arithmetic coder is a generic, adaptive coder with the seed-state being a binary tree of sufficient depth to cover all pertinent entries with a starting count of the one used for both zero and one states in all sub-states.

II.5. Test images

The test images used for the evaluation were provided by WG-IV. The image test suite represented five imaging modalities: computed radiography (CR), computed tomography (CT), magnetic resonance (MR), nuclear medicine (NM), digital subtraction angiography (SP) and ultrasound (US). The table at the right shows the typical matrix size and bit depth of the image suite. The images were compressed to four levels (5:1, 10:1, 20:1 and 40:1) calculated from average bit depth. Bit-rate was controlled to ±5%. Following compression, the images were restored to their original resolution.

Image type	**Matrix size**	**Bit depth**
CR	1760 x 2140	10
CT	512 x 512	12
MR	256 x 256	10
NM	128 x 128	10
SP	512 x 512	10
US	480 x 488	8

II.6. Metrics

Image degradation was quantitated using absolute and squared error criteria. Metrics calculated from the absolute error included the peak absolute error (PAE) and mean absolute error (MAE). Metrics calculated from the squared error included the root mean squared error (RMSE) and peak signal-to-noise ratio (PSNR). The code to calculate these metrics was provided by WG-IV.

The metrics for each compressed image were determined from an error image. The error image was the difference between the original image and the compressed image at each pixel location. The PAE and MAE were simply the absolute maximum and the average pixel value of the error image, respectively. The sum total of all pixels in the error image was squared, divided by the total number of pixels, and the square root taken to yield the RMSE. The PSNR was calculated by dividing the maximum (nominal) pixel value by the RMSE, then converting to decibels.

To compensate for variations in image bit depth, normalized values of the PAE, MAE, and RMSE were also calculated. The normalized PAE (NPAE) was calculated as the PAE divided by the absolute range of pixel values in the original image. Normalized MAE (NMAE) was calculated by dividing MAE with the sum total of the pixel values in the original image. Normalized RMSE (NRMSE) was calculated by dividing the RMSE by the squared sum total of the pixel values.

II.7. Joint Photographic Experts Group compression

For comparison, the test suite images were also compressed using a version of the standard discrete cosine transform method described by the Joint Photographic Expert Group (JPEG). Release 6 (August 2, 1995) of the Independent JPEG User's Group implementation was obtained via anonymous ftp and compiled on a Sun Sparc 20 (SunOS 4.1.3, Mountain View, CA). Two versions of the executables (cjpeg and djpeg) were compiled; one for 8 bit images and the other for 9 to 12 bit images. This release allows the user to select an optimized Huffman table, which was used for all images. To get compression ratios of the target bit rate each image was compressed at many quality factors (QF). The target rate was selected from the resulting "QF to bit rate" tables.

III. Results

In general, the wavelet algorithm outperformed the JPEG codec in all cases for all metrics, with the sole exception of PSNR for the MR images where the performance was similar. The tables below show the relative advantage of the wavelet algorithm for PSNR and PAE error metrics. PSNR and PAE were chosen as representative metrics where the wavelet advantage was smaller (PSNR) and one for which the metrics clearly favored the wavelet algorithm (PAE).

PSNR comparison of the wavelet and JPEG algorithms (values in dB).

Algorithm	Comp. ratio	CR	CT	MR	NM	SP	US
Wavelet	**5**	58.48	63.92	59.77	62.07	55.75	50.76
JPEG	**5**	54.82	64.85	58.95	58.34	52.82	48.35
Wavelet	**10**	52.68	59.14	52.18	52.46	48.79	41.73
JPEG	**10**	51.15	56.66	52.63	48.21	49.62	40.35
Wavelet	**20**	50.61	53.92	48.04	43.75	48.39	35.75
JPEG	**20**	49.13	50.05	48.29	41.55	46.08	35.02
Wavelet	**40**	48.48	48.02	44.48	38.00	45.35	30.33
JPEG	**40**	47.82	44.71	44.62	35.78	41.45	31.02

PAE comparison of the wavelet and JPEG algorithms.

Algorithm	Comp. ratio	CR	CT	MR	NM	SP	US
Wavelet	5	6.83	17.83	22.50	15.36	5.33	4.17
JPEG	5	15.50	27.83	28.83	42.58	10.33	9.00
Wavelet	10	15.71	41.86	78.14	60.75	14.00	18.00
JPEG	10	32.67	90.83	84.83	171.92	31.33	34.00
Wavelet	20	23.83	89.33	128.17	209.58	20.67	52.50
JPEG	20	62.67	306.00	151.50	349.92	76.17	76.00
Wavelet	40	45.67	272.67	241.83	423.50	49.83	93.00
JPEG	40	104.33	661.33	258.50	536.08	160.67	108.50

PSNR was essentially the same for the MR images for either wavelet or JPEG compression, but was better for the wavelet for all other image types (>1% difference). The remaining metrics found the wavelet algorithm to result in up to 177% better performance (PAE for US images), with several metrics having greater than 100% better results for the wavelet relative to JPEG. PAE tended to show the most significant advantage for the wavelet algorithm, while MAE and NMAE were typically closer. The metrics also tended to show and greater advantage for the wavelet algorithm with the larger image formats (CR, SP, US and CT).

The table below summarizes the percent difference in the wavelet and JPEG metrics. Note that for PSNR a positive value indicates an advantage for wavelets, while for all other metrics a negative value indicates an advantage for the wavelet algorithm.

Percent difference in mean image metrics for wavelet and JPEG.

Image type	PSNR	RMSE	NRMSE	PAE	NPAE	MAE	NMAE
CR	3.4	-19.3	-19.2	-131.5	-135.3	-18.6	-18.1
CT	4.2	-28.7	-27.7	-139.5	-141.3	-20.9	-21.1
MR	-0.1	-1.2	-0.7	-15.5	-15.4	-0.7	-0.3
SP	6.2	-41.5	-40.6	-113.4	-113.4	-29.9	-29.7
US	4.2	-29.8	-18.6	-177.1	-139.8	-19.2	-12.0
NM	2.0	-12.5	-13.2	-66.6	-61.5	-0.7	-3.4

IV. Discussion

A new wavelet based compression algorithm has been developed specifically for medical image compression. This algorithm uses efficient spline wavelet filters and optimized quantization and encoding techniques. Although the algorithm is immature, it already outperforms the industry standard JPEG implementation across a broad spectrum of radiologic imaging modalities. Further optimization of the quantization process is possible and promises to improve the performance of the algorithm.

References

Chui, C.K., Wang, J.Z. Computational and algorithmic aspects of cardinal spline wavelets, Center for Approximation Theory Report #235, Texas A&M University, College Station, TX, 1990.

Chui, C.K. An introduction to wavelets, Academic Press, San Diego, 1992.

Chui, C.K. Wavelets: A mathematical tool for signal analysis, SIAM Publ., Philadelphia, PA, 1996.

Daubechies, I. Orthonormal bases of compactly supported wavelets, Comm. Pure and Appl. Math. 41:909-996, 1988.

Said, A., Pearlman, W.A. A new fast and efficient image codec based on set partitioning in hierarchical trees, IEEE Trans. Circuits and Sys. for Video Techn., 1993.

Online PACS Data Archiving Using Redundant Array of Inexpensive Disk (RAID) Technology

James L. Lear, Jonathan P. Pratt and Nelson P. Trujillo
Division of Nuclear Medicine, University of Colorado
Health Sciences Center, Denver, Colorado

Background

Personal computer-based networks for acquisition, distribution, and archiving of nuclear medicine image data have been available for several years (1). The use of such systems over standard film-based systems offers several advantages. These advantages include the accurate preservation of the data in a manner which facilitates comparison of old and new studies and the ability to reprocess data using newer methods as they are developed.

A problem with the use of all digital data acquisition is how to store the data. A busy nuclear medicine department may perform 5,000 to 10,000 cases per year with an average requirement of approximately one megabyte of storage per study. Therefore, over a period of ten years, 100 gigabytes of data may be generated.

Such quantities of data can be stored on magnetic tape, optical disks, or CD ROM disks However, these methods have limitations. Magnetic tape is inexpensive, but data access times are very long (hours). Optical and CD ROM disks are faster, but present disks are limited to approximately 1 gigabyte each. While jukeboxes help reduce this limitation, they are fairly expensive and mechanical problems can occur.

Redundant arrays of independent disks (RAID) have been developed to facilitate data storage on magnetic drives. RAID uses multiple disks to store data, so potential storage space is greater than with single disk systems.

For several years, RAID systems have been available in two configurations known as Levels 0 and 1. With Level 0, information is split between two disks. This approach allows data to be stored or retrieved at a rate approximately twice that of a single disk system. However, a disadvantage is that if one disk of the pair fails, all data is lost. In other words, system failure will occur at twice the frequency of a single disk system. Also, as the data transfer speeds of single disk drives are increasing continually, this year's Level 0 speed is usually achieved by next year's single disks.

With Level 1, information is mirrored onto two disks. Thus, data is stored in a redundant fashion. If one disk fails, the other preserves the data. However, this approach has limited speed and requires twice the disk space of a single disk system to store data. Also, the added expense of the RAID control system is difficult to justify in comparison to inexpensive software that can write information onto two standard single disks, albeit more slowly.

RAID Levels 3 and 5 have been recently introduced to solve the problems associated with Levels 0 and 1. While Levels 3 and 5 differ slightly between each other, they provide similar functionality. Data is stored in a redundant manner, but not mirrored as with Level 1. Rather, data and parity information are spread across several disks. If a single disk fails, data can be reconstructed from the information on the other disks. Therefore, this approach supports both rapid data transfer and redundancy, while requiring only an additional 25% of disk space compared to single drive systems.

One potential disadvantage with most RAID 3 and 5 systems with respect to their use with personal computers is that they require the use of one computer address per disk. Personal computers have only a limited number of addresses available, usually 5 or 6 SCSI addresses. Thus, the total number of disks that can be used in standard RAID systems is limited. Also, personal computers generally cannot directly access data stored in drives with greater than 4 gigabytes of space.

We developed a modified approach to RAID Level 5 data storage for use with nuclear medicine image archiving. The approach was intended to allow the use of vast, redundant disk storage space on a standard personal computer, the POWER Macintosh 8100/80.

Materials and Methods

Ten high speed disk drives, each with nine gigabytes storage capacity, were assembled into two systems of five disks each. Proprietary controllers (MegaDrive, Inc.) that permitted the use of multiple disks per SCSI address were used as opposed to standard controllers. This approach required the use of two SCSI addresses. Importantly, the controllers also supported "hot-swapability"; if a disk failed, another could be inserted in its place while the system was running.

Software was used to segment the 72 available gigabytes (90 gigabytes x 80%) into 3 gigabyte partitions. The software caused each 3 gigabyte partition to appear to the computer as a single disk drive. Each "pseudo-disk" appeared on the computer desktop so that all 72 gigabytes of space could be accessed.

After the system was assembled, it was tested by performing continual data storage and retrieval for 10 days. Simulated failures (removal of disk drives) were performed twice daily.

After testing, the system was optimized for our caseload. Eight years of digital data that we had previously stored on optical disks were loaded into the system. Data was stored in the 4 gigabyte partitions based on the dates the studies were acquired. Within each partition, the studies were stored in one-month folders. Within each one-month folder, the data was arranged according to study type, e.g. thallium scans, bone scans, etc. Individual studies were placed within the appropriate study-type folder and labeled by patient name, patient number, study type, and date using a maximum of 31 characters (the Macintosh limit).

Results

The system passed all initial tests without problems. After simulated failures, data could be reconstructed in less than 45 minutes (while the system remained in use).

By compressing only cardiac first pass data, we could store our 7,000 annual cases using approximately 6 gigabytes of disk space. Data was therefore stored in six month blocks using one 3 gigabyte partition per block, e.g. 1/88 - 6/88, 7/88 - 12/88, etc.

The time to locate a file and retrieve data was very rapid. A study could be located within any partition in approximately 20 seconds using the standard Macintosh Finder. Retrieval of the study and display upon a monitor required less than 5 seconds.

No failure occurred during six months of clinical use.

Discussion

RAID technology has reached a level which can support long term archiving and rapid retrieval of nuclear medicine image data. The cost of a practical system is reasonable. For example, the complete system (computer, controllers, and drives) used in this study was assembled at a cost of approximately $40,000. Importantly, this cost will drop by greater than 50% by late 1996 with the commercial release of 18 gigabyte drives.

In addition to its use in nuclear medicine, RAID Level 5 will likely have important use in storage of digital information in a general radiology department. A system with 250 gigabytes of redundant data storage capacity can be assembled using twenty, eighteen gigabyte drives at a cost of approximately $100,000. Assuming an average file size of 10 megabytes, more than 25,000 studies can be stored in such a system. This number of cases represents a month of all studies in a busy department. Thus RAID can be used as a buffer between immediate and long term storage in a complete PACs network.

Reference

1. Lear JL, Pratt JP, Roberts DR, et al. Gamma camera image acquisition, display, and processing with the personal microcomputer. Radiology 175: 241-245, 1990

Electronic Archiving of Radiology Images: A Comparison of Storage Technologies

Tim Chunn, Senior Health Industry Consultant
Storage Technology Corporation, Louisville, Colorado

Overview: Electronic archiving of radiology images from a busy department over many years will require several terabytes of digital storage and fairly rapid access to all of the images. Several technologies are available today to store large amounts of image data. However, there are many tradeoffs and architectural considerations when designing an archive system.

Recent advances in storage technologies have drastically reduced the cost of storage as well as improved access performance. This presentation will look at the requirements for long term storage of radiological images, primarily from a cost, capacity and performance standpoint. The reduction in cost has been a key to the justification of electronic radiology image archives.

The ability to capture large amounts of data as well as retrieve the information quickly and in a random basis is critical in this application. A number of different technologies are now available for short-term, intermediate and long-term storage of medical images. Magnetic direct access storage devices (DASD), redundant array of inexpensive disks (RAID), automated optical discs and very inexpensive automated magnetic tape technologies are all available in commercial systems. The significance of these new technologies in a radiological archive system will be addressed.

Currently, automated high-speed magnetic tape storage offers the capability of storing thousands of gigabytes of image data in a format that allows retrieval of selected images in an average time of 1 to 2 minutes. Configurations start with enough capacity for an average x-ray department to keep 5 years of storage in only 20 sq. ft. of floor space. The system is comparable in speed and reliability to the other systems mentioned above. In terms of cost, it offers a significant advantage. We anticipate seeing this type of high-speed magnetic storage assume an ever-increasing role in future PACS systems.

Medical Image Application Requirements

When designing a medical image archive system, it is important to consider the following:

- Number of users who will simultaneously access the archive
- Volume of Retrievals (Batch and Interactive - images per hour)
- Planned Pre-fetch of images (queuing)
- Batch Processing Window (hours)
- Network and Storage Device Data Transfer Rate
- Image File Size

These parameters all affect the cost and performance of the system and should be well understood before implementing a PACS system.

Medical image archives have two major operational storage environments to consider: first the picture capture phase (or record/write) where the following are important:

- Data Rate (images directly captured or converted and stored per hour)
- Total Capacity – what is the maximum storage needed

Second, the retrieval of the stored images where these items are important:

- Time to display image (Ad hoc, interactive – i.e. emergency room)
- Images processed per hour, or batch processing of several images (pre-staging based on next day appointments),

Other issues are important as well, such as: Media Standards and Interchange, Durability, Longevity, Reliability, Legality/Admissibility, and Data Protection. However, these issues will not be discussed in detail in this paper.

Computer Based Storage Options

Rotating magnetic disk (Direct Access Storage Device - **DASD**) is the fastest form of storage that is suitable for image archives. Device access speeds are typically in the 5 to 10 msec range and with suitable network and processing power, present images to a user within a few seconds. This type of storage typically costs between $.50 to $1.00 per MB.

RAID (Redundant Array of Inexpensive Disks) DASD is one type of magnetic disk storage that is commonly used today. RAID is a way of inexpensively protecting the data on this storage platform in case of device failure, but usually costs more than non-RAID magnetic disk (10 to 20% more). RAID technology insures very high availability of data to end users. RAID is discussed in further detail in a paper by Mr. James Lear. The focus of this paper will be with removable storage media.

Removable storage media consists primarily of optical and magnetic tape. **Optical disks** come in several formats today. 5 1/4" media holds from 1.3GB to 2.6GB per platter, and platters typically cost $50 to $60. There are several vendors who manufacture these devices (HP, Sony, Panasonic, Maxoptic, Olympus, IBM, etc.). Most 5 1/4" optical data transfer rates are between 1 and 2 MB per second, with the newer 2.6GB drives advertising 2 to 4 MB per second. Using multi-function optical drives, you can take advantage of WORM storage (Write Once Read Many) and rewriteable storage (MO - Magneto Optical), depending on the type of platter that is used. Currently, 5 1/4" technology is being squeezed from two sides due to tremendous competitive pressure from rapidly decreasing costs of magnetic disk and rapidly increasing capacity and performance from CD R and tape technology.

Higher capacity optical formats use 12" & 14" platters. Phillips LMS, Sony, ATG Cygnet and Hitachi are the primary vendors with 12". These larger platters hold between 12 and 15GBs and cost $500 to $600 each. Kodak makes the 14" optical drives which hold 15GBs today and cost about $600 each. The Phillips drive reads data at 2.7MB per second and writes at 1.3MB per second.

Optical archives usually are cost effective for small to medium sized archives, i.e., 10s to 100s of GBs. The largest 5 1/4" jukeboxes today hold approximately 650GBs (HP and Sony). On the very high end, with 12" optical in a Cygnet jukebox (141 platters), 1,440GBs is possible.

CD-R (Compact Disk, Recordable) fills out the optical storage platform. CD is the least expensive optical media ($1,000 - $1,500 per drive and about $15 per 600MB platter), but the slowest performing (only 0.6MB per second data transfer rate). CD is commonly used for applications where distribution of large amounts of data is required (catalog, manuals, check images for large commercial banks, etc.). There are now large CD jukeboxes that can hold up to 500 platters. Because of the performance and mechanical design of CD drives (primarily for desk top PC use), this storage platform is only applicable for low access applications.

Magnetic tape is the other very common removable media storage platform. Magnetic tape has been around for decades, with newer square cartridge formats (3480 type 1/2" tape) common for the last 10 years. Tape traditionally has been used for backups of magnetic disks and batch/sequential data processing applications due to its high data transfer speed and low cost. Many tape formats are available today. Low to medium performance and capacity formats are: QIC (Quarter Inch Cartridge), 4mm, and 8mm. High performance and capacity formats are: DLT (Digital Linear Tape), 3490 and Timberline, RedWood, and Magstar.

The high performance tape devices typically have very fast data transfer rates: IBM and STK's 3490 devices are 3MB per second, STK's Timberline is 6MB per second, IBM's Magstar is 9MB, STK's RedWood is just over 11MB per second. However, because of the sequential nature of tape, random access of data from any place on the tape is much slower than optical devices. For example, even with the industry's fastest tape drive (Timberline), average load, thread and seek time is about 20 to 25 seconds (to middle of tape). Higher capacity devices, such as DLT, take longer: 70 seconds to load, thread and seek half way down the tape.

Tape reliability and performance are much improved in the last 5 years. Tape media has improved due to new chemical processes and techniques. Media life can be 15 years and beyond, with 10s of thousands of loads and read write passes occurring with no data loss. Error correction routines also find "soft" errors on the media and correct them without the host computer even knowing about them. New software techniques (within the tape control units) allow applications to fast forward through the hundreds of feet of tape at a very high speed until the tape is positioned at the beginning of a file. Random retrievals from high performance tape such as Timberline can be done, as long as the end user is satisfied with 20 to 30 second retrieval times.

Tape storage is very cost effective when coupled with DASD and appropriate software so that large batch retrievals of images can be done the night before images will be needed. Patients scheduled for appointments the next day can have their images pre-fetched from tape to fast DASD storage when PACS applications are coupled with Radiology Information Systems software. Once the patient images are no longer needed, software can also delete the copied image from more expensive DASD, with the permanent image still residing on tape.

Storage and Retrieval Performance and Cost Trends

In today's health services office environment, about 90% of all information is stored on paper or film. Typically only about 5% is stored in a computer system and 5% is stored on some sort of microfilm or microfiche. All but computer stored data is retrieved manually and requires considerable time and labor and often is not in the right place at the right time to be of great value to the person who needs the information. The following chart illustrates the dramatic decrease in cost of various types of computer storage over the last several years as compared to manual methods of storage and retrieval.

Most people do not realize that due to increasing costs of labor and floor space, manual methods of storing and retrieving information now cost as much if not more than much faster computerized methods. This chart graphically illustrates the rapidly declining price of magnetic disk and how optical is being squeezed from above.

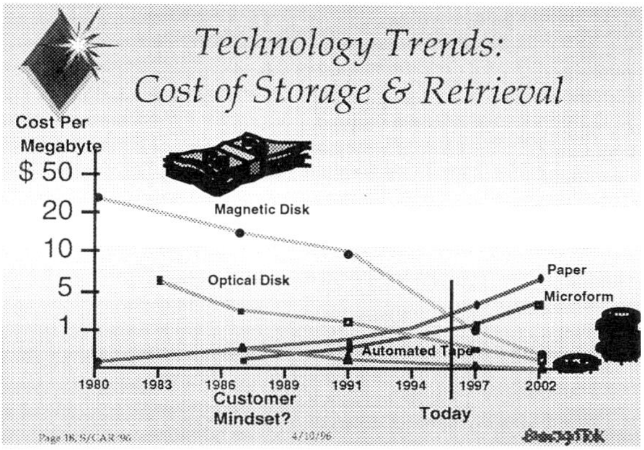

Medical information also has a very definite life cycle. Early in an images life, quick access is critical and often needed by several people in many different places within a medical facility. Access to a critically injured person's x-ray within minutes if not seconds can be a key factor in the diagnosis and treatment of the patient. However, after the patient has been treated and discharged, this same x-ray may rarely be accessed again, and if it does, minutes or hours to retrieve this x-ray are normally acceptable. The requirement for fast retrieval of information initially, then slower retrieval later suggests that different types of storage devices could be used over time to store an image with considerable savings in storage cost. As fast retrieval times grow less and less important, the image could be migrated to less costly storage devices to minimize the cost of storage over the life of the image. The following chart illustrates this concept.

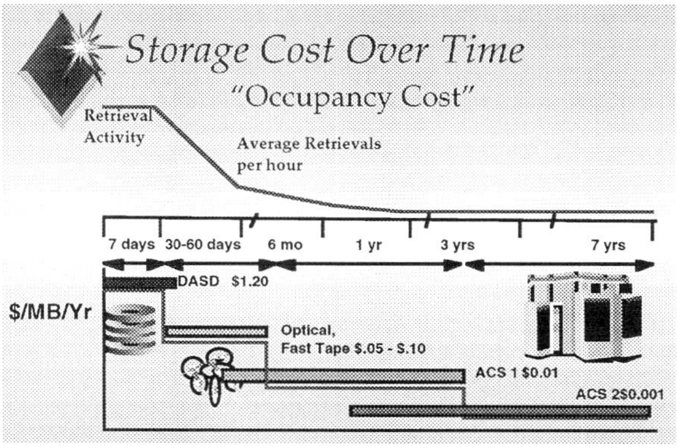

The longer images are kept on DASD, the more it costs. The total cost of storage over time would be the area under this step curve. Once an image no longer requires fast retrievals, total cost can be minimized by migrating data from faster, more expensive storage platforms to slower, less expensive storage. The above step curve is not drawn to scale. With today's technology, it is not unusual to see an order of magnitude difference in cost between storage platforms. The sample costs shown on the chart are for actual configurations and include acquisition cost, maintenance, media, floor space and power/cooling costs over a 5 year time frame.

Performance and Cost Modeling

Now that you know that you have a broad range of choices for image storage, you also now have the responsibility of determining what storage will best suit the needs of your organization. There are several ways of doing this. One very helpful way is to model your storage requirements before purchasing any products and be able to simulate your actual working environment to determine if a proposed configuration will actually meet your needs. StorageTek has developed several of these tools. The Nearline® Performance Estimator (NPE) will be discussed here as well as a pricing and configuration tool called Image Sizer.

The NPE model considers all mechanical and electronic performance within a removable storage media subsystem such as a robotic tape library or an optical jukebox. Variables such as robotic speed (media exchanges per hour), data channel speed (data path between the storage device and the host computer), read/write data speed from the media itself and all of the mechanical times associated with the read/write device (time for media load/unload, tape thread, platter spin up/down, and search time primarily) are all considered in the model.

Configuration variables are then input into the model. These are: File size (determines the amount of time it takes to actually read and write data from media), number of read/write devices (determines the number of simultaneous or parallel accesses to data) and for tape, the actual length of tape being used (in feet/meters). For image storage modeling, it is assumed that the image already comes compressed and the storage device does no additional compression.

For the purposes of this paper, I only consider random retrieval patterns, i.e., ad hoc requests for information directly from the removable media device. Also, the retrieval times that are calculated do not include any host computer processing times nor does it consider network transmission times. These random retrieval times also reflect averages for the tape devices, meaning seek times include the time to get to the middle of the tape (for example, for Timberline this would add 21 seconds to the fastest time, for RedWood this would add 53 seconds, both reflect times for the longest tape available).

The following charts show sample outputs from NPE. These charts show the price/performance combination together. The vertical axis is response time in seconds, the horizontal axis is exchanges or retrievals per hour. As you can see, these curves are classic "hockey stick" curves that exhibit fairly flat characteristics until some bottleneck is reached, at which time, response time increases significantly. The lower curve on both charts is the performance of both 5 1/4" and 12" optical technology, and on the first chart, the second curve is how 4 DLT drives perform. The DLT subsystem can support up to about 50 requests per hour in less than 2 minutes average retrieval time. On the second chart, the middle curve is Timberline's (TL) performance and the top line, RedWood (RW). For up to about 150 requests per hour, optical achieves about 30 second retrieval times, Timberline has about 35 second response up to 100 requests per hour and RedWood has about 90 second response up to 40 retrievals per hour.

The boxes on the charts describe the costs for each type of storage device. These costs were calculated based on the Image Sizer model and include hardware acquisition cost, maintenance, media, floor space and environmental costs over a 7 year period. The DLT/Optical configuration has 7 years of images on tape and 5 months of images on optical, providing an average of 2 minute and 30 second retrieval times respectively. Over the 7 year period, DLT costs less than a penny per MB per year, optical costs about 6.5 cents per MB per year. Total 7 year cost for the storage system would be $450K. If this entire archive were on optical, the storage cost would be 4 cents per MB per year, or $1.37 million dollars over 7 years, about 4 times the cost of tape & optical solution. This is the cost/performance tradeoff - you would pay an additional $920K to have 30 second access to your entire 7 year history as compared to 2 minute response from DLT tape after the image is 5 months old.

The second chart illustrates a tape configuration that is based on 5 months of storage on Timberline ("fast tape") and the entire 7 years on RedWood 50 GB tape cartridges. The combined cost of both tape technologies is shown in the Total Tape Cost box. The tape solution costs 1 1/4 cents per MB per year, or $1.86 million over 7 years. If the entire 20TBs of images were stored on 12" optical, 12 jukeboxes would be required, at a cost of 5 cents per MB per year, or over 7 years, $7 million dollars. Again, this is the cost/performance tradeoff - to have 25 second access to all of your images, it would cost over $5 million more, or almost 4 times the cost of tape.

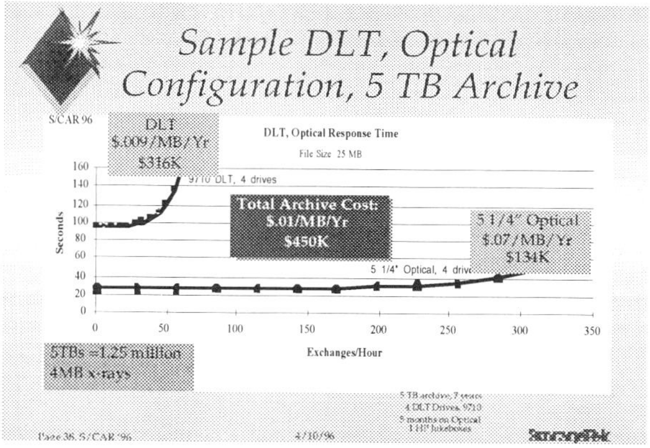

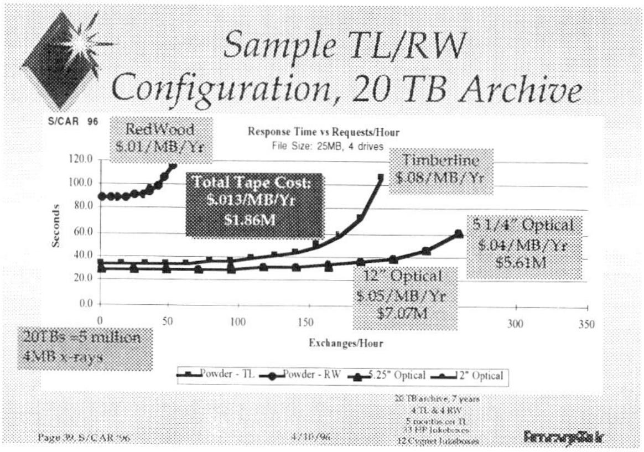

For comparison, based on a 1993 IEEE Symposium on Mass Storage Systems paper by Samuel J. Dwyer, et al, UCLA Medical Center produces about 49,000 films per month. This archive would represent about 20 TBs of digitized data over 5 years. UCLA's cost to maintain 3 film libraries is over $2.4 million per year or about $16.8 million over 7 years. The savings of digitized storage as compared to traditional film libraries are obviously very great.

Bi-directional Multi-Modality Integration of the Samsung PACS and the Loral PACS

Chul Hwa Paik, Tae Woo Kim, Myung Jin Song, and Won Ky Kim
Samsung Biomedical Research Institute, Seoul, Korea

Introduction

The Loral PACS was installed at the Samsung Medical Center(SMC) in Seoul and has been expanded to the full-PACS up to 150 viewing stations by the end of this year. The hospital own PACS is being developed for archiving and displaying the unconventional modalities such as a PET image, a SPECT image, an ultrasound image, a 3-D reconstructed image and an endoscopic image. The development of the bi-directional multi-modality interface between two PACSs with retrieval and storage functions may eventually integrate two PACS databases and make all kinds of the image modalities scanned in the hospital be in one PACS environment.

Methods

All image modalities except MR and CT images archived into the Loral PACS database are transferred from scanners directly, converted into a DICOM 3.0 format and archived into the Samsung PACS database. The Samsung PACS can retrieve the image data from the Loral PACS database as well as the Samsung PACS database for displaying on the Samsung viewing station called the Advanced Multi-modalities Image Station(AMIS), and also archive the image data into the Loral PACS database through a bi-directional image gateway for displaying on the Loral viewing station. The AMIS viewing software is developed in a X-window environment and runs on a workstation(Sun Sparc-20, ICS-Motif, ISG's IAP) with a VGA color monitor and two 2Kx2K B/W monitors. A PET image, a SPECT image and an endoscopic image are viewed on the color monitor and a MR image and a CT image are viewed on two high resolution B/W monitors. The AMIS has a multi-planar reformat(MPR) viewer which is a cost-effective implementation in a viewing station, as well as a 2-D viewer, zoom, etc.

The 35 axial [^{18}F]FDG PET images (128x128 resolutions, 4.25mm thickness) acquired on a GE Advance PET scanner are shown in a MPR mode in the figure 1. The laparoscopic images of cholecystectomy and endometriosis are shown in the figure 2. The 32 optic nerve images scanned by the optic disc analyzer are shown in the figure 3. These data sets are converted into DICOM 3.0 format, archived into the Samsung PACS database, transferred into the AMIS workstation and visualized interactively in the 2-D viewer or the MPR viewer. The overall Samsung image management network is also shown in the figure 4.

Discussion

A key advantage of the integration for two PACS databases is their independence to each database. In addition, it has been found that the logical integration of the database is particularly conducive to easy image management in a PACS environment. The multi-modality image display on the same viewing station may also provide a speedy diagnosis to a physician due to being in the integrated database.

References

1. Chen D., Ho B., Chao W., Taira R., "Image Flow Management in a PACS Network", SPIE Medical Imaging, Vol. 2165, 1994.
2. Behlen F., Hoffmann K., MacMahon H., "Long Term Strategies for PACS Archive Design", SPIE Medical Imaging, Vol. 2711, 1996.
3. Wong E., Hoo K., Huang H., "Empower PACS with Content-Based Queries and 3D Image Visualization", SPIE Medical Imaging, Vol. 2711, 1996.

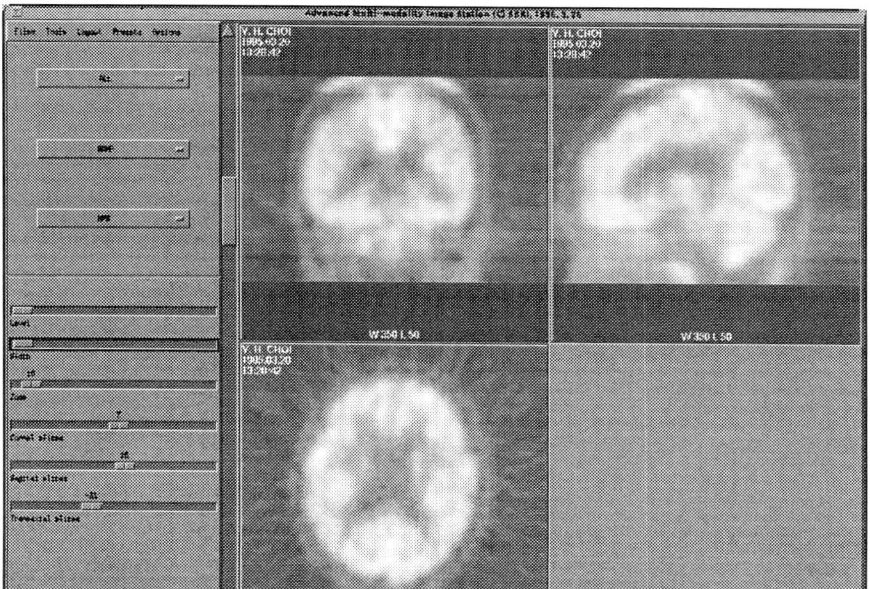

Figure 1. The 35 [^{18}F]FDG PET images are visualized interactively in the multi-planar reformat viewer.

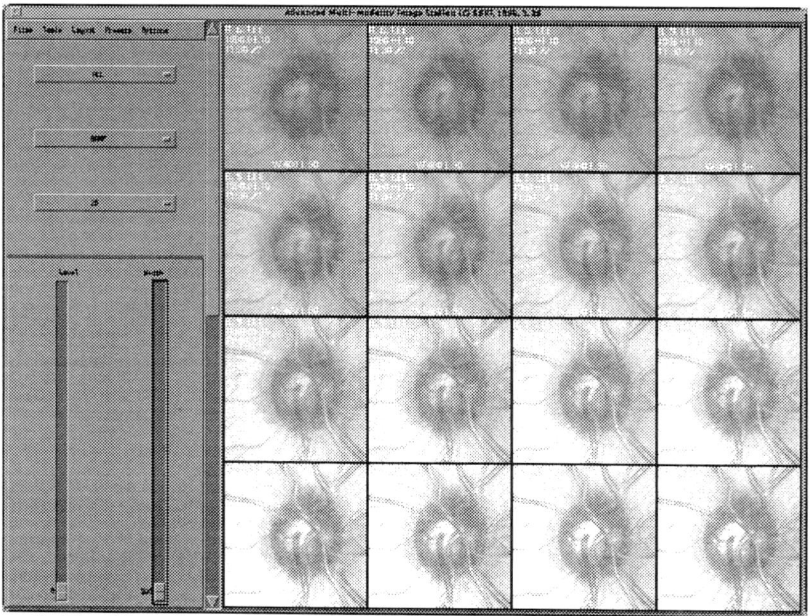

Figure 2. The 32 optic nerve images scanned by the optic disc analyzer are shown in the 2-D viewer. The images are scanned in a sequence with varying a focal plane.

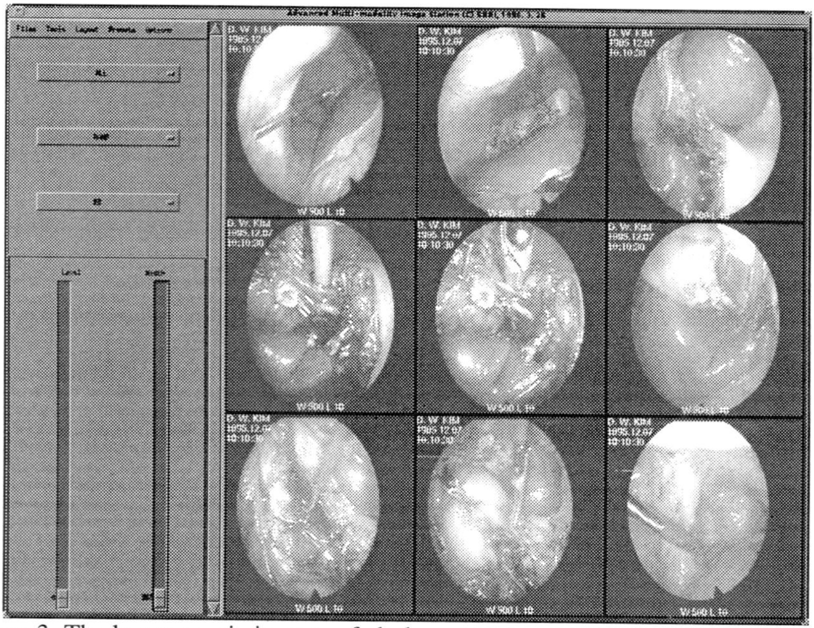

Figure 3. The laparoscopic images of cholecystectomy and endometriosis are shown in the 2-D viewer.

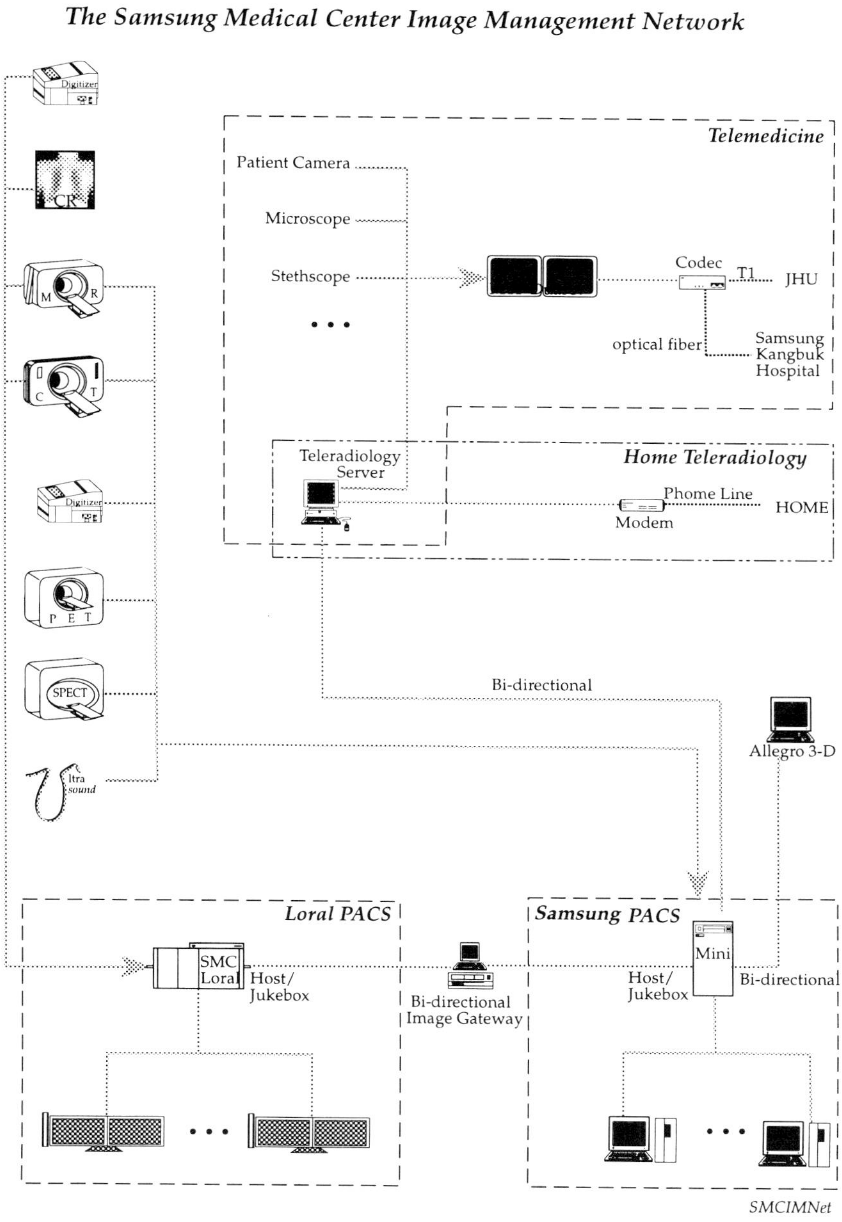

Figure 4. The diagram shows the overall Samsung Image Management Network including the telemedicine system with a foreign hospital and a local branch hospital.

Design and Implementation of the First Filmless Children's Hospital

Dr. Merl de Silva
Director Imaging Department, Royal Alexandra Hospital for Children, Westmead, Australia
Wil Van Den Berg
Client Manager, Electromedical Section, Department of Public Works & Services, Sydney, Australia
David Brown
Product Manager PACS, Medical Applications Pty Ltd, Gladesville, Australia

1. INTRODUCTION:

The Royal Alexandra Hospital for Children is the major paediatric facility of the University of Sydney, Australia, having been established in 1880. The hospital has just been relocated to a "greenfield" site at Westmead, located at the population centre of Sydney, Australia. The facility provides tertiary care services with 350 in-patient beds and out-patients departments for all paediatric sub-specialities. The case load has dramatically increased since the opening of the new facilities, and is anticipated to be 45,000 for the 1996 year, based upon the past five months work.

2. PROCUREMENT PROCESS:

A business case was undertaken in August to September 1993, and was completed in October 1993. The conclusion provided an cost analysis for the various options open to the Hospital at that time, from No PACS, fully film based, through a phased implementation over time, and the full PACS installation as part of the "green fields" relocation of the Hospital. The full PACS option was ranked number 1 in the analysis, in terms of cost effectiveness for the new site, with a break even(or return on investment) on the differential with a conventional system, of around 3 years.

A strategic study was undertaken for the Hospital (by Simson and Bowes) to determine the future direction of the Hospital's information network and technology. The report highlighted the unique concentration of paediatric subspecialties within the Hospital, and recommended that access to such expertise from other locations (intra hospital), via national and international links be established. These type of links would enhance the education of paediatric radiologists and raise the level of available paediatric radiology expertise. It would have the benefit of "morale" boosters for doctors who were located remotely, and in addition would provide a potential "export" market to SE Asian countries.

Prior to gaining formal approval from the Health Department, Public Works on behalf of the Hospital, called an Expression of Interest (EOI), to prepare possible contenders for what lay ahead and to canvass our developing design philosophy in the market place, to see if a system was available that would come close to meeting the overall design criteria laid down for the full hospital PACS. As a result of the EOI, an approved tenderer "short" list was established.

As part of defining the tender specifications a decision was required regarding functional design concepts for the proposed system. At this time two types of PACS architecture were being considered. Centralised image archival and processing versus distributed image archival and processing. Both forms of architecture had advantages and disadvantages and it was the Hospital's intention to ensure that neither option would be disadvantaged by the forthcoming tender specification, consideration was given to "accessing speed", "random" versus "planned" or the prefetched approach, networking design alternatives, and cost. The Hospital also sought independent expert advise from Mr. Fred Pryor, who was involved in the DICOM standard formulation. He provided an "arms" length review of the specification to ensure that it was understandable and was achievable.

An important consideration was the PACS to Radiology Information System (RIS) interface. The hospital realised its existing RIS was inadequate therefore it was decided to include the RIS as a separable part in the PACS technical specification, however it was procured later in a separate tender. The Hospital was anxious to ensure that both the RIS and PACS vendors would have sufficient expertise and resources, to guarantee a high level of bidirectional communication between the two domains, to provide advanced facilities such as organ and modality specific pre-fetching and autorouting of reported studies to their final destinations. The features were regarded by the hospital as mandatory for systems using distributed architecture. Determining the size of the archive for the tender specification was a relatively easy task. The New Children's Hospital Westmead is a Hospital for seriously ill children and it was determined that the typical confinement could be as long as five months. These children, many suffering from congenital illnesses will continue to present at the hospital for follow up procedures and further treatment often into their teenage years.

Based on background requirements we decided that the short term archive should hold up to five months of patients images corresponding to current patients being treated in the hospital. This period would also minimise the pre-fetching requirement for current patients. With regard to the long term archive it was decided to seek eight years on line storage.

On the issue of user interaction with workstations, there was a desire to keep user interfaces as simple as possible whilst maintaining the functionality required on a PACS diagnostic workstation. It was hoped that this issue would be addressed by specifying different types of workstations for different applications eg diagnostic, clinical, etc, whilst maintaining some degree of standardisation between the user interfaces. The specification was kept fairly general in the area of workstation interfaces, specifying the fundamental requirements but leaving the final form of the interface open in the belief that it would encourage innovation within the offers. The network infrastructure was part of the building design by PWD, based upon a structured network approach. The PACS network was separate from the hospital PC based network for reasons of network loading and to ensure overall contractual responsibility of the PACS provider.

Tenders were called in February 1994, with the tender closing in April 1994. The tender covered both the imaging modalities and the PACS as one integrated whole, and provided opportunities for companies to work together as partners with one company appointed as prime contractor. The prime contractor was responsible for the coordination and project management of the project for the various companies. A hospital procurement committee had been formed to oversee the procurement of the imaging equipment and it was clear from the outset that there were potentially two major obstacles to the success of this project:

1. The relocation time frame was such that all patients from the old hospital had to be transferred to the new site within a 4 week period. This meant that all new equipment should be installed and all relevant staff trained in the function of this new equipment before patient transfer commenced. These dead lines were clearly specified to ensure that tenderers understood their task clearly. In addition substantial completion penalties in the form of liquidated damages, were included in the specification, again in an effort to guarantee completion of the installation by the required transfer dead line.
2. The successful tenderer had to possess the necessary capabilities and strengths to install what was shaping up to be the largest clinical PACS systems to date. Furthermore the equipment procurement committee was anxious to ensure that they obtained value for money.

A baseline study was performed by an independent consultant prior to the move from the old hospital. The base line study was aimed at providing indicators which could be used in the post relocation study to see how successfully the PACS equipment had been integrated into the working life of the new hospital.

3. PROJECT DELIVERY:

Part of the tender specification stipulated the need for a qualified project manager dedicated to this project. The project's success depended on the cooperation from all the project team members; the selected prime contractor, Medical Applications, appointed a local manager to take advantage of the know-how of the local environment and culture. Every member of the team took complete ownership of the project to ensure timely completion of their part.

Siemens commitment to the project included the provision of one of their factory PACS engineers, Mr. Michael Jonas, who was seconded to Medical Applications for at least an eighteen month period to provide PACS expertise, not available locally, to ensure the system was configured correctly and to provide a factory link.

The system was acceptance tested by Public Works in conjunction with hospital staff. As part of the introduction of this new technology within the hospital, the responsibility within the tender also included a comprehensive training program.

Recently a visit from a Siemens CR specialist saw the reprogramming of the CR filtering and processing parameters, programs and protocols, to improve the image quality and reduce the patient radiation dose. Initially many of the "test" exposures were taken utilising a (dead) chicken model to approximate paediatric chests. Included in the evaluation was the value of lead backed cassettes.

4. USAGE AND EXPERIENCE:

The system provides the only means for reporting for all procedures undertaken at the New Childrens Hospital. Reporting is currently done on workstations with High Lux 1K X 1K high resolution screens. The tender specified 2K X 2K workstations for CR reporting, which remain on back order, and are one of the few outstanding hardware items with Siemens, Erlangen.

With CR reporting it was found that 2 monitors were not sufficient for effective reporting, and the workstations were upgraded to provide 3 monitors. This allows one monitor to be used for the 'tokenview' sketch view and the other two for comparison of images from different folders. The 2 on top of 2 monitor arrangement was found to be ergonomically unacceptable for CR reporting, however it proved to be satisfactory for conferencing and MRI reporting. A two bay workstation was found to be adequate for CT reporting. Each radiologist and visiting consultants were provided with a single bay diagnostic workstation in their office, to enable them to report on urgent cases from their offices and provide consultations with physicians over the phone.

The present folder management system allows the images to be sorted by patient modality and organ, however it is not possible, on most of the connected modalities to specify the organ examined. A desire to group images on organ based grouping would provide the required flexibility for reporting and for conferencing (including clinics). The system needs the facillity of a "conference-folder" for clinical meetings where these images can be arranged, plus the pulling together of images from various patients with the same or similar morphologies. Arrangements where worklists can be setup for multiple workstations or for specific (but separate, multiple) collections of images, would be considered useful but is presently not yet available. Presently available are "reference" folders where images are stripped of all header information, reducing it usefulness in a teaching or conferencing setting. New workstation software is to be released in July 1996 which apparently introduces a totally new concept in lieu of the worklist philosophy. A pre-release version of the new software is to be demonstrated to the New Childrens Hospital staff in April for user comments and evaluation.

For report dictation the hospital installed Phillips digital dictation system (system 4000). The reports are transcribed on a CERNER RADNET (RIS) screen and once verified are accessible from an inquiry on the PACS workstations. Currently the report and the images are not exactly (one to one) matched. The last five reports are made available and the user has to find the matching report from this selection. Siemens and Cerner are currently working to provide this feature. The next phase in this process will be the introduction of a Phillips voice recognition reporting system (system 6000), as the beta site evaluation for the English language version, commencing May 1996.

5. TELERADIOLOGY:

The hospital carried out 2 pilot programs in 1993. Each program was for a three month period. The films were transmitted from hospital sites 55 km and 400 km away, using ISDN 128 Kbit lines. For paediatric radiology the quality of the transmitted images were evaluated against original films. No significant lack of image quality was detected. Transmission times were in the order of 5 minutes for a chest X-ray, and the costs were approximately $1.00 per megabyte with off-peak tariffs, or $2.30 during peak times.
The new hospital has been selected as one of 12 sites for state wide Teleradiology/ Tele-medicine/ video conferencing trials for Teleradiology and Tele-psychiatry. One of the hospitals involved in the previous trial 400km away, plus another remote located hospital approx 1200km away, will be involved. These projects will commence in May 1996 for paediatric patients, and will be expended to other areas dependent upon the clinical evaluation. The hospital is investigating the use of satellite lines for this project. A PC based image review station will be evaluated during this project, for use by general practitioners. Other speciality areas are also included in this state wide evaluation, eg: Tele-ophthalmology, and Tele-pathology.

6. OTHER SYSTEMS

In addition to the PACS installation as part of the move to the new location the Hospital also implemented an EMTEK CONTINUM 2000 computerised charting system (CCIS) for the Paediatric and Neonatal ICU areas. The Intensive Care Units were converted to "paperless" 6 weeks after the relocation of the Hospital. The two information systems are linked through a PACS/CCIS interface that will allow the viewing of radiology images at the bedside. At present only an alpha software version of the interface is implemented on selected non-bedside non-primary care workstations.
The hospital has established a department of multimedia education to provide such services to other paediatric centres and to the general practitioners. The multimedia department has been equipped with facilities for developing CD-ROM based educational programs in areas such as child Asthma, child abuse, child development, etc for distribution to parents and the wider community.

NEW CHILDRENS HOSPITAL WESTMEAD

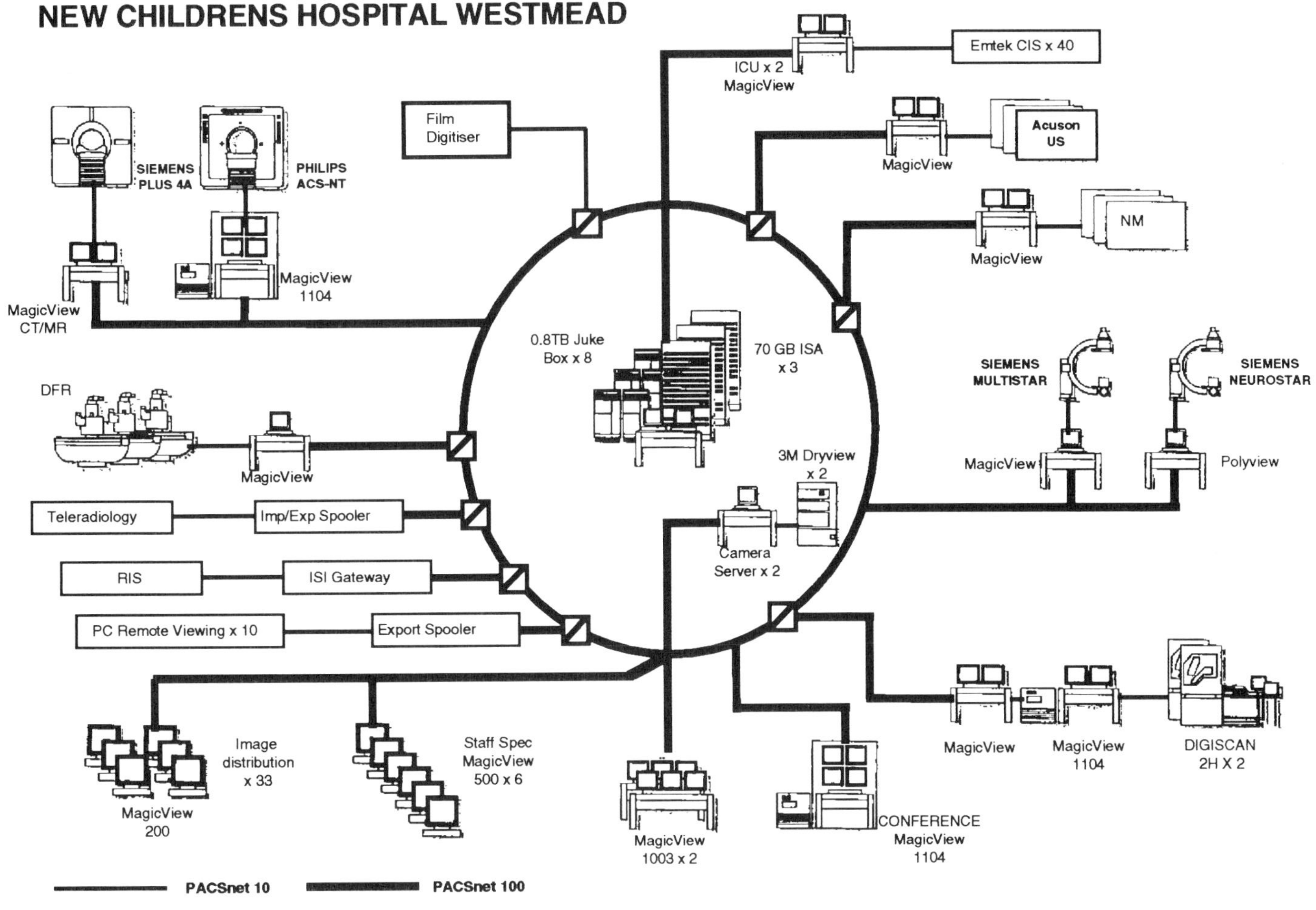

The Mayo Clinic Jacksonville Electronic Radiology Practice

Richard L. Morin and Thomas H. Berquist
Department of Radiology, Mayo Clinic Jacksonville, Jacksonville, Florida
Wolfgang Rueger
Siemens Medical Systems, Inc., Iselin, New Jersey

I. INTRODUCTION

The current Radiology practice at Mayo Clinic Jacksonville is very efficient from the referring physicians point of view. On average the films with the final (authenticated) report for a chest examination are delivered to the referring physician in about 45 minutes following x-ray exposure. For other conventional radiographic examinations the turnaround is approximately 60 min and about 120 min for Computed Tomography, Magnetic Resonance, Ultrasound, and Nuclear Medicine. This efficiency is achieved with personnel intensive effort. For a typical examination about 8 persons handle a radiograph and envelope from exposure to referring physician delivery. Hence, the motivation for the implementation of the Electronic Radiology Practice (ERP) was firstly to maintain our efficiency in an ever increasingly cost conscience environment and secondly to increase the productivity at all staff levels while preparing for the further changes in the practice of Medicine in general and Radiology in particular. The ERP implementation parallels an institution-wide project to eliminate the circulation and archival of the paper medical record.

II. PRACTICE PARAMETERS

Mayo Clinic Jacksonville is staffed by 170 physicians in 23 medical and 12 surgical specialties and includes two additional off-campus Family Medicine practice sites with Radiology facilities (approximately 40/exams/day/site). Clinic patient visits are approximately 200,000 per year with about 14,750 Comprehensive History and Physical Examinations and 15,000 Specialty Consultations per year. St. Luke's Hospital is a 289 bed facility located approximately 10 miles from the Clinic. The Radiology department currently performs about 180,000 examinations annually at both clinic and hospital sites, with a staff of 16 Radiologists, 2 Fellows, 1 Resident, and 117 Technologists. The imaging equipment includes about 65 x-ray Tubes, 4 CT scanners, 3 MR Systems, 10 Nuclear Medicine Systems, 7 Ultrasound systems, and 2 Cardiac Catherization Systems. Current electronic systems include the automated PACS archive of CT and MR images, Teleradiology applications to 14 radiologists' homes, and a Family Practice site.

III. THE AUTOMATED CLINICAL PRACTICE

The usual patient flow through the Clinic is an entry Comprehensive History and Physical (CHP). This examination may result in one or more Specialty Consultations (SPEC) and tests (Lab and Radiology). The diagnosis and treatment regimen are finalized by the Physician who first examined the patient following the analysis of all consultations and tests. The patient is then dismissed and after a period of time may be seen again for a Return Examination (RTNV).

During the course of these interactions the patient's medical record is circulated to all involved with the patient. Hence, the number of steps involved in these activities is substantial. The number of manual processing steps for a CHP Examination is 55, for a SPEC Consultation 40 and for a RTNV Examination 29. The personnel associated with each of these steps is formidable. Thus the motivation for the design and implementation of the ACP was to maintain patient satisfaction and Physician efficiency while increasing cost effectiveness and management of resources. In addition, the project was felt to be an asset in enabling Clinical Pathways and Managed Care settings with the ability to adapt to the changing healthcare environment. The ACP is designed to increase patient satisfaction by decreasing waiting time, improve efficiency of appointment scheduling, and increase timeliness of correspondence and response to patient queries. The primary benefits to Physicians center on increased productivity through increasing the availability of patient information by eliminating the time spent waiting for the paper record.

Implementation of the ACP has reduced the manual processing steps for CHP Examinations, SPEC Consultations and RTVN Examinations by 55%, 58%, and 35% respectively. Physician acceptance has been remarkably high and implementation is nearly complete.

The ACP was developed in conjunction with Cerner Corp. and is based on their Open Clinical Foundation (OCF) system. The ACP is integrated with a Cerner PathNet Laboratory System, an IMNET Document Scanning System, a CyCare Billing System, a Sudbury Dictation system, and an institutionally developed Radiology

Information System (RIMS). Over 500 PC based workstations are installed throughout the Clinic.

IV. ELECTRONIC RADIOLOGY PRACTICE

The ERP was conceived to enhance our Radiology practice and provide the means to further enhance the capabilities of the ACP. The fundamental features of the ERP were an outgrowth of separate discussions over the last two years which developed seven projects utilizing different aspects of Electronic Imaging and PACS to improve our Radiology practice while maintaining the level of quality felt to be essential for our patients. The ERP includes interfaces to the ACP, the RIMS Radiology Information System, and the existing Mayo/IBM PACS system the AEGIS Ultrasound Network and Medasys and ADAC Nuclear Medicine Networks. In addition, implementation includes the use of Computed Radiography and interfaces to all present imaging equipment, through DICOM. The network, workstations and most importantly interfaces and system integration is in collaboration with Siemens Medical Systems.

In order to accomplish this level of integration the development of many interfaces is necessary. Ideally, we wish to have all devices communicate fully with the RIS; however, it is not always possible to establish such complete connections. Hence, some interfaces (particularly for demographics at an imaging modality) consist only of reading bar-codes to complete demographic fields at the modality console. While not the most elegant solution, this does eliminate the manual entry of the Clinic Identification Number. This feature is crucial to maintain database integrity in the totally electronic environment. Our previous experience with PACS for CT and MRI has shown us that substantial numbers of errors occur with manual entry, requiring intervention and considerable personnel time to rectify. The importance of this feature is often not appreciated if one is using a local or modality specific PACS (particularly if film is used as the archival material or backup).

The methodology for presentation of prior examinations for comparison during image interpretation is a particularly interesting problem. There are many approaches to this activity ranging from loading all old images into the electronic archive to having film and viewboxes available beside the workstation. There are tremendous tradeoffs involved among time required, personnel cost, and convenience At the current time we have adopted the approach of selective digitization of certain examinations organized by medical specialty (Targeted Load).

The Clinic implementation includes a Digital Chest X-ray System, 4 dedicated CR readers (2 off-campus), 18 workstations, 11 servers, 4 optical libraries, 4 film digitizers, 3 laser printers, and interfaces to 2 CT systems, 2 MR systems, 2 Fluoroscopic systems, and Ultrasound and Nuclear Medicine Networks. File servers will accommodate a 3 day capacity (the average length of activity during a patient visit) and optical libraries will maintain about 2 years of storage on-line

All communication within the Radiology Department will occur via FDDI. Images will be transmitted via FDDI to dedicated servers on each Clinical floor. Image review will then occur on the ACP workstation by Ethernet transmission from the server. These data will be provided in compressed, 8-bit formats. Servers will be populated overnight with all images for patients scheduled to be seen by a physician on the floor.

The Hospital implementation includes a Digital Chest X-ray System, 3 dedicated CR readers, 17 workstations, 10 servers, 3 optical libraries, 2 film digitizers, 4 laser printers and interfaces to 2 CT systems, 1 MR system, and 2 Interventional systems, 2 fluoroscopic systems, 3 mobile C-arms, and Ultrasound and Nuclear Medicine Networks.

Interestingly, we believe that production of hard copy will still be important. We intend to produce hard copy (film or paper) for referral purposes in the Operating Rooms, on certain specialty floors (e.g., orthopedics, oncology, neurology, etc.), and for patient physician copies. However, these sites of remote copy production will not use conventional printers and chemistry. Most importantly we shall not maintain an archive or record which would involve personnel and supervision. The initial production of this type will occur using DryView 8700 printers (3-M Corp)..

V. Summary

The design, specification, and early implementation of the ERP at Mayo Clinic Jacksonville has been an exciting and interesting endeavor. We believe many more aspects of Radiology Practice will shift as implementation proceeds. For example, we are in the process of re-design of reading rooms to more fully realize the benefits attainable with electronic imaging.

The hallmark of our project lies in the integration of the Radiology Electronic Imaging and PACS components with the institution-wide systems. The overall impact of the project is dependent upon this integration to produce ubiquitous access and seamless us

Cost of Film: Purchasing, Processing, Packaging, Storing and Disposal Over the Lifetime of a Film Examination in a Large Radiology Department

B.F. King, M.D., S. Ward, B.A., R. Bruesewitz, R.T., R. Feia, R.T., W. Webbles, R.T., Scott Seinola, B.A., N.J. Hangiandreou, Ph.D. and B. Williamson, M.D.

Mayo Medical Center, Rochester, Minnesota

In order to more fully understand the costs of existing technology to capture images on film and to transport these images on film, we determined the annual cost per x-ray examination to purchase, process, package, transport, store, and dispose a film examination over its lifetime. We divided the cost evaluation into four categories: 1) the average cost per sheet of film and the average sheets of film per examination, 2) the costs of building space and supplies that are a 100% related to film management, 3) the costs of personnel who are 100% related to film management in the Department of Radiology, and 4) the costs of personnel who are 100% related to film management in other clinical departments. These costs were evaluated for one year and were divided by the number of examinations performed at our institution each year. It was determined an average radiology exam contains an average of 3.53 films per examination. In a 5-state area, it was determined that the average purchase price of a sheet of film was $1.77. Therefore, the average cost of film per examination was $6.25. The average cost of supplies and building space directly related to film management was $1.46 per x-ray examination. The average cost of personnel 100% related to film management in the Department of Radiology was $5.91 per x-ray examination. The average cost of personnel 100% related to film management outside of the Department of Radiology was $2.20 per examination. This resulted in an average cost of $15.82 per x-ray examination to acquire and maintain diagnostic radiology images on film each year. This cost estimate is most likely an underestimate of cost compared to smaller institutions in light of greater efficiencies at our institution because of its large size. Other studies have estimated this cost to be even higher ($25-30 per examination). Therefore, we believe the average cost to an institution to acquire and store an x-ray examination on film is somewhere between $15-20 per examination each year.

This figure underscores the significant cost institutions endure for x-ray film and its management. Cost justification for conversion to a total electronic imaging department and possibly a "film-least" or "filmless" department can be undertaken in light of these figures.

I. Introduction

In the early part of this century, x-ray images were captured on glass plates covered with a silver emulsion. Later, cellulose film was substituted for glass plates. Since then, x-ray film has been the main means of capturing, storing, and displaying diagnostic imaging examinations.

There are many limitations to x-ray film as a means of image capture and storage. The major limitation of film is that it can only be at one place at one time. This major limitation can affect clinical efficiencies in all types of medical practice. Many physicians or health care providers often need simultaneous access to a diagnostic imaging examination to provide better quality of health care as well as more efficient health care.[1]

In light of the new cost restraints facing health care today, many are looking for more efficient and higher quality methods of practice. It is believed that electronic imaging will allow for ubiquitous access to diagnostic imaging for multiple different sites and/or locations instantaneously. This will allow medical practices to become faster and more efficient in delivering health care and also providing higher quality care by allowing consultation and/or interpretation of certain images remotely by highly specialized radiologists.

However, the cost of electronic imaging today is very high and converting to a totally electronic digital practice often seems prohibitive.[2] Therefore, we need to determine what we currently spend on film and film management each year. This study was performed to provide a clear understanding of the exact cost of current image management with film.

II. Methods and Materials

To estimate the cost of film and film management in our large institution, we proceeded to estimate the cost of film and film management over a 1 year period. We accomplished this by evaluating our 1994 budget expenditures.

We broke the cost of film and film management down into four categories (Table 1).

We first needed to determine the average cost of film. In doing this, we asked all of the major x-ray film vendors to give to us the list price of all of the varieties of film available through their organization. We then asked each firm to give us the average discounted price in the five state area surrounding Minnesota. We determined the percentages of the various kinds of films used in our practices. From this usage percentage, we applied an appropriate percentage weighting for each type of film at its average discounted price. The average discounted cost per sheet of film then was determined.

We then turned to space and supply costs. All supplies that were purchased during 1994 that were directly related to film and film management were totaled. Items such as developer and fixer fluids were included. In addition, the cost of film developers was prorated over a seven year depreciation schedule and included in the cost of supplies. Finally, the cost of space was calculated relating to buildings that were dedicated fully to film developing and film storage. Space costs were prorated over a 30 year depreciation schedule.

The personnel costs in 1994 that were 100% related to film management within the Department of Radiology were also determined. These individuals were darkroom personnel and file room clerks.

Finally, personnel costs outside of the Department of Radiology that were totally related to film management were calculated for 1994. These individuals were "film runners" that were primarily in the departments of orthopedics and oncology.

III. Results

We determined that the average x-ray examination (chest x-rays, bone x-rays, CT, MR and ultrasound) averaged to be 3.5 films per examination. The average cost of a sheet of film in the 5-state area surrounding Minnesota was determined to be $1.77 per sheet of film. Therefore, the average cost of film per examination was $1.77 x 3.53 which is equal to $6.25 per examination.

After totaling the cost of supplies (film developers, chemicals, film jackets, etc.) and space costs (darkrooms, file rooms and warehouses) it was determined that the cost of supplies and space per examination per year was $1.46.

The cost of personnel who were totally related to film or film management in the Department of Radiology was divided by the number of examinations each year. This resulted in a figure of $5.91 which was the cost of radiology personnel per x-ray examination each year. In the same light, personnel costs that were 100% related to film or film management outside the Department of Radiology resulted in a figure of $2.20 per examination per year.

The final, total estimate of cost of film per examination per year at our institution was $15.82 (Table 2).

IV. Discussion

Evaluating the cost of film and film management is a very difficult task. Each institution has its own unique methods of film purchasing and film management. Often radiology jackets are shared between institutions thus adding to the complexity. Our estimated cost of film per examination per year of $15.82 is most likely an underestimation of real costs when compared to other institutions. Some estimates have been as high as $25-30 per examination. At our institution we perform approximately 800,000 x-ray examinations each year. This allows us to operate efficiently in terms of film purchasing, supplies and space and dedicated personnel. Although it would be difficult to translate our cost estimates to other institutions, it would be safe to assume that film management costs to smaller institutions would be higher, possibly between $15-20 per examination per year.[4,5]

This study did not address other potential factors such as those relating to film loss and subsequent costs of "re-takes" and costs to clinical areas for delays and inconveniences. These unique costs need to be calculated for each institution and added to the estimates in this study.

As stated earlier, at our institution we perform approximately 800,000 x-ray examinations per year. All exams are archived for at least five years. All positive examinations are held for ten years. The average cost of $15.82 per x-ray examination times the number of exams per year of 800,000 results in an estimated cost of $12,656,000 per year to our institution that we spend on acquiring, maintaining and storing x-ray images on film.

As we all move to an electronic digital environment in the future, many of us are faced with the initial investment costs of digital acquisition devices such as computed radiography (CR) machines, picture archiving communication systems (PACS) to network and store these images, and the personnel costs (computer and engineering) needed to maintain such complex systems.[6-8] Because technology is changing rapidly, it appears that the cost of electronic imaging equipment will come down.[9-12] As we face the inevitable conversion to an electronic environment, we all need to understand our current expenditures related to film. In doing so, our conversion to an electronic environment can be done in a logical, fiscal manner that will allow the electronic imaging departments of the future to become a reality.[13-14]

References

1. Craig O. Diagnostic radiology without films. *The Practitioner*, 229 (1985) 1011-1015.

2. Crowe BL, Hailey DM, Carter R. Assessment of costs and benefits in the introduction of digital radiology systems. *Int J Biomed Comput* 1992 Jan; 30(1):17-25.

3. Cywinski JK, van den Brink JA, Hagen J. Experience with a cost justification model for evaluating acquisition of a radiology information management system. In *Computer Applications to Assist Radiology* (Eds: RL Arenson and RM Friedenberg), Symposia Foundation, Carlsbad, California. 1990.

4. Elliott LP, Mun SK, Horri SC, Benson H. *Digital Imaging Network System* [DINS] *Evaluation Report*, Georgetown University Medical Centre, Washington, DC, 1990.

5. Eusek J. Cost savings: through the use of digital angiography. *Administrative Radiology* 1995 Feb; 25-28.

6. Glazer HS, Muka E, Sagel SS, Jost RG. New techniques in chest radiography. *Radiol Clin North Am* 1994 Jul; 32(4): 711-29.

7. Hansell DM. Digital chest radiography. *Br J Hosp Med* 1993 Jan 20-Feb 2; 49(2):117-20.

8. Luck D. Commentary on Crowe BL and Hailey DM: Cost and benefit considerations in the introduction of digital radiology systems to Australian hospitals. In *Economics and Health:* 1990 (Ed: C Selby-Smith), Monash University, Melborne 1991 p. 285.

9. Powe NR. Economic and cost effectiveness investigations of radiologic practices. *Radiology* 192:11-18, 1994.

10. Stabb EV, Stewart DA. FutuRAD: Work in progress. *Radiology* 190:43A-49A, 1994.

11. Thrall JH. The radiologist in the1990s: New practice expectations and management responsibilities. *AJR* 163:11-15, 1994.

12. Van Gennip EMSJ, Ottes FP, van Poppel BM, Andriessen JHTH. Why do cost-benefit studies of PACS disagree? *Medical Imaging IV*: (1990) 1234.

13. Warburton RN, Fisher PD, Nosil J. Digital diagnostic imaging with a comprehensive PACS: hypothetical economic evaluation at a large community hospital. *J Dig Imag.* 3 (1990) 101-107.

14. X-ray angiography systems. *Health Devices* 1993 Nov; 22(11):507-54.

Table 1.

Categories of Film and Film Management Costs

1. Average Cost of Film
2. Supplies and Building Space
3. Personnel - Radiology
4. Personnel - Nonradiology

Table 2.

Film Cost Study

Total Cost/Examination

		Cost/Exam
1.	Film/exam	$ 6.25
2.	Supplies & space	$ 1.46
3.	Personnel - Radiology	$ 5.91
4.	Personnel - Nonradiology	$ 2.20
		$15.82

SESSION 4

Digital Mammography

Co-Chairs:

John Boehme, III
Hamid Jafroudi

Advanced Digital Mammography

Ronald B. Schilling, John D. Cox, S.R. Dev Sharma and S. Gaalema
PGI Corporation, Los Altos Hills, California

Currently the lifetime risk of breast cancer for women is one in nine. The annual death rate from breast cancer in the United States is estimated to be approximately 44,000 women per year [1]. Several Studies have shown that asymptomatic screening with mammography can reduce mortality from breast cancer by 20-40% [2-4]. Based on these studies, the American Cancer Society and other medical associations have recommended mammographic screening for women over the age of 40. Consequently, mammography may become one of the largest volume radiographic procedures interpreted by radiologists.

Mammography is the most demanding of all clinical imaging applications. It requires high contrast, high spatial resolution and high signal to noise ratio at the minimum possible x-radiation dose to the patient. Fundamentally, it is often the minimum contrast of the cancer, relative to its surroundings, which determines the detection of the breast cancer. This can be as low as 0.1%, and averages 6 to 8% at the 18 to 20 KeV x-ray beam energies employed in mammography. The detectable contrast of a cancer is inversely proportional to the signal-to noise ratio of the imaging system. Clusters of much higher contrast microcalcifications are a frequent mammographic presentation of breast cancer requiring high image resolution.

Diagnosing cancer from a mammogram requires skillful and meticulous interpretation. The two primary indicators of breast cancer in a mammogram are the presence of a mass and clustered microcalcifications. Microcalcifications are an important indication of breast cancer because they are present in 30-50% of all cancers found mammographically. Further, microcalcifications are often visible in the mammogram before a mass can be detected clinically by physical exam.

However, microcalcifications are often difficult to detect because, radiographically they appear as tiny areas (as small as 0.2 mm in diameter). Although radiologists do find microcalcifications in 30-50% of cases with breast carcinoma, as much as 80% of breast carcinomas reveal microcalcifications in pathologic examination.

Mammography is the most effective method for early detection of breast cancer [5-6] and yet, 10-30% of women who have breast cancer and undergo mammography have negative mammograms. Furthermore, of the women who are sent to biopsy, only 20-40% actually have breast cancer. Quantitative analysis of the radiographic features of microcalcifications and masses may help radiologists improve their specificity.

Recent work in CAD has demonstrated significantly improved accuracy, mainly due to improved computer vision [7], better methods for film digitization [8] and an increase in the image quality of mammograms [9]. It is for this reason, that CAD is expected to enjoy improved accuracy with the advent of digital imaging systems for mammography, because these systems are expected to be superior to conventional film-screen in image quality.

The current state-of-the-art in screening and diagnostic mammography is still conventional film-screen mammography. However, the efficacy of film-screen mammography is limited by its dynamic range, low contrast resolution, film noise, dose-inefficient scatter reduction and film processing artifacts. It offers low diagnostic specificity in the range of 20% to 30% resulting in a high number of false-positive film-screen initiated biopsies, the cost of which alone is estimated at several hundred million dollars. It is currently estimated that one out of every four women screened annually for ten years by film-screen mammography will experience the anxiety and cost of a screening initiated false-positive mammogram (benign biopsy).

Solid-state x-ray sensor technology has the potential to improve the diagnostic quality of mammograms through higher quantum efficiency and spatial resolution than screened film can provide. These improvements in performance can be obtained while lowering the patient exposure dose.

The first x-ray sensors to have found application in commercial mammography equipment are the Charge-Coupled Device (CCD) based systems [10-12]. Currently, however, these systems lack adequate spatial resolution for commercial full-field mammography. Other similar systems using linear photodiode arrays to scan image intensifier tubes have also been reported [13,14]. Proposed x-ray area sensors include an amorphous selenium (a-Se) primary sensor [15]; reusable flat plate storage phosphor screen [16-19] that can be fitted into a film cassette (with limited spatial resolution, 4-5 lp/mm); systems using a transparent phosphor [20]; and a photoconductive a-Se plate readout either with an electrometer array or a laser [21-23].

PGI is currently developing two primary x-ray, slot-scanned digital mammography (DXM-1) prototype units based on high performance direct x-ray detection hybrid sensors. The system is schematically shown in Figure 1. The heart of this system is the semiconductor x-radiation sensors. As shown in Figure 1, the transmission is similar to a conventional (screen-film) mammography system except for a moving aperture. It consists of a x-ray tube and a beam collimating aperture that rotates about the tube focal spot. The moving aperture protects the patient from 'unsensed' x-rays by providing a fan shaped beam synchronous in its motion to the sensor assembly on the receptor side.

The key system specifications include:

Field of View - the system must image an area of similar size to that of a conventional mammography system (180 x 240 mm) and must be able to record this image with sufficient pixels to maintain the desired resolution.

Exposure time - the image must be acquired in a time consistent with reasonable comfort for the patient and in a way that the susceptibility to patient motion is no worse than a conventional film-screen system.

Image Quality - the quality of the image produced (sharpness, contrast, SNR) should be significantly superior to conventional film-screen systems at moderate and high spatial frequencies, and at a minimum, equal to conventional systems at low spatial frequencies.

Dose Efficiency - system should have high DQE to reduce dose to the patient without sacrificing image quality.

Roehrig et al [24], using two digital imaging systems used for mammographically guided stereotactic breast biopsy, concluded that the improved DQE of one of the digital imaging systems over the DQE of the conventional screen-film permitted an improved signal-to-noise ratio. Therefore, the digital system was capable of resolving an object of about 100 microns. Had the digital imaging system been "ideal" in terms of DQE, it would have been able to resolve an object ("microcalcification") of 70 microns in diameter at the above mentioned x-ray fluence. The modulation transfer function for this system at 10 line-pairs/mm should be almost 3 times better than film-screen systems. Predicted detective quantum efficiency (DQE) at 15 line pairs/mm is about 15 times better than that of film-screen at 15 lp/mm.

The high predicted DQE of the DXM-1 system allows x-ray exposure to be reduced by a factor of up to 5 from the typical film-screen exposures while maintaining the same signal to noise ratio at low spatial frequencies. Even at this reduced exposure, this system will have a better signal to noise ratio at 13 lp/mm than film-screen at 10 lp/mm.

Figure (2) shows assembly of a direct x-ray sensing hybrid semiconductor sensor employed in the DXM-1. The sensor is a hybrid structure incorporating a detector and a readout/multiplexer. The detector is a silicon PiN diode array with a thickness of 1.5 mm. Each sensor is about 6 mm wide and 23 mm in length. As shown in Figure 3, eight of these sensors are aligned to form a staggered array for a cross-scan dimension of about 180 mm. With an in-scan motion for four seconds, it provides a normal size mammogram (180 mm by 240 mm).

Prototype hybrid sensors designed specifically for applications in screening and diagnostic mammography were fabricated and tested by PGI[25]. Figure (4) shows the predicted and measured values of quantum efficiency for 1.0 mm and 1.5 mm thick detectors with molybdenum and tungsten x-ray spectra. As shown in this figure, the measured DQE data are consistent with the predicted values. As shown in Figure (5), the PGI direct x-ray sensing system DQE is significantly better than the film-screen system. The measured quantum efficiency of a 1.5 mm thick detector is over 80%. On the other hand, scatter and grid effects reduce the film-screen system DQE to about 7% to 20%. Figure (6) shows that the MTF data approaches the predicted values. At 10 line pairs/mm, the system MTF is 20%

when the sensor is operated in one sample per dwell mode and almost 40% when the sensor is operated in the two samples per dwell mode. This MTF performance is far superior to a film-screen system.

Initial testing of the prototype version of the DXM-1 has demonstrated a detective quantum efficiency greater than 80% and a Nyquist image resolution limit of greater than 17 line pairs per millimeter. Images of the ACR/RMI-156 quality assurance breast phantom acquired using these prototype sensors demonstrate image quality superior to film-screen even at exposure levels one-fifth to one-half the normal for film-screen. These results were exhibited and presented at the 1994 RSNA meeting in Chicago[26].

PGI has recently been awarded a contract from the US Army Medical Research and Materiel Command through a Broad Agency Announcement for Breast Cancer Research. The 3-year contract is expected to begin on July 1, 1996 and will provide funding to complete the development of the prototype DXM-1 low-dose digital mammography system and pursue a vigorous technical and clinical evaluation. The clinical evaluation will evaluate film screen versus digital mammography using 1,000 women as volunteers.

References:

1. Silverberg E., Boring C.C., Squires, T.S.: Cancer Statistics, 1990. CA, 1990; 40: 9-27.
2. Andersson I., Aspergren L., Janzon L., et al. Br. Med. J., 1988; 297: 943-948.
3. Shapiro S., Venet W., Strax P.H., et al. JNCI, 1982; 69: 349-355.
4. Tabar L., Gad A., Holmberg L.H., et al. Lancet, 1985; 1: 829-832.
5. Bassett L.W., Gold R.H. Breast Imaging. New York: Grune and Stratton; 198. 82.
6. Lissner J., Kessler M., Anhalt G. J. Zander and J. Baltzer, eds., Early Breast Cancer. Berlin: Springer-Verlag: 1985; 93-123.
7. Jain, AK: Fundamentals of Digital Image Processing; Englewood Cliffs, NJ; Prentice Hall; 1989
8. Cook LT, Giger ML, Banitzky S. Invest. Radiol. 1989; 24:910-916
9. Haus AG. Radiol. Clinics of North America, 1987; 25:913-928
10. Piccaro, M. F. and Toker, E. SPIE 1901, 1993.
11. Toker, E. and Piccaro, M. F. SPIE 2009, 1993.
12. Karellas, A. and Harris, L. J. Med. Phys., 1992. 19(4), 1015-1023.
13. Nishikawa, R. M., Mawdsley, G. E., Fenster, A., Yaffe, M. J. Med. Phys., 1987. 14(5), 717-727.

14. Munier, B., Prieur-Drevon, P., Roziere, G. and Chabbal, J. Medical Imaging VI: Instrumentation, SPIE 1651, 1992, 106-115.
15. Zhao, W. and Rowlands, J. A. Medical Imaging VI: Instrumentation, SPIE 1651, 1992, 134-143.
16. Korn D. M., Lubinski, A. R. and Owen, J. F. Applications of Optical Instrumentation to Medicine XIV, SPIE, 626, 1986. p. 108(1) and 120(2).
17. Hillen, W., Schiebel, U. and Zaengel, T. Med. Phys., 1987. 14, p.744.
18. Fujita, H., Ueda, K., Morishita, T., and Ohtsuka, A. Med. Phys, 1989. 16, p. 52.
19. Miyahara, J. Chemistry Today, Oct. 1989, 29-36
20. Korn D. M., Lubinski, A. R. and Owen, J. F. US patent # 4762998 (1988)
21. Hillen, W., Schiebel, U. and Zaengel, T. Medical Imaging II, SPIE 914, 1988, p. 253.
22. Schiebel, U., Hillen, W., and Zaengel, T. Applications of Optical Instrumentation to Medicine XIV, SPIE, 626, 1986. p. 176.
23. Rowlands, J. A., Hunter, D. M. and Araj, N. Med. Phys., 18, 1991, 421-431.
24. Roehrig H, Krupinski E, Yu T. SPIE 2436:124-134;(1995)
25. Roehrig H, Yu T, Gaalema S, Sharma SR, Minteer JA, Yorke WE. SPIE 2519, 118-126, (1995)
26. S. R. Dev Sharma. Inforad, RSNA, 1994.

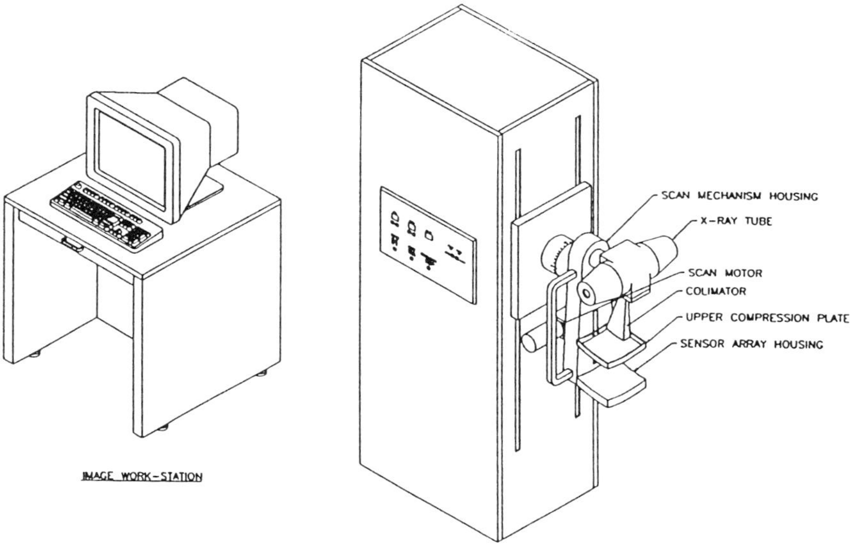

Figure 1. Slot-scan and semiconductor detectors replace film in otherwise conventional system configuration.

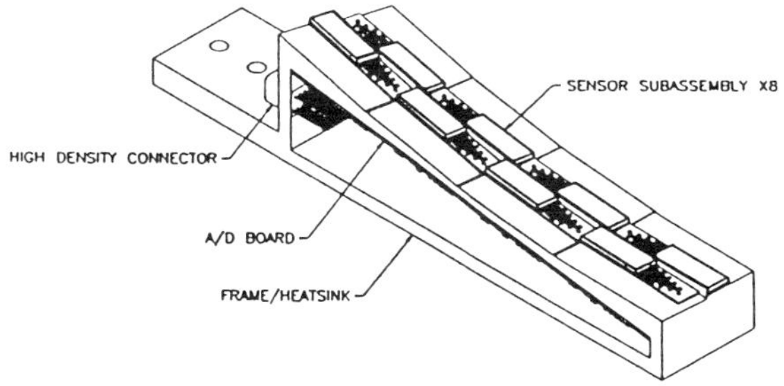

Figure 3. Eight hybrid sensors in cross-scan give a normal size mammogram. (180mm x 240mm)

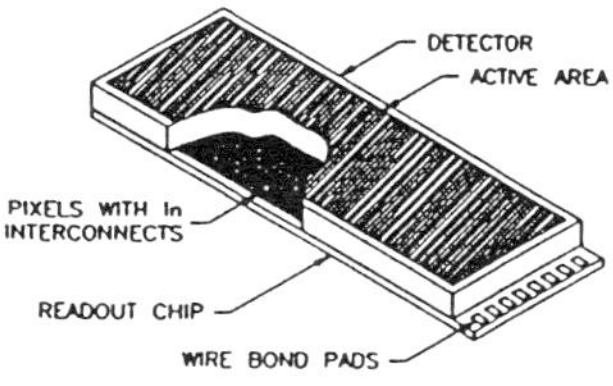

Figure 2. Hybrid radiation sensor allows for optimization and fabrication of the detector and the readout/multiplexer IC's seperately.

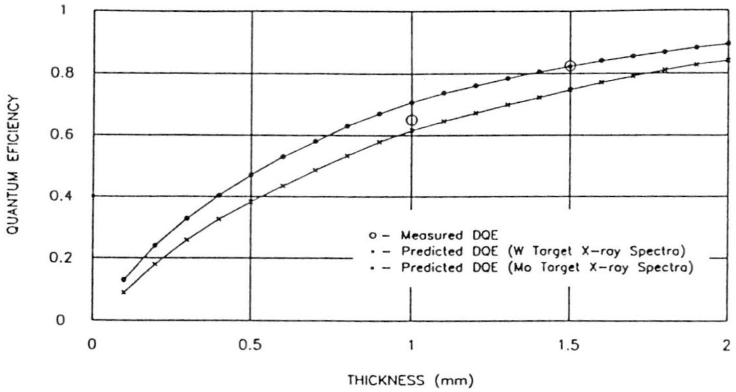

Figure 4. The measured and predicted quantum efficiency data is consistant with predicted values.

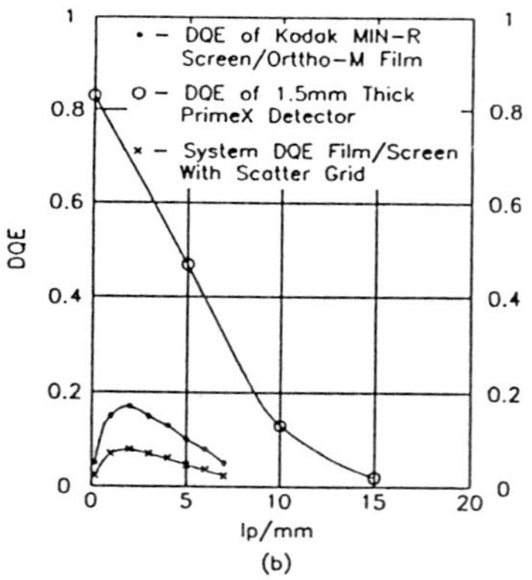

Figure 5. Primary slot scan system DQE is significantly higher than the film-screen mammography system.

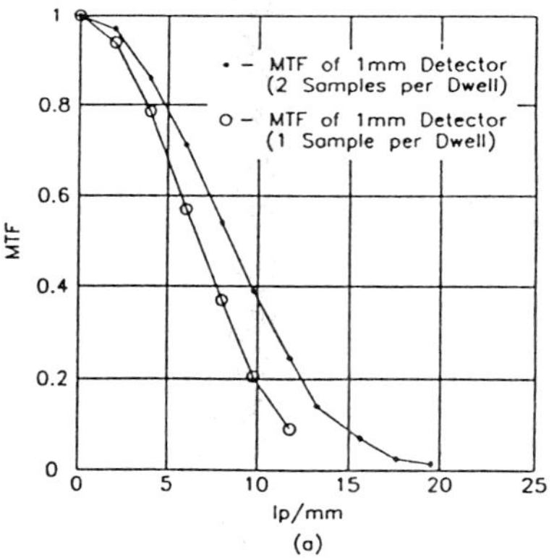

Figure 6. Measured MTF data is consistant with the predicted values.

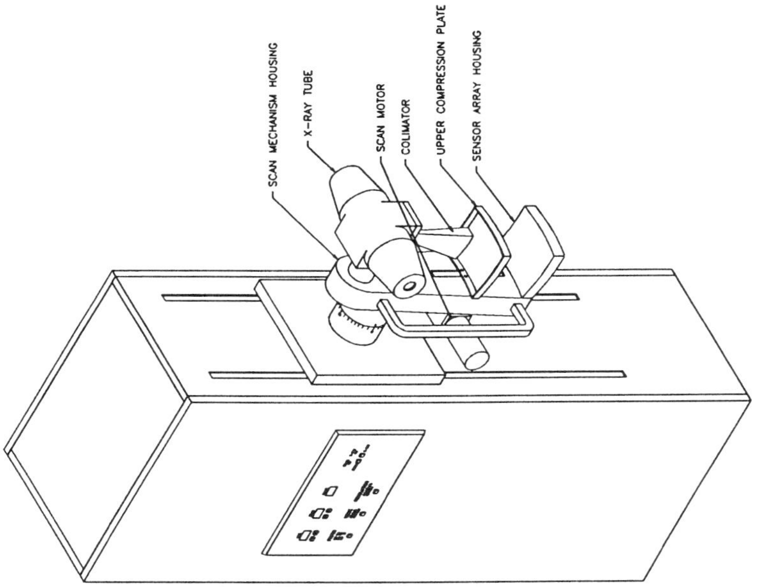

DIGITAL SLOT SCAN MAMMOGRAPHY UNIT

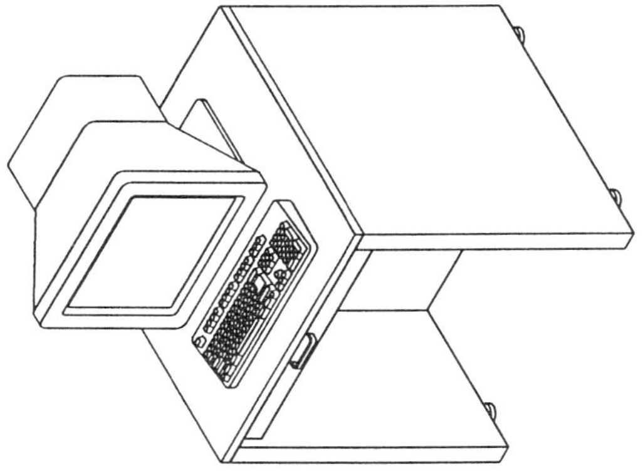

IMAGE WORK-STATION

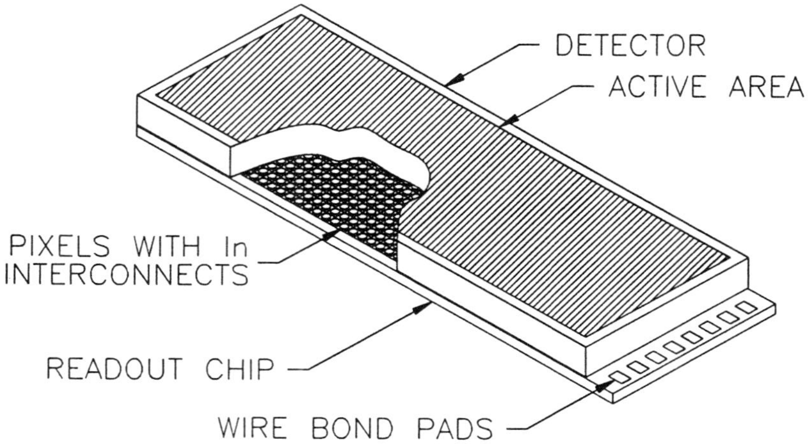

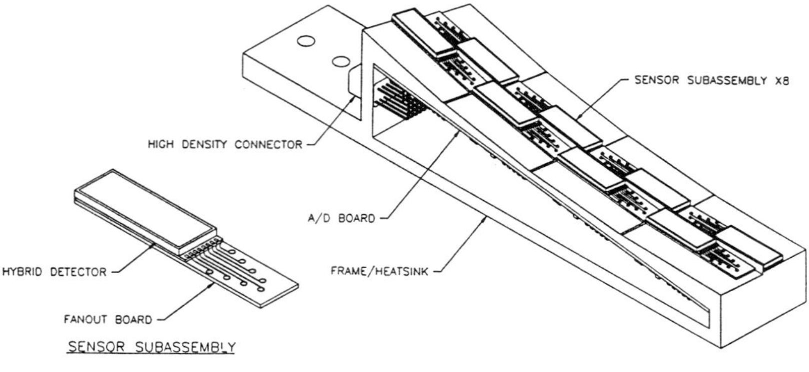

SLOT SCAN SENSOR ARRAY FOR PRIMARY X-RAY DETECTORS

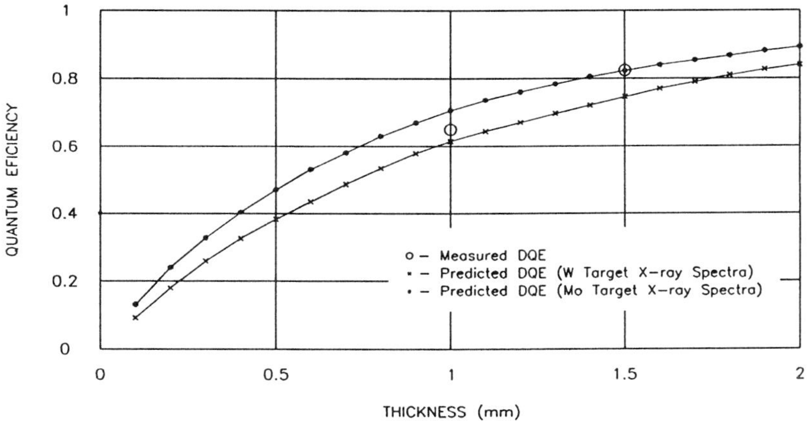
QUANTUM EFICIENCY
THICKNESS (mm)
o – Measured DQE
▪ – Predicted DQE (W Target X-ray Spectra)
• – Predicted DQE (Mo Target X-ray Spectra)
0
0.2
0.4
0.6
0.8
1
0
0.5
1
1.5
2

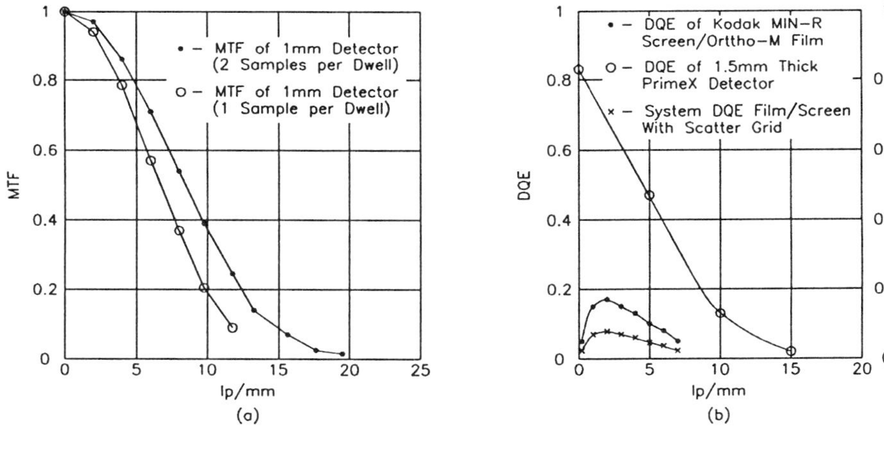
MTF
lp/mm
• – MTF of 1mm Detector (2 Samples per Dwell)
O – MTF of 1mm Detector (1 Sample per Dwell)
0
5
10
15
20
25
DQE
• – DQE of Kodak MIN-R Screen/Orttho-M Film
O – DQE of 1.5mm Thick PrimeX Detector
× – System DQE Film/Screen With Scatter Grid
0
5
10
15
20

(a)

(b)

Wavelet-Based Computer-Aided Diagnosis for Screening Mammography

Howard C. Choe and Andrew K. Chan
Department of Electrical Engineering, Texas A&M University, College Station, Texas
Hsien-Hsun S. Wu
Department of Computer Science, Texas A&M University, College Station, Texas
Charles K. Chui
Department of Mathematics, Texas A&M University, College Station, Texas

I. INTRODUCTION

A new detection algorithm that takes advantages of wavelet multi-resolution analysis (MRA) and synthesis is proposed to assist the radiologists in looking for small clusters of microcalcifications as well as mass lesions in digital mammograms. The new algorithm combined with a conventional clustering algorithm will reliably detect suspicious microcalcification cluster and/or mass lesion regions in ambiguous mammograms.

The majority of early breast cancers are indicated by the presence of one or more clusters of microcalcifications on a mammogram[1]. Although breast cancer can become fatal, it has the highest chances of survival among cancer types in women if it can be found in an early stage[2]. Thus, detection of micro-calcifications without false negative with minimizing false positive is critical to breast cancer patients. Microcalcifications are small deposits of $Ca_5(PO_4)_3OH$ in breast tissue with size ranging from 0.05 to 1.0 mm in diameter, which appear as bright specks on the photo-negative x-ray film[3,4]. Individual microcalcifications are difficult to detect because: (1) they vary in size and shape; and (2) they are embedded in and camouflaged by varying densities of parenchymal tissue structures[4]. Mass lesions can be missed mainly due to human fatigue, clutter and intensities surrounding the masses.

To complement human errors - 10-20% misdiagnosis of patients whose mammograms show some evident of microcalcifications or masses in retrospect[5,6] - in breast abnormality detection, there have been a great deal of interest to develop a computer-aided diagnostic (CAD) tool using various image processing techniques and pattern recognition to help the radiologist's diagnostic efforts[1-5,7-11]. These continuing efforts are still in need of innovative approaches for early detection of microcalcification clusters as well as mass lesions.

The multiresolution analysis technique has been one of the most successful tools not only for detecting microcalcification clusters and masses in mammograms but also for enhancing mammogram contrast for further processing[6,12]. By using wavelet MRA, a mammogram is decomposed into a set of subband images (images in separate frequency bands) using tree-structured filter banks. Mathematical operations on the images in separate frequency bands result in a very effective feature extraction[13] especially when analyzing non-stationary signals as shown in mammograms. Of course, MRA should be combined with other processing techniques to be useful for breast cancer detection.

Our new algorithm successfully unmasks the complexity and rejects the false positives by combining wavelet MRA with several image processing techniques. Initial evaluation of this algorithm using various test mammograms demonstrated a reliable detection of microcalcifications and masses in various situations and surroundings without *a priori* knowledge of their locations within the mammograms. For the test images, we used Mammographic Image Analysis Society (MIAS) Digital MiniMammogram Database. This algorithm can become an effective mechanism to localize suspicious microcalcification regions and masses for further inspection by the radiologists.

In Section II, we will discuss our method and approach to the detection of microcalcifications and mass lesions used in this algorithm. We will provide the results in Section III, by including several mammogram input and output images from the algorithm. The conclusion is also given in Section III. Section IV lists the references. To facilitate the description of our method, we use Figure 1 to show the overall algorithm architecture in a flow diagram. We will describe our method according to the blocks in the flow diagram.

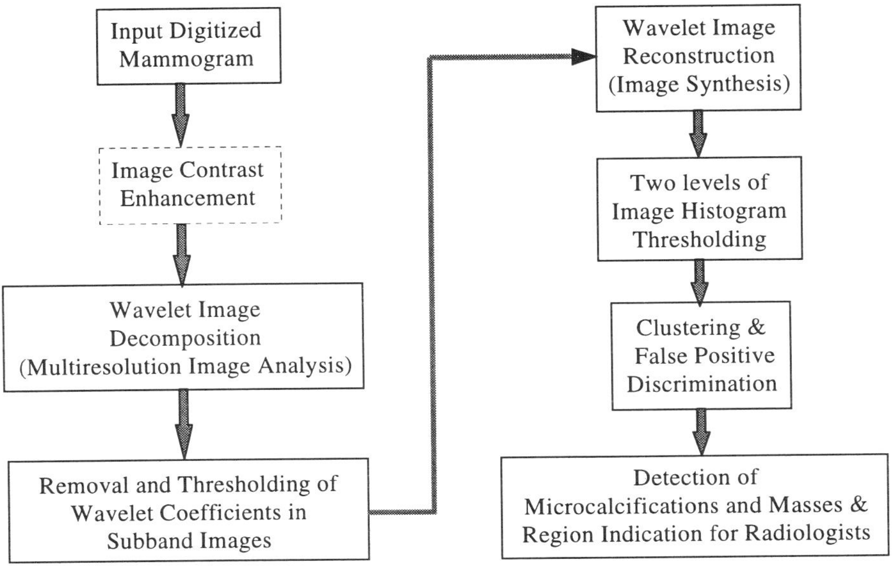

Figure 1. Overall Algorithm Architecture.

II. METHODOLOGY

In this section, we will briefly describe each process shown in Figure 1. We will provide illustrations whenever possible.

II.1. Image Contrast Enhancement

Image contrast enhancement is considered as preprocessing[14] that is useful to bringing out microcalcifications or masses whose pixel intensities are compatible to their surroundings. In Figure 1, this block is depicted with a dotted line because we did not use this block for our results generated for this paper. Normally, this processing is to map the original gray scale values to a different set of gray scale values. This operation include non-linear filtering[15] using systematic mathematical transforms[6,12] and/or a non-linear mapping similar to an expander often used in non-linear quantization[16] in data compression.

II.2. Wavelet Multiresolution Image Decomposition and Reconstruction

We use a tree-structured MRA to decompose the input digitized mammogram and to reconstruct it after wavelet-domain operations. In this paper, we used the Daubechies 20 tap and spline wavelets to decompose the images into subbands. We decomposed the image to, at least, three levels for the given mammogram to have the maximum flexibility in wavelet coefficient thresholding and removal described in the next section.

The one-level decomposition and reconstruction process is depicted in Figure 2. In this figure, $I(x,y)$ represents the input digitized mammogram, which is then decomposed into $I_{LL}(x,y)$, $I_{LH}(x,y)$, $I_{HL}(x,y)$, and $I_{HH}(x,y)$. Here, *G and *H mean convolution with high-pass and low-pass filers, respectively. $2\Downarrow x$ and $2\Downarrow y$ represent down-sampling (decimation) by 2 in the x and y directions, respectively. $2\Uparrow x$ and $2\Uparrow y$ represent upsampling in the x and y directions, respectively. The hat, ^, indicates modification as a result of the wavelet domain operations.

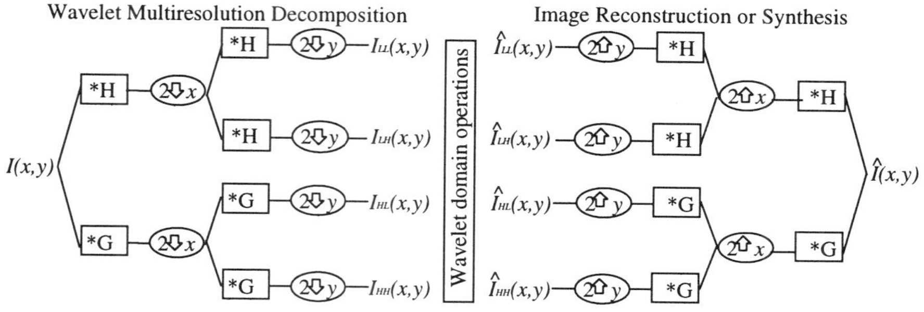

Figure 2. Wavelet MRA decomposition and reconstruction.

When microcalcifications are considered as a non-stationary high frequency signal in a digital mammogram, masses can be considered as localized low frequency signal with high amplitude or intensity. These characteristics of microcalcifications and masses lead to the motivation of using wavelet MRA or the discrete wavelet transform (DWT)[17,18] to enhance mammograms and to detect abnormalities in them.

II.3. Wavelet Domain Operations - Coefficient Removal and Thresholding

For microcalcification detection, we remove the wavelet coefficients in lower resolution subbands and threshold the coefficients in the higher resolution subbands. For mass detection, we remove the wavelet coefficients in the higher resolution subbands and threshold the coefficients in the lower resolution subbands. The former is to retain most of the high frequency changes and to eliminate all low frequency components; the latter is to remove all of the high frequency components in the mammogram but to retain most of the low frequency components. The removal is equivalent to setting the coefficients to zero. The thresholding is performed for each subband independent of other subbands. The threshold applied is $\mu + k\sigma$, where μ and σ are the mean and the standard deviation of a subband, respectively, and $k \geq 1$. In this paper, $k = 1$ is used.

II.4. Image Histogram Thresholding

When the wavelet-domain operations are completed, reconstruction of the mammogram using the modified wavelet coefficients is performed as shown in Figure 2. Once this is completed, image adjustment and histogram thresholding are performed. The image adjustment is to remove the remaining d-c bias in the reconstructed image. The pixel values less than the d-c bias are set to zero. An image histogram is generated with the adjusted image. From this histogram, we assign the minimum gray scale values by evaluating 66% of the area under the histogram curve from the left of the histogram. We set a bound for all the gray scale values in the adjusted image by the minimum gray scale value. The bounded image can be multiplied by the input image to enhance the gray scale expansion. We then generate another histogram based on the bounded image. Based on this histogram, we perform some hard thresholding; Set the pixels greater than or equal to the hard threshold to 1 (or 255 gray scale value) and the pixels less than the threshold to 0 (or 0 gray scale value).

II.5. Clustering, False Positive Discrimination, and Region Indication

We are currently surveying clustering algorithms that can be used in our application. One of the candidates is the *k*-means or *c*-means clustering algorithm. It is simple and yet effective and allows many variations to tailor to micro-calcification cluster and mass lesion detection. The procedure is as follows:

(1) Choose an initial assignment for cluster representations: $\mu_1^0, \mu_2^0, \ldots, \mu_L^0$.

(2) Reassign each detected pixel to the class corresponding to cluster $w_i(\mu_i)$ by the minimization criteria: $\| x - \mu_i \|^2 > \| x - \mu_j \|^2$.
(3) Recompute $\mu_1^+, \mu_2^+, \ldots, \mu_L^+$.
(4) Compare μ_i and μ_i^+. If no change, stop iteration; otherwise, go to step (2).

In the course of this process, a suspicious microcalcification cluster is detected if 3 or more detections appear in an area about 1 cm$\times$1 cm[2], which is about 50$\times$50 pixels for our test images. Those clusters with less than 3 detections will not be considered as microcalcification clusters and will be labeled as false positives. For mass lesions, the same clustering algorithm can be used for clustering of pixels in a confined region by growing the distance from the mean to the sample pixels.

Once the detection and the discrimination are completed, the detected suspicious regions of microcalcifications and mass lesions are outlined with either a rectangular box or circular line enclosing the area. To provide the most information to the radiologists, the detection and the original image are to be displayed side by side.

III. RESULTS AND CONCLUDING REMARKS

The images before and after this process are illustrated in Figures 3-5. As aforementioned, our test images were downloaded from the MIAS Mini-Mammographic Database whose images have 200 μm pixel edge and a size of 1024$\times$1024 pixels. We processed the full size image up to the detection; neither clustering nor region indication is performed on the detection image. For the display in this paper, we clipped the region of interest from the original and the detection images in the size of 256$\times$256 pixels. The detailed information about each image is provided in the figure captions.

The wavelet multiresolution analysis that decomposes the input digital mammogram imagery, combined with other processing techniques, provides an attractive capability for the detection of suspicious microcalcification and mass lesion regions. Based on our initial assessment of the proposed algorithm, this wavelet-based algorithm can become an effective computer-aided diagnostic (CAD) tool to assist the radiologists by improving the detection performance and throughput of screening mammography. We plan to process mammograms from several different databases to gain performance statistics of our algorithm.

IV. REFERENCES

[1] F. Aghdasi, R.K. Ward, and B. Palcic, "Classification of Mammographic Microcalcification Clusters," IEEE ECECC 1993, pp. 1196-1199.
[2] I. N. Bankman, W.A. Christens-Barry, I.N. Weinberg, et al., "An Algorithm for Early Breast Cancer Detection in Mammograms," 5th Annual IEEE Symp. on Computer-Based Medical Systems, 1992, pp. 362-369.

[3] D. Nesbitt, F. Aghdasi, R. Ward, and J. Morgan-Parkes, "Detection of Microcalcifications in Digitized Mammogram Film Images using Wavelet Enhancement and Local Adaptive False Positive Suppression," IEEE Communications, Computer and Signal Processing, 1995, pp. 594-597.
[4] R.N. Strickland and H.I. Hahn, "Wavelet Transforms for Detecting Microcalcifications in Mammography," IEEE International Conference on Image Processing 1994, pp. 402-406.
[5] D.A. McCandless, S.K. Rogers, J.W. Hoffmeister, et al., "Wavelet Detection of Clustered Microcalcifications," SPIE Proceedings on Wavelet Applications III, Vol. 2762, 1996, pp. 388-399.
[6] L. Chen, C.W. Chen, and K.J. Parker, "Adaptive Mammographic Image Feature Enhancement Using Wavelet-Based Multiresolution Analysis," SPIE Proceedings on Wavelet Applications III, Vol. 2762, 1996, pp. 400-411.
[7] I.N. Bankman. J. Tsai, D.W. Kim, et al., "Detection of Microcalcification Clusters Using Neural Networks," IEEE International Conference on Engineering in Medicine and Biology 1994, pp. 590-591.
[8] J.L. Solka, W.L. Poston, C.E. Priebe, et al., "The Detection of Micro-Calcification in Mammographic Images Using High Dimensional Features," Symposium on Computer-Based Medical Systems 1994, pp. 139-145.
[9] Y. Jiang, et al., "Mammographic Feature Analysis of Clustered Micro-calcifications for Classification of Breast Cancer and Benign Breast Diseases," Internat'l Conf. on Engr. in Med. & Biology 1994, pp. 594-595.
[10] D. Betal, "Extraction of Microcalcifications from Digital Mammograms Using Mathematical Morphology," IEEE Colloq. (1993) No. 145: Morphological and Nonlinear.
[11] R. Nishikawa, Y. Jiang, M.L. Giger, et al., "Computer-Aided Detection of Clustered Microcalcification," International Conference on Systems, Man, and Cybernetics 1992, pp. 1375-1378.
[12] W. Qian and L.P. Clarke, "Adaptive Multistage Nonlinear Filtering and Wavelet for Medical Image Enhancement," International Conference on Image Processing 1994, pp. 711-715.
[13] H.C. Choe, et al., "Wavelet-Based Ground Vehicle Recognition Using Acoustic Signals," SPIE Proceedings on Wavelet Applications III, Vol. 2762, 1996, pp. 434-445.
[14] L.W. Estevez and N.D. Kehtarnavaz, "Computer Assisted Enhancement of Mammograms for Detection of Microcalcifications," Symposium on Computer-Based Medical Systems 1995, pp. 16-23.
[15] W. Qian, L.P. Clarke, M. Kallergi, and R.A. Clark, "Tree-Structured Nonlinear Filters in Digital Mammography," IEEE Transaction on Medical Imaging, March 1994, pp. 25-36.
[16] K. Sayood, *Introduction to Data Compression*, MK Publishers, Inc., 1996.
[17] B.J. Lucier, "Wavelet Compression and Segmentation of Digital Mammograms," Journal of Digital Imaging, Vol. 7, No. 1, 1994.
[18] W.B. Richardson, "Applying Wavelets to Mammograms," IEEE Engineering in Medical and Biology Magazine, Vol. 14, No. 11, 1995.

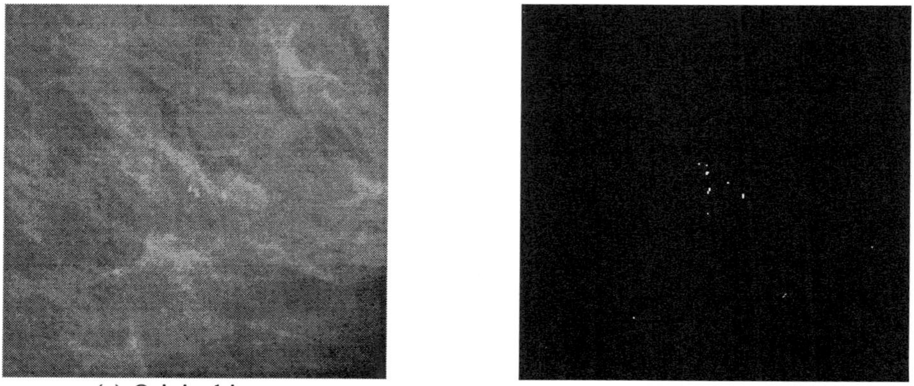

(a) Original image (b) Detection image

Figure 3. mdb249 - Background tissue: Dense-glandular; Malignant calcification.

(a) Original image (b) Detection image

Figure 4. mdb252 - Background tissue: Fatty; Benign calcification.

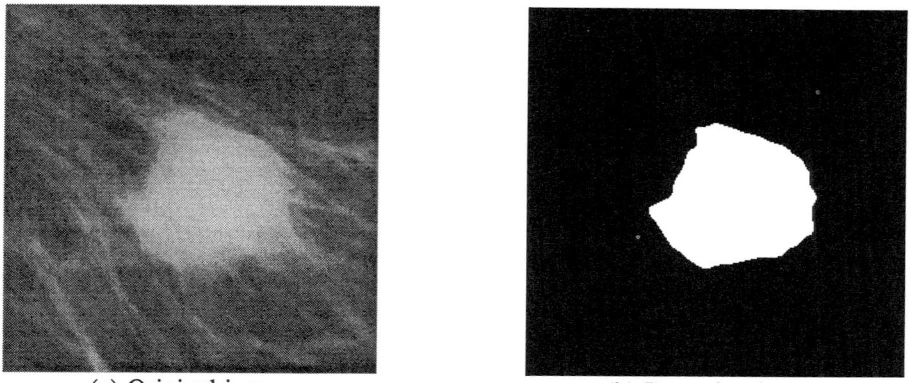

(a) Original image (b) Detection image

Figure 5. mdb028 - Background tissue: Fatty; Malignant circular mass.

ROC Study of An Adaptive Image Enhancement for Mammography

J.K. Kim, K.H. Kim, Y.J. Lee and H.W. Park
Dept. of Information and Communication Eng., KAIST, Seoul, Korea

J.M. Park and K.S. Song
Dept. of Diagnostic Radiology, Asan Medical Center, and
College of Medicine, University of Ulsan, Korea

Abstract

This paper evaluates the clinical performance of an adaptive image enhancement method, which is based on the first derivative and the local statistics of a mammographic image. The adaptive enhancement method consists of three processing steps. The first step is to remove the film artifacts which are like impulse noise. The second step is to compute the gradient image by using the first derivative operators. The third step is to enhance the important features of the mammographic image by applying the local statistics in conjunction with the thinning process of the edge points. The performance of the algorithm was evaluated by means of receiver operating characteristics (ROC) analysis for seventy-eight digitized mammograms including fifty mammograms with microcalcifications.

Keywords : *Receiver operating characteristics (ROC) curve, First derivative operator, Local statistics, Mammographic image enhancement*

1. INTRODUCTION

Breast cancer is one of the major causes of mortality increase to middle aged women, especially in developed countries. Currently, it is well known that the mammography is the best method for early detection of breast cancer. However, it is very difficult to interpret the mammogram because of the small differences in image density of various breast tissues, especially for dense breasts.[1]

Calcifications in the breast are tiny granular deposits of calcium. These calcifications can have benign or malignant characteristics. Some of those have indeterminate appearances in the mammogram. For diagnosis of the indeterminate ones, biopsy is required. A sign of breast cancer is the appearance of clusters of microcalcifications whose individual particles are usually under 0.5 *mm* in diameter with irregular and heterogeneous shape.[2] Individual microcalcifications are difficult to be detected because they are variable in shape as well as in size and may be embedded in areas of dense parencymal tissues. Therefore, careful diagnosis should be performed for the clustered microcalcifications that may herald an early-stage cancer. To improve the visibility of these cancerous features on a computer monitor, image enhancement techniques for digital mammograms have been attempted by several researchers.[3-6] The digital image enhancement of the mammograms can allow more confident interpretation to radiologists without increase of the caseload and the improper diagnosis.

An adaptive image enhancement method for digital mammograms was submitted previously,[7] which exploits the first derivative operators such as the gradient operator[8,9] and the compass operator[10], and the local statistics of a mammographic image. The purpose of this paper is to evaluate the clinical performance of the adaptive image enhancement method by means of ROC analysis. ROC analysis is based on statistical decision theory and has been applied extensively to diagnostic system in clinical medicine[11]. The ROC curve represents the relationship between the true-positive fraction (TPF) and the false-positive fraction (FPF) as the decision threshold varies. The area under the fitted ROC curve, A_z, was used as an index of detection accuracy.

2. IMAGE ENHANCEMENT METHOD

A simple artifact removal filter is applied to the digitized mammograms to remove the film artifacts. There are small processing artifacts on the X-ray films, which look like microcalcifications.[2] These artifacts are usually sharply defined, and brighter than the microcalcifications. Let us consider two windows centered on a current pixel *(x,y)* as shown in Fig. 1. In Fig. 1, R_1 is the inner region and R_2 is the surrounding region. The output of the filtering, *S(x,y)* is defined as

$$\begin{cases} S(x',y')\big|_{(x',y')\in R_1(x,y)} = \overline{E}(x,y), & \text{if } \; [I(x,y) - \overline{E}(x,y)] > T \\ S(x,y) = I(x,y), & \text{otherwise} \end{cases} \tag{1}$$

where *I(x,y)* is the digitized original image and $\overline{E}(x,y)$ is the mean value of the surrounding region. In eq. (1), the threshold value, *T*, had a value of 320 empirically in the ROC study.

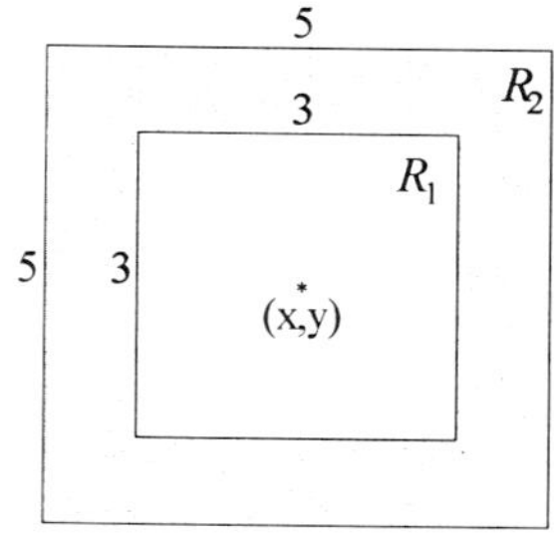

Fig. 1. Configuration of artifact removal filter

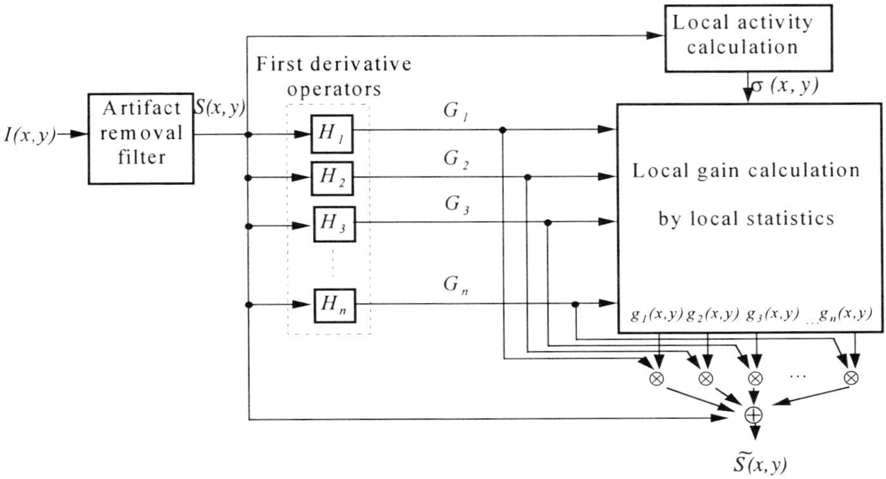

Fig. 2. Block diagram of the adaptive enhancement algorithm.

Figure 2 shows the block diagram of the adaptive enhancement algorithm. The enhanced image $\tilde{S}(x,y)$ is obtained by adding the adaptively enhanced gradient images to the image $S(x,y)$ as follows,

$$\tilde{S}(x,y) = S(x,y) + \sum_{k=1}^{n} \tilde{G}_k(x,y) \tag{2}$$

where n is the number of first derivative operators. In eq.(2), the enhanced gradient images, $\tilde{G}_k(x,y)$, were defined by

$$\tilde{G}_k(x,y) = \begin{cases} g_k(x,y)G_k(x,y) & if \;\; e(x,y) > 0 \\ G_k(x,y) & if \;\; e(x,y) = 0, \;\; for \; k = 1,2,\ldots,n \end{cases} \tag{3}$$

where $G_k(x,y)$ is the gradient image of $S(x,y)$ with respect to kth derivative operator, and edge value, $e(x,y)$, is defined by using the nonmaximum deletion algorithm[12] as follows,

$$e(x,y) = \begin{cases} M(x,y), & if \; M(x,y) \; is \; maximum \; in \; the \; 3 \times 1 \; window \\ 0, & otherwise \end{cases} \tag{4}$$

where $M(x,y)$ is the magnitude of gradient images obtained by the first derivative operators. In eq.(3), the local gain $g_k(x,y)$, which adaptively weights the gradient images, is given as

$$g_k(x,y) = -\frac{g_k^{max} - g_k^{min}}{\sigma_0^{max}} \sigma(x,y) + g_k^{max}, \qquad for \; k = 1,2,\ldots,n \tag{5}$$

where $\sigma(x,y)$ is the local standard deviation of the filtered image with the proper window size centered at the current pixel (x,y) and σ_0^{max} is the maximum value of the local standard deviation, and g_k^{max} and g_k^{min} are the maximum gain and the minimum gain at each gradient image, respectively. This local gain is large for the nonbusy regions where standard deviation is small, whereas the local gain is small for the busy region. Therefore, the local gain can improve the image quality in the viewpoint of human visual concept.

An effective strategy is proposed to adaptively select the maximum gain, g_k^{max}, of each gradient image. It is defined by using standard deviation σ_k of gradient image as follows,

$$\sigma_k = \sqrt{\frac{1}{N^2}\sum_{x=0}^{N-1}\sum_{y=0}^{N-1}[G_k(x,y) - m_k]^2}\,,\ for\ k = 1,2,\ldots,n \tag{6}$$

where m_k is the mean value of $G_k(x,y)$ and N x N is the size of the gradient image. If the gradient value is within one-sigma region for each gradient image, it can be regarded as the uniform region. Thus, each gradient image is classified into two cases as follows,

$$\begin{aligned} &CASE\ 1: m_k-\sigma_k \le G_k(x,y) \le m_k+\sigma_k \\ &CASE\ 2: G_k(x,y) < m_k-\sigma_k\ \ or\ \ G_k(x,y) > m_k+\sigma_k, \qquad for\ k=1,2,\ldots\ldots,n \end{aligned} \tag{7}$$

For each gradient image, the maximum gain is computed as follows,

$$\begin{aligned} g_k^{max} &= \frac{\sigma^{max}}{\sigma_k} && for\ CASE\ 1 \\ g_k^{max} &= \frac{\sigma^{max}}{\sigma_k} + \lambda_k && for\ CASE\ 2 \end{aligned} \tag{8}$$

where $\sigma^{max} = max\{\sigma_k,\ 1 \le k \le n\}$, and

$$\lambda_k = \frac{\sigma_k}{\sigma_1 + \sigma_2 + \cdots + \sigma_n}$$

As shown in eq. (8), the gradient values of busy region are more amplified than those of uniform region, so that the image details can be enhanced and noise can be reduced. The maximum gain g_k^{max} in eq. (8) is defined to equalize the energy of each gradient image. The minimum gain, g_k^{min}, has a value of 1 for each gradient image in our experiment. The first derivative operator used in our ROC study is a compass operator.

3. ROC RESULTS AND DISCUSSIONS

For the study of ROC, seventy-eight mammograms, among which fifty mammograms had microcalcifications, were used. All mammograms were digitized with 180 microns pixel size and 12 bits per pixel using Lumisys laser film digitizer.

The digitized mammograms is cropped to a matrix size of 900 x 580 including breast region. Mammograms with microcalcifications in the database were verified subjectively by an experienced radiologist. These digitized images were displayed on 21" high contrast monochrome monitor which had a display resolution of 1760 x 2180.

The ROC evaluation was accomplished by three experienced radiologists. The ROC curves for the visibility of detection of microcalcifications are shown in Fig. 3. According to the area A_z under the ROC curve of Fig. 3, the adaptive enhancement method improves the diagnostic performance of mammogram. A_z of the digitized original mammograms (case A) is 0.73, whereas A_z's of the enhanced mammograms without and with film artifact correction are 0.76 and 0.86, respectively. Because the film artifacts are the cause of improper detection as shown in Fig. 3, the artifacts have to be removed before the image enhancement.

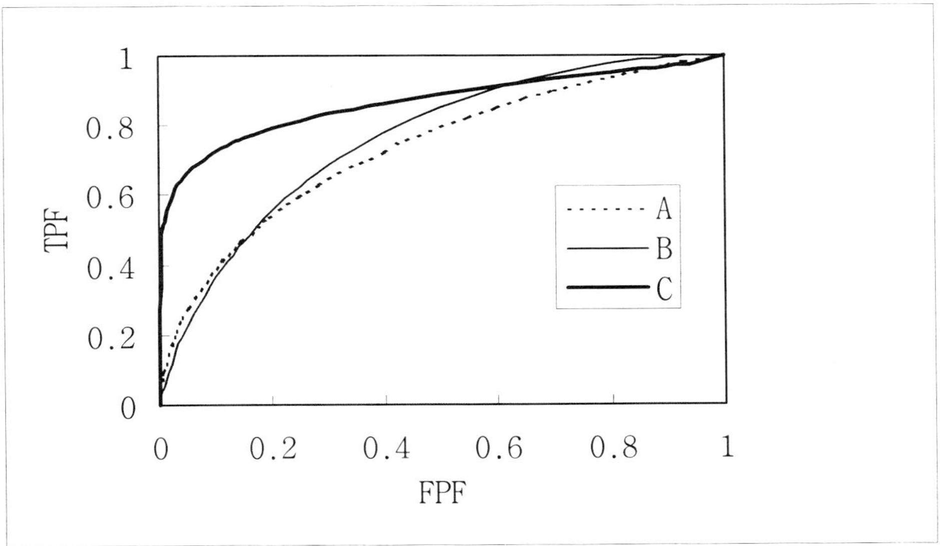

Fig. 3. ROC analysis of the adaptive image enhancement for mammograms. Case A, B, and C are the ROC curves for the digitized original mammograms, the enhanced mammograms with film artifact, and the enhanced mammograms with film artifact correction, respectively.

4. CONCLUSIONS

In this paper, we evaluated the clinical performance of an adaptive image enhancement method by means of ROC analysis. The enhancement method also shows the image to appear 3-D, which is useful in discriminating the cancerous lesions from normal parenchymal tissues in a mammographic image.[7] Hence, it may improve chances of early detection of breast cancer. This ROC study shows that the adaptive image enhancement is very effective in identifying the microcalcifications on mammograms.

REFERENCES

1. P. C. Johns and M. J. Yaffe, "X-ray characterization of normal and neoplastic breast tissues," Phys. in Med. and Biol., vol. 32, no. 6, pp. 675-695, 1987.
2. D. B. Kopans, Breast Imaging, J. B. Lippincoff company, Philadelpia, 1989.
3. A. P. Dhawan, G. Buelloni, and R. Gordon, "Enhancement of mammographic features by optimal adaptive neighborhood image processing," IEEE Trans. on Med. Imag., vol. MI-5, no. 1, pp. 8-15, 1986.
4. P. G. Tahoces, J. Correa, M. Souto, et. al., "Enhancement of chest and breast radiographs by automatic spatial filtering," IEEE Trans. on Med. Imag., vol. 10, no. 3, pp. 330-335, 1991.
5. W. M. Morrow, R. B. Paranjape, R. M. Rangayyan, et. al., "Region-based contrast enhancement of mammograms," IEEE Trans. on Med. Imag., vol. 11, no. 3, pp. 392-406, 1992.
6. A. F. Laine, S. Schuler, J. Fan, and W. Huda, "Mammographic feature enhancement by multiscale analysis," IEEE Trans. on Med. Imag., vol. 13, no. 4, pp. 725-740, 1994.
7. J. K. Kim and H. W. Park, "Adaptive mammographic image enhancement using first derivative and local statistics," submitted to IEEE Trans. on Med. Imag., 1995.
8. A. K. Jain, Fundamentals of Digital Image Processing. Englewood Cliffs, NJ, Prentice-Hall, 1989.
9. R. C. Gonzalez and R. E. Woods, Digital Image Processing. Reading, MA, Addison-Wesley, 1992.
10. G. S. Robinson, "Edge detection by compass gradient masks," Computer Graphics and Image Processing , vol. 6, pp. 492-501, 1977.
11. C. E. Metz, "ROC methodology in radiologic imaging," Investigative radiology, vol. 21, no. 9, pp. 720-733, 1986.
12. V. Lacroix, "A three-module strategy for edge detection," IEEE Trans. on Pattern anal. Machine Intell., vol. 10, no. 6, pp. 803-810, 1988.

Derivation of a Novel Neural Network Error Function and a Learning Rule and their Application to the Detection of Microcalcifications in Digitized Mammograms

Daniel Rosen
Sage Diagnosis, Mountain View, California
Rosenstiel Basic Medical Sciences Research Center, Brandeis University, Waltham, Massachusetts

Benjamin Martin, Mark Monheit and Greg Wolff
Sage Diagnosis, Mountain View, California

1 INTRODUCTION

In the last decade the field of computer aided diagnosis (CAD) in mammography has grown at a furious pace (Vybomy and Giger, 1994). Neural networks have proved to be particularly popular tools among researchers attempting to detect signs of cancer in digitized mammograms. These researchers have shown that neural networks can accurately analyze mammographic images (Sahiner et al., 1995, Chan et al.,1995, Zhang et al., 1994, Lo et al., 1995), or features extracted from those images (Wu et al., 1993, Floyd et al., 1994), and improve the diagnostic accuracy of the mammographic exam. Common to this work has been the use of the standard backpropagation learning rule, or a slight variant of it, to train the networks.

In this paper we describe the development of a neural network to detect microcalcifications that differs from the previous work in two ways. First, we choose a novel error function and a learning algorithm that are derived specifically to solve binary classification problems (Rumelhart et al., 1995). Second, we do not use preprocessing algorithms as part of our detection scheme. In the following sections we describe the network's error function, learning rule, architecture and training scheme.

2 DERIVATION of the ERROR FUNCTION

Our task is to design a neural network to predict the location of mirocalcifications based upon information it gleans from digitized mammograms. We may think of a neural network as performing a type of non-linear regression, with the network weights corresponding to the fitted parameters of the regression model. One trains a network in much the same way that one updates a regression model. We first choose a set of weights (or regression parameters), then measure how accurately the network (or the regression model) performs at the assigned prediction task. Next we choose a new set of weights, and again measure the network's performance. If the network with the second set of weights is a better predictor of the relationship between the images and the existence of microcalcifications, we say that this is the more probable network. We repeat this process until we have found the *most* probable network – the one that best accounts for the relationship between the input images and the location of microcalcifications. This is the standard task of regression. We formalize this goal by stating that we wish to find the most probable model (network), given the data (the images and the known locations of the microcalcifications). Using Bayes' rule we write this probability as:

$$P(\mathcal{M}|\mathcal{D}) = \frac{P(\mathcal{D}|\mathcal{M})P(\mathcal{M})}{P(\mathcal{D})}.$$

Here $\mathcal{M}$ represents the network model and $\mathcal{D}$ represents the data. In the rest of this section we modify this equation in order to derive an error measure, similar to the standard sum-squared error measure used in linear regression, that allows us to compare one model with another.

We simplify the previous equation by taking the natural logarithm of each side:

$$\ln P(\mathcal{M}|\mathcal{D}) = \ln P(\mathcal{D}|\mathcal{M}) + \ln P(\mathcal{M}) - \ln P(\mathcal{D}).$$

Since the natural log is a monotonic transformation, if our model is the most probable according to the second equation it will also be the most probable according to the first. The final term, $\ln P(\mathcal{D})$, is the probability of the data. It is constant across models and we may safely discard it from the equation. The second term in the equation, $\ln P(\mathcal{M})$, represents the probability of the model. This is the *prior* term in Bayesian analysis and estimates how likely it is that a particular model is true, independent of the data. Researchers have established numerous methods to maximize this term (Rumelhart et al., 1995), but we do not employ them in this paper – we simply consider all models to have equal priors. This simplifies the equation to $\ln P(\mathcal{D}|\mathcal{M})$.

We use paired input–target data to train the network and therefore write the equation as:

$$\ln P(\mathcal{D}|\mathcal{M}) = \sum_i \ln P(<\vec{x}, y>_i |\mathcal{M}),$$

where $\vec{x}$ is the input image and y is the target value – our knowledge of whether or not a microcalcification exists in the input image. The i subscript denotes the training pair. We assume the data are independent, and expand the term above to:

$$\sum_i \ln P(<\vec{x}, y>_i |\mathcal{M}) = \sum_i \ln P(y_i|\vec{x}_i \wedge \mathcal{M}) + \sum_i \ln P(\vec{x}_i).$$

Once again we can ignore the last term, since the inputs are not dependent on the model. We are left with the task of finding the most probable model according to the equation: $\sum_i \ln P(y_i|\vec{x}_i \wedge \mathcal{M})$.

This equation tells us that there is a probabilistic relationship between the input vector, $\vec{x}_i$, and the target, y_i – that for a given input there exists a distribution of possible target values. In the case of microcalcifications we assume this distribution is binomial – that a microcalcification did or did not give rise to the input signal.

We can now clarify our interpretation of the network output, $\hat{y}_i$. (Our network will have only one output unit.) As in a standard regression problem, we assume that the network's output estimates the mean of a probability distribution, in this case the binomial. The value of the output unit therefore represents the probability that a microcalcification occurs in the input region. We now write the probability of the data given the network as:

$$P(y_i|\vec{x}_i \wedge \mathcal{M}) = \hat{y}_i^{y_i}(1 - \hat{y}_i)^{1-y_i}.$$

Taking the natural log of this probability and summing over all data pairs we get:

$$C = \sum_i P(y_i|\vec{x}_i \wedge \mathcal{M}) = \sum_i y_i \ln \hat{y}_i + (1 - y_i)\ln(1 - \hat{y}_i).$$

In the neural network literature C is known as cross-entropy error, and we want to find a model that maximizes this term. We can easily measure this term since it depends only upon the output of the network ($\hat{y}_i$), given a particular input ($\vec{x}_i$), and upon the target value that is paired with that input (y_i).

3 DERIVATION of the LEARNING RULE

Having established that we will use the cross-entropy error measure, we now derive a learning rule that allows us to repeatedly choose new weights such that each new network performs better than the previous one. The general backpropagation learning rule states that we should update the network weights according to:

$$\Delta w_{ij} = -\rho \frac{\partial C}{\partial \eta_j} o_i,$$

where ρ is the learning rate, η_j is the net-input to a unit and o_i is the output of the unit sending activation along that weight. Therefore, we need to compute $\frac{\partial C}{\partial \eta_j}$ which we write as:

$$\frac{\partial C}{\partial \eta_j} = \frac{\partial C}{\partial \mathcal{F}(\eta_j)} \frac{\partial \mathcal{F}(\eta_j)}{\partial \eta_j} = \frac{(y_j - \hat{y}_j)}{\hat{y}_j(1 - \hat{y}_j)} \frac{\partial \mathcal{F}(\eta_j)}{\partial \eta_j},$$

where $\partial \mathcal{F}(\eta_j)$ is the derivative of a unit's activation function evaluated at its net input.

Now we must choose an appropriate activation function for the output unit. The logistic,

$$\mathcal{F}(\eta_j) = \frac{1}{(1 + e^{-\eta_j})},$$

has two properties which make it a good choice. First it is bounded by zero and one. Second, we notice that the derivative of the logistic function:

$$\partial \mathcal{F}(\eta_j) = \mathcal{F}(\eta_j)(1 - \mathcal{F}(\eta_j)) = \hat{y}_j(1 - \hat{y}_j),$$

equals the variance of a binomial distribution. When we insert this variance term into the equation describing the derivative of the error function, the equation simplifies to:

$$\frac{\partial C}{\partial \eta_j} = (y_j - \hat{y}_j).$$

We then update the weights of the network according to:

$$\Delta w_{ij} = \rho(\hat{y}_j - y_j) o_i,$$

which ensures that the network performs gradient descent in its error space.

4 APPLICATION to MICROCALCIFICATION DETECTION

We use a two layer fully connected neural network, with a 9x9 grid of input units, eighteen hidden units, and one output unit. We train the network on a set of 40 images from 21 different patients, digitized at 100 microns and 12 bits, made available by the Department of Radiology, University Hospital Nijmegen, The Netherlands. Two experienced radiologists recorded the position and size of microcalcification clusters in the images. From this data we located over 1000 individual microcalcifications. The network inputs were regions centered on the individual microcalcifications, grouped with with roughly 10000 similarly sized regions chosen at random from sections of the images that did not include microcalcifications.

4.1 Training

We begin by training nine sub-networks, each with 9x9 input units and one output unit. There are no hidden units in these networks. We use the weights from these sub-networks as the initial first layer weights of the larger network. We train both the sub-networks and the large network under a modified jackknife procedure, using 80% of the images during the training phase, while saving 20% for testing.

4.2 Rule Based Clustering Algorithm

After completing training we convolve the network with each of the test images. This creates an output image in which the value of each pixel represents the probability that the pixel is in a region that includes a microcalcification. We then threshold this image so that all but the highest-valued pixels are excluded from the set of possible microcalcifications. We label groups of adjacent pixels as potential microcalcifications, after excluding those groups that are either too large or too small.

Once we have identified potential microcalcifications, we apply a simple rule-based algorithm to determine the location of microcalcification clusters. Under this scheme, if two or more microcalcifications fall within a region scored by the radiologists as a cluster, we record a true positive finding. If two or more microcalcifications are found in a 1cm square area not scored by the radiologists, we record a false positive.

We chose a rule-based clustering algorithm over a neural network method because the clustering problem is easily solved by a rule-based algorithm, and there are too few clusters in our data set to adequately train a network.

5 RESULTS

Using the algorithm described above we are able to find 91% of the clusters with a false positive rate of 0.13 clusters per image. Figure 1 shows a graph of the FROC we record using different threshold values to filter the output of the neural network. While the use of different image databases makes it difficult to compare various algorithms, these results are on par with those obtained by others in the field, and compare favorably with the one published algorithm that uses the same image database (Karssemeijer, 1993).

The cross-entropy network also learns faster than the network trained under a standard backpropagation learning rule. Figure 2 shows how the network error decreases as training time increases. The standard network takes roughly 60 times as long as the cross-entropy network does to reach the same error level.

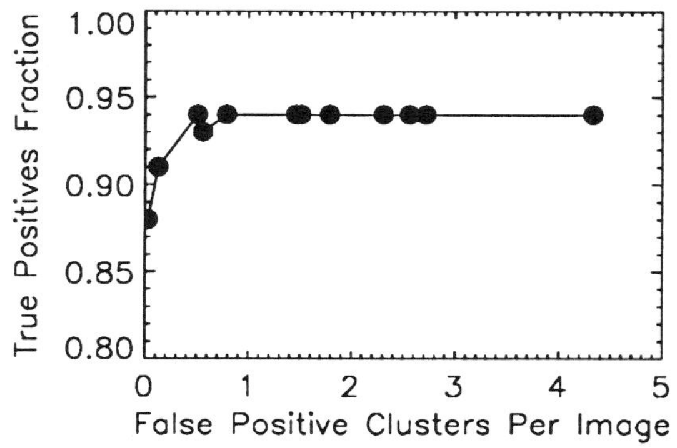

Figure 1: FROC curve for the network described in text. This figure shows the percentage of microcalcification clusters correctly detected versus the average number of false positive clusters found per image.

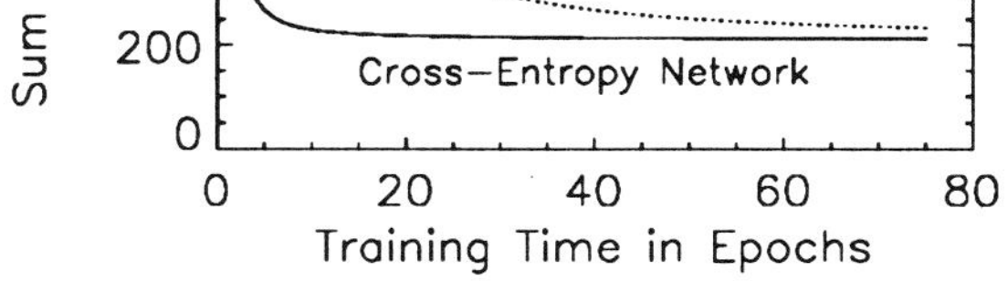

Figure 2: Change in SSE over the course of learning under two training schemes. This figure shows the rate at which both the standard backpropagation network and the cross-entropy error network improve, as shown by the decrease in sum-squared error over the course of learning.

6 DISCUSSION

Recent advances in the field of neural networks have provided us a deeper understanding of these systems, and we are now able to design networks that are appropriate for the specific task we set them. We hope that this work shows that neural networks need not be considered as mysterious black boxes, but rather as well-defined and clearly interpretable statistical tools. When applying neural networks to mammography, we enjoy significant benefits by using an error function and a learning rule appropriate to the task at hand: we are able to improve the speed and accuracy with which the network learns, and provide a principled interpretation of the network output.

In addition, our system does not use pre-processing algorithms and therefore is not limited to searching through a pre-defined set of features when analyzing the image. When detecting simple and well described features, such as microcalcifications, this method may be of limited value. However, when searching for less well characterized features such as masses, anatomical asymmetries or spiculated lesions, this method may provide much benefit.

This work was supported in part by NIH Grant CA66202

References

Chan, H. P., Lo, S. C. B., Sahiner, B., Lam, K. L., & Helvie, M. A. (1995). Computer-aided detection of mammographic microcalcifications: Pattern recognition with an artificial neural network. *Medical Physics*, *22*(10), 1555–1567.

Floyd, Carey E., Jr., Lo, J. Y., Yun, A. J., Sullivan, D. C., & Kornguth, P. J. (1994). Prediction of breast cancer malignancy using an artificial neural network. *Cancer*, *74*(11), 2944–2948.

Karssemeijer, N. (1993). Adaptive noise equalization and recognition of microcalcification clusters in mammograms. *International Journal of Pattern Recognition and Image Analysis*, *7*(6).

Lo, S. C. B., Chan, H. P., Lin, J. S., Lai, H., Freedman, M., & Mun, S. K. (1995). Artificial convolution neural network for medical image pattern recognition. *Neural Networks*, *8*, 1–14.

Rumelhart, D. E., Durbin, R., Golden, R., & Chauvin, Y. (1995). Backpropagation: The basic theory. In Y. Chauvin & D. E. Rumelhart (Eds.), *Backpropagation: Theory, architectures and applications*. Hillsdale, N.J.: Lawrence Earlbaum Associates.

Sahiner, B., Chan, H.-P., Petrick, N., Wei, D., Helvie, M. A., Adler, D. D., & Goodsitt, M. M. (1995). Image classification using artificial neural networks. *SPIE*, *2434*, 838–845.

Vyborny, C. J., & Giger, M. (1994). Computer vision and artificial intelligence in mammography. *American Journal of Roentgenology*, *162*, 699–708.

Wu, Y., Giger, M., Doi, K., Vyborny, C. J., Schmidt, R., & Metz, C. (1993). Artificial neural networks in mammography: Application to decision making in the diagnosis of breast cancer. *Radiology*, *187*, 81–87.

Zhang, W., Doi, K., Giger, M., Wu, Y., Nishikawa, R. M., & Schmidt, R. (1994). Computerized detection of clusterd microcalcifications in digital mammograms using a shift-invariant artificial neural network. *Medical Physics*, *21*(4), 517–524.

Monotonicity and Logical Analysis of Data: A Mechanism for Evaluation of Mammographic and Clinical Data[1]

Boris Kovalerchuk and Evangelos Triantaphyllou
Department of Industrial Engineering, Louisiana State University, Baton Rouge, Louisiana

James F. Ruiz
Department of Radiology, Woman's Hospital, Baton Rouge, Louisiana

1. INTRODUCTION

Computer assisted diagnosis has become one of the promising methods for improving the accuracy and early detection of breast cancer. Standard back-propagation neural networks are presently very popular diagnostic tools, but this approach does not inform the physician user on how a conclusion was reached. Some promising results have obtained with rule based techniques[3]. This method has the advantage of providing the physician with a tool that promotes consistency and accuracy. However, these (and most other) models suffer from relatively small training sample sets which in turn limit statistical significance.

An approach called logical analysis of data (LAD), and which is based on inferring discriminant Boolean functions, has the potential to overcome these weaknesses. By discovering logical relationships in existing classes of disjoint observations, the method can improve the understanding of the diagnostic process The statistical significance problem is eliminated by exploiting the property of monotonicity that exists within mammographic evaluation and interpretation.

The resultant discriminant functions could be used many ways. In the evaluation of a new *"problem case"* the radiologist could use these function for that case to draw a diagnostic conclusion. Alternatively, with a set of *"gold standard"* test cases, the functions could be used as a reproducible testing mechanism. Each radiologist could determine his/her own function, compare it to the gold standard and thereby identify areas of strength or weakness. Progress or improvement over time could then be objectively measured.

2. BACKGROUND

Currently methods of computer-aided diagnostics include neural networks, nearest neighbor methods, descriminant analysis, cluster analysis, and linear programming based methods.[3,11] These techniques attempt to generalize from collections of available training data. Therefore, they rely on the fact that the more representative the data are, the more accurate the performance of these methods will

---

[1] *The first two authors gratefully acknowledge the support from the Office of Naval Research (ONR) grant N0014-95-1-0639*

be. However, there **are some basic weaknesses** in using these techniques. For example, according to Jonson[6] the use of Baysian models in medical diagnosis is controversial, if not unethical, because the fundamental requirement of **strict randomness** rarely occurs in reality. Standard back-propagation neural networks techniques are problematic because they do not provide **bio-medical explanations**[4]. While newly developed intelligent hybrid systems, and in particular knowledge based neural networks[4], appear to be more promising, these systems have the potential to create too many (i.e., an exponential number) of rules[12]. In summary, there are two closely related difficulties with these methods as they may be applied to breast cancer diagnosis:

(i) **The available training data are often insufficient to guaranty statistically significant results by using ordinary mathematical methods.**

(ii)**The way these computerized diagnostic tools work and produce recommendations, is not appealing to medical doctors**.

The diagnostic problem considered in this research is a **nested** one. That is, it is composed of two interrelated sub-problems. The **first sub-problem** is related to the clinical question of whether a biopsy or short term follow-up is necessary or not. The **second sub-problem** is related to the question whether the radiologist believes that the current case is highly suspicious for malignancy or not. It is assumed that if the radiologist believes that the case is malignant, then he/she will also definitely recommend a biopsy. Formally, these two sub-problems are defined as follows:

The Clinical Management Sub-Problem: One and only one of two disjoint outcomes is possible. That is: 1) *"biopsy/short term followup is necessary"*; or 2) *"biopsy/short term followup is not necessary"*.

The Diagnosis Sub-Problem: Similarly as above, one and only one of two disjoint outcomes is possible. That is, a given case is: 1) *"highly suspicious for malignancy"*; or, 2) *"not highly suspicious for malignancy"*.

The above nested sub-problems provide a natural area for the application of a recent development in artificial intelligence. The technique aims at to discovering **logical relationships** which may be present in classes of disjoint observations. Each observation is described in terms of a number of characteristics or features. Then, the challenge is to find patterns which can be used to explain which features, or combinations of features, are present in each class. This development is called ***Logical Analysis of Data (or LAD)*** and consists of a group of methods.[2,7,8] The proposed logical analysis of data approach has several unique advantages related to: (1) the understanding/comprehension of the diagnostic process and recognition of sources of uncertainty in existing knowledge, (2) overcoming the statistical significance problem mentioned earlier by utilizing the ***property of monotonicity,*** (3) resolving differences arising in conclusions that are based upon the same premises, (4) developing AI-based expert systems to assist in the diagnosis of breast cancer.

The validity and accuracy (reliability) of a classifier should be reasonably high for clinical applications. Many, if not the majority, of the pattern recognition studies in radiology operate with approximately 80 training cancer cases. To explore the issue of **reliability**, assume that $f(x_1,x_2,...,x_{11})$ is some discriminant function in the space of 11 binary (i.e., with 0 or 1 value) indirect diagnostic features (vectors,) see section 5. Also assume that this discriminant function was constructed by using a sample of 80 cases (many studies consider sample sizes around 80). Next, suppose that the function f discriminates the entire state space (which is of size: $2^{11} = 2{,}048$) by describing 2,048 distinct binary vectors (combinations of 11 features). The vectors are as follows: 1,600 (i.e., about 80%) of them are features suggestive of cancer and 448 (i.e., about 20%) are negative for cancer. A description of suspicious/benign features is given in section 5. Thus, in this illustrative scenario, at most 80 different vectors (5% of 1,600) were used to learn to discriminate 1,600 cancer vectors. At this point one may wish to ask the question: "Is this function (which was inferred by using a training sample of 5% of the combinations of features suggesting malignancy) sufficiently reliable to require a patient to undergo a surgical procedure ?" While this function can be useful, its statistical significance is very questionable for the reliable diagnosis of cancer. Observe that the concept of **state space** is different than the concept of **population**. The state space expresses all possible combinations of features. However, the actual population may not exhibit all these combinations of features (i.e., some combinations may be impossible) and these can be eliminated from consideration. We consider the ratio *S/N* (where *S* is the sample size and *N* is the size of the state space) as the index of the potential reliability.

In the light of the above considerations, consider the published data[11]. We estimated the sample/space ratio (i.e., the *S/N* value) for these data. That is, for 43 features $S/N = 133/10^{43} = 1.33\times10^{-41}$. This means that the available sample is 1.33×10^{-39} % of the total possible number of different vectors in the state space. Therefore, the question which is naturally raised is: *"Can this small number of training cases be considered as reliable in order to assist in accurately diagnosing new (and thus unknown) cases?"* According to some estimations[5] the recommended value of the *S/C* ratio (where *C* is the number of connections in a neural network) must be no less that 10:1 for potentially reliable learning of a neural network. (Note that this ratio is similar but not identical to the *S/N* ratio).

The 10:1 ratio is debated by Boon[1]. He compares the neural network with biological networks (e.g. radiologists), showing that for them the ratio of sample/connections is much worse, over 10^{10} times less, than the ones presented in studies which were criticized by Gurney[5]. Thus, Boone asks: "Is there any reason that we should hold a computer to higher standards than a human?" Maybe not, but we should ask of both systems: "Is learning based on small subsets sufficiently reliable to distinguish suspicious from not suspicious given the vast diversity of all potential mammographic images?" The Machine Learning Theory[10] shows that there are relatively simple concepts that no algorithm is capable of learning in a reasonable amount of time (polynomial time). **Therefore, the question about reliability is among the most fundamental questions of scientific rigor of mammographic diagnosis**. Thus, in this study we explore the question: "Are accessible, relatively small samples sufficiently representative for learning how to evaluate the broad range of mammographic appearances?".

3. THE REPRESENTATION HYPOTHESIS

One of the most common fundamental hypotheses supporting the usage of small samples in pattern recognition is the hypothesis that a small sample is representative for the whole population (the *representation hypothesis*): *"The training data must still form a representative sample of the set of all possible inputs if the network is to perform correctly"*[9]. Therefore, without confirmation of the representation hypothesis as it applies to mammography, all pattern recognition work with small samples will be extremely heuristic and of questionable reliability. Specifically, we study the following version of the representation hypothesis: the *hypothesis of narrow vicinity.* According to the hypothesis of narrow vicinity (the NV hypothesis): ***All real possible cases are in the narrow vicinity of an accessible small training sample.*** The NV hypothesis means that we can generalize a training sample with 80 vectors, for instance, for an additional 40-80 vectors, but not for an additional 1,600 vectors. It also means that we may exclude those 1,520-1,560 vectors from 1,600 that do not represent possible cases.

4. TASKS

Let us consider how one can confirm the narrow vicinity (NV) hypothesis when a small sample is available. This is a difficult methodological question. If one has a large sample available, then he/she does not need the NV hypothesis. On the other hand, without a large sample, one does not have direct data to confirm the hypothesis.

We develop a new methodology to avoid these difficulties. The main idea is to **extend insufficient clinical cases with information from an experienced radiologist**. Another approach is mentioned by Miller et al.[9]: "One obvious solution to the problem of restricted training and testing data is to create simulated data using either a **computer based or physical model.**" Unfortunately this way is still a theoretical possibility. There is no such model. We will use experienced experts as a **"biological"/expert model to generate new potential cases**. One can ask a radiologist to evaluate a particular case when a number of features take on a set of specific values. A typical query will have the following format: "If feature *1* has value V_1, feature 2 has value V_2, ..., feature n has value V_n, then should biopsy/short term follow-up be recommended or not? Or, does the above setting of values correspond to a highly suspicious case or not?"

The above queries can be defined with artificially constructed vectors or with artificially generated new mammograms by modifying existing ones. In this way one may increase a sample size but not as much as may be necessary. The technical weakness now is, roughly speaking, the same as before. It is practically impossible to ask a radiologist to generate many thousands of artificial, new mammographic appearances.

A logical analysis approach can avoid these difficulties in two possible ways. First, if the features can be organized in a **hierarchical manner,** then a proper exploitation of this structure can lead to a significant reduction of the needed queries. Second, if the property of monotonicity is applicable, then the available data can be generalized to cover a larger training sample[7,8].

5. METHODS AND RESULTS

We construct a hierarchy of medically interpretable features from a very generalized level to a less generalized level. For example, we consider the generalized binary feature x_1--*"Shape and density of calcification"* with grades (0-*"contra cancer"* and 1-*"pro cancer"*). On the second level we consider the feature x to be some function of five other features: $y_1, y_2, .., y_5$. That is, $x = \psi(y_1, y_2, .., y_5)$, where: y_1-- *"Irregularity in shape of individual calcifications"*; y_2--*"Variation in shape of calcifications"*;y_3-- *"Variation in size of calcifications"*;y_4-- *"Variation in density of calcifications"* and y_5-- *"Density of calcifications"*.

Monotonicity in Boolean functions is the core of a powerful mathematical theory, which we applied in the breast cancer problem. For instance, consider the evaluation of calcifications in a mammogram. For simplicity and illustrative purposes assume that x_1 is the number and the volume occupied by calcifications, in a binary setting, as follows: (0-*"contra cancer"*, 1-*"pro cancer"*). Similarly with the same values we used features:x_2--{shape and density of calcifications}, x_3--{ductal orientation}, x_4--{comparison w. previous examination}, and x_5--{associated findings}.

Given the above definitions we can represent clinical cases in terms of binary vectors with these five features as: $(x_1, x_2, x_3, x_4, x_5)$. Next consider the two clinical cases which are represented by the two binary vectors: (00111) and (10100). If one is given that a radiologist correctly diagnosed (10100) as a malignancy, then, by utilizing the monotonicity property, we can also conclude that the second clinical case (10110) should also be malignancy.

A detailed description of the method and the specific steps can be found in [7,8] we show that the descriminant monotone Boolean functions for features on the upper level of the hierarchy are as follows. For the **Biopsy**/Short term followup Sub-Problem: $f_1(x)=x_2x_4 \vee x_1x_2 \vee x_1x_4 \vee x_3 \vee x_5$. Similarly, for the second sub-problem (**highly suspicious for cancer**) the function which we found was: $f_2(x)=x_1x_2 \vee x_3 \vee (x_2 \vee x_1 \vee x_4)x_5$ Regarding the second level of the hierarchy (which recall has 11 binary features) we interactively constructed the following functions (interpretation of the features is presented below): $x_1 = \varphi(w_1, w_2, w_3) = w_2 \vee w_1 w_3$ and $x_2 = \psi(y_1, y_2, y_3, y_4, y_5) = y_1 \vee y_2 \vee y_3 y_4 y_5$. By combining the previous functions we obtained theformulas of all the 11 features for **biopsy**/short term followup:

$$f_1(x)=(y_2 \vee y_1 \vee y_3 y_4 y_5)x_4 \vee (w_2 \vee w_1 w_3)(y_2 \vee y_1 \vee y_3 y_4 y_5) \vee (w_2 \vee w_1 w_3)x_4 \vee x_3 \vee x_5$$

and for **highly suspicious for cancer**: $f_2(x) = x_1x_2 \vee x_3 \vee (x_2 \vee x_1 \vee x_4)x_5 =$

$$=(w_2 \vee w_1 w_3)(y_1 \vee y_2 \vee y_3 y_4 y_5) \vee x_3 \vee (y_1 \vee y_2 \vee y_3 y_4 y_5) \vee (w_2 \vee w_1 w_3 \vee x_4)x_5$$

To construct these functions with usual methods one needs more than **4000 training cases**[8] or to ask an experienced radiologist to diagnose these 4000 cases, presented as binary vectors. We constructed these discriminant functions for one hour in dialog with a radiologist. Our approach allowed to ask only **42 questions, i.e., about 100 times less diagnostic questions than the number of all possible cases.**

An analysis of these functions and real statistics has shown that that, in general, the hypothesis of narrow vicinity (NVH) is not valid for mammographic evaluation. **Recall, that this is exactly the hypothesis implicitly used by all traditional pattern recognition methods in breast cancer diagnosis!**

We have done this study for binarized the features presented below:
x_1-amount & volume of calcifications , w_1 - number of calcifications/sm^2; w_2 - volume, cm^3 w_3-total number of calcifications; x_2-shape & density of calcifications.

Note, we consider x_2 as a function (y_1,y_2,y_3,y_4,y_5) of y_1,y_2,y_3,y_4,y_5,.
y_1 - irregularity in shape of individual calcifications; y_2 - variation in shape of calcifications; y_3 -variation in size of calcification; y_4 - variation in density of calcification; y_5 - density of calcification; x_3 - ductal orientation; x_4 - comparison with previous exam ; x_5 - associated findings.

We assume that radiologists implicitly use monotone regularities when they learn to diagnose breast cancer. This gives them a chance to be more successful than computer programs learning just by positive and negative examples. Incorporation of these verified regularities in computer learning programs opens a new direction of improvement in mammographic evaluation.

REFERENCES

1. J.Boon "Sidetracked at the Crossroads", Radiology, v. 193, n. 1, 28-30, 1994.

2. E.Boros, P. Hammer, T. Ibaraki, "Predicting cause-effective relations from incomplete discrete observations", SIAM J. on Discrete Mathematics, v. 7, n.4, 1994, 531-534.

3. C.D'orsi,D.Getty,J.Swets,R.Picket,S.Seltzer,B.McNeil, "Reading and decision aids for improved accuracy and standardization of mammographic diagnosis", Radiology, v. 184, 619-622, 1992.

4. L.M.Fu, "Knowledge-based connectionism for revising domain theories". IEEE Transactions on Systems, Man, and Cybernetics, v. 23, n. 1, 173-182, 1993.

5 J.Gurney "Neural Networks at the crossroads: caution ahead", Radiology, v. 193., n. 1, 27-28, 1994.

6 N. Jonson, "Everyday diagnostics-- a critique of the Bayessian model". Med. Hypotheses, v. 34, n. 4, 289-96, 1991.

7. B.Kovalerchuk, E.Triantaphyllou, E.Vityaev, "Monotone Boolean functions learning technique integrated with user interaction". In: Proc. of Workshop "Learning from examples", 12-th International Conference on Machine Learning, Tahoe City, CA, 41-48, 1995.

8. B.Kovalerchuk., E.Triantaphyllou, A. Deshpande, and E. Vityaev, "Interractive learning of a monotone Boolean function". Information Sciences, 1996 (in print).

9.A.Miller, B.Blott, T.Hames, "Review of neural network applications in medical imaging and signal processing", Medical & Biological Engineering & Computing, v. 30, 449-464, 1992.

10.R.Schapire, The design and analysis of efficient learning algorithms. MIT Press, 1992.

11.Y.Wu,M.Giger, K.Doi.C.Vyborny, R.Schmidt, C.Metz, "Artificial neural networks in mammography: application to decision making in the diagnosis of breast cancer", Radiology, v. 187, n. 1, 81-87, 1993.

12 .J.Shavlik, "Combining symbolic and neural learning", *Macine Learning,* v.14, 1994, .321-331.

Detection of Abnormal Changes in Mammograms by Comparing Different Screenings

D. Brzakovic, N. Vujovic and P. Bakic
Department of Electrical Engineering and Computer Science
Lehigh University, Bethlehem, Pennsylvania

P. Brzakovic
Serbian Cancer Society, Belgrade, Yugoslavia

1. INTRODUCTION

Routine mammogram screening is recommended for a large percentage of the female population as the most reliable means for detecting early cancer. Two of the most important requirements to make massive screenings possible are improving efficacy and reducing the cost of the current procedure. A viable means of achieving simultaneously both objectives is using computer technology to substitute part of manual readings. Many recent studies have attempted to develop a computer-based aid for mammogram screenings. Usually, the proposed approaches consider a single mammogram and utilize complex image processing and/or pattern recognition methods to enhance, detect, and/or characterize two most common manifestations of cancer [1], masses and microcalcifications.

The approach proposed in this paper is different: it performs mammogram followup, i.e., detection of abnormalities is based on the comparison of different screenings of the same patient. The major advantage of this approach is that the analysis is adaptive because abnormality is determined using the older mammogram as a reference. Furthermore, the approach has the potential to provide for very early cancer detection, possibly earlier than presently possible. However, the problem of automated mammogram followup is very complex and requires solving a number of subproblems, including standardizing screening procedures, registering mammograms, and characterizing minor changes in texture patterns. This paper focuses on mammogram registration, which is technically one of the most difficult subproblems. Precise registration, which is intractable, is surmounted by establishing regional correspondence between images. The regions are compared in terms of intensity and texture characteristics to determine existence of abnormal changes. The algorithm's performance is evaluated at different phases based on human/expert performance.

2. PROBLEM DESCRIPTION AND APPROACH

Comparison of mammograms acquired in different screenings requires solving the registration problem. Registering mammograms is a very difficult task because the two images may differ significantly and the differences cannot be modeled. The primary sources of differences are (i) variations in positioning, (ii) variations in compression, and (iii) changes normally encountered in breast tissue. The premise behind the solution to the registration problem proposed in this work is that there is no rational basis to develop registration techniques that counter-affect 3-D positioning differences by precise 2-D image registration. In view of this, we propose an alternative approach which surmounts the problem of precise mammogram registration and performs regional registration instead.

In this approach, mammograms are compared regionally. In order to compensate for 2-D rotational distortions arising from digitization, the regions are circular. Each circle is defined by the location of its center relative to the control points and its radius, which is determined by intensity characteristics of two mammograms. Both mammograms are covered, without gaps, by corresponding overlapping circles. Regions are compared in terms of their intensity statistics and texture characteristics; the ongoing study concentrates on developing appropriate characterization methods (the preliminary results are described in [2]).

3. MAMMOGRAM REGISTRATION AND COMPARISON

In the following we first describe methodology employed to register the two mammograms and then briefly summarize approaches under consideration for regional comparison.

3.1 Determination of control points

The control point selection requires identification of unique points in two mammograms whose correspondence can be established. Identification of such points is a difficult task because mammograms are in essence non-structured texture patterns. After considering different approaches the following two step protocol was adopted:

- *Step 1: Selection of candidate control points in two mammograms.* Intersections between elongated structures (such as ducts and blood vessels) are selected to be candidate control points. Relative locations of cross-sections may vary in two images due to positioning differences and compression; however, these variations are minor and the cross-sections are reliable in establishing regional correspondence.

  The intersections between elongated structures are detected utilizing modified monotony operators. Monotony operators were originally developed to identify points which were used to derive displacement vector fields in image sequences [4]. The monotony operator compares the gray level of an image pixel with its eight neighbors and assigns to it a value 0-8, according to the number of neighbors that have smaller gray values than the central pixel. In this work we utilize a modification of the monotony operators designed to detect narrow elongated structures (ridges) in reduced resolution mammograms. Two operators are designed, one to detect predominantly horizontal and the other to detect predominantly vertical ridges. Intersections between the outputs of the two operators define potential control points. Modified monotony operators are applied to reduced resolution mammograms in order to reduce the number of potential control points by limiting the analysis to the most prominent structures. Details of the algorithm are described in [3].

- *Step 2: Establishment of correspondence between a common subset of control points.* Given two sets of potential control points, the objective of the correspondence algorithm is to identify the common subset and within it individual point correspondence. The algorithm for establishing point correspondence utilizes accumulator matrix (based on work described in [5]) which is used to tally votes for a particular match. Given a set of m potential control points in the older mammogram, M_o, and a set of n potential control points in the newer mammogram, M_n, the accumulator matrix is an $m \times n$ array, where an entry $e(p,q)$ corresponds to points labeled p and q in M_o and M_n, respectively. The entry $e(p,q)$ is updated every time when a match between p and q is established. In this work, the matching is based on signatures which are designed to capture the local arrangements of the elongated structures in the neighborhoods of the control points. At the end of the voting process, the accumulator matrix is thresholded to eliminate inconsistent matches and then scanned to determine the best (most reliable) matches.

3.2 Regional correspondence and comparison

Regional correspondence involves defining corresponding circular regions. The centers for these regions are determined based on distances from a subset of control points which are initially assumed to be approximately the same in two images. Transformations that relate distances are under consideration. In order to reduce the effects of variations in breast tissue density on the subsequent analysis, the regions are selected such that each region contains primarily a single tissue type. For this purpose, we utilize image partitioning described in [2] and constrain regions to belong to a single partition. Corresponding regions have the same radius, which is determined by segmentation of the older mammogram. Both mammograms are covered, without gaps, by corresponding overlapping circles. The procedure used to define circular regions is illustrated in Figure 1, and an example of obtained regions is shown in Figure 2(a).

Differentiation between normal and abnormal changes in mammograms is based on intensity statistics and textural characteristics. The premises behind current work are as follows. Normally, there are significant differences in intensity ranges between mammograms of the same individual taken at different times. Most of the normal differences between two mammograms are expected to be evenly distributed over the whole intensity range or are expected to be localized at low intensities because of changes such as increase in percentage of fat. Abnormal changes considered in this study are masses and microcalcifications. In both cases, changes are expected to show statistical difference only in specific regions and with high intensities. To evaluate differences in mammograms two types of measurements are considered: (i) intensity statistics and (ii) texture characterization. The preliminary results for the first type are reported in [2]. These measurements are useful in detecting some changes associated with masses. Texture measures are in general more powerful since they can be insensitive to intensity changes due to the acquisition conditions, and as an additional tool improve the intensity analysis performance.

Comparison of different screenings considered in this work is based on multiresolution analysis that employs overcomplete wavelet decomposition. The decomposition includes the approximation and the detail images of a mammogram pair, all of which are further processed using B-spline filtering as described in [6]. The preliminary evaluation of the approach employs thresholding and clustering. An example of regions labeled suspicious for regions shown in Figure 2(a) is shown in Figure 2(b).

Further development of the mammogram comparison includes local linear transforms, fractal texture measures, and features derived from the texture spectrum.

4. PRELIMINARY RESULTS AND DISCUSSION

The algorithm for control point extraction described in this paper was tested on 29 mammogram pairs acquired in the time span of six months to two years. The spatial resolution of digitized mammograms varied from $.1 - .5mm$. Using the algorithms described in Sections 3.1, an average of 70 potential control points was detected per mammogram. Using these points the correspondence algorithm has established an average of 5 correspondences per mammogram pair. Since there is no precise knowledge on location of control points, the algorithm performance was validated by visual inspection. The validation was performed independently by three unbiased observers (i.e., observers who had no knowledge about the algorithm), an experienced radiologist, and two casual observers. The evaluation procedure compared the points obtained by the algorithm with points identified by observers. Based on the spatial resolution, the algorithm and an observer were considered to be in agreement if the distance between the two points was less than 10 pixels. The results of evaluation are as follows: the agreement between the casual observers and the algorithm was about 70% and the agreement between the radiologist and the algorithm was a little over 90%.

The control points are used to identify regions, as described in Section 3.2. Currently we are investigating methods for characterizing abnormal vs. normal changes in mammograms. The algorithms under development are being compared with three independent readings by radiologists and results of biopsy.

REFERENCES

[1] B.D. Stewart, D.A. Folkes, A.Y. Cairns, I.W. Ricketts, P.E. Preece, and A.J. Thomson, "Computer Image Processing in Mammographic Screening: A Re-

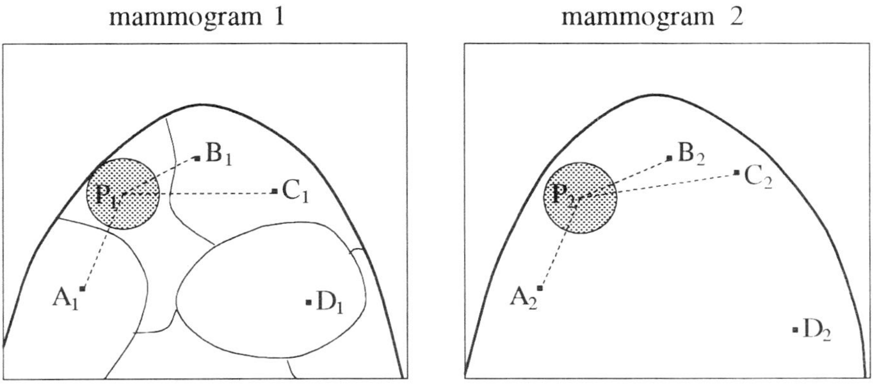

A_i, B_i, C_i, D_i = control points, $i = 1, 2$
P_i = circle centers, $i = 1, 2$

Figure 1: Determination of circular regions.

view," *Automedica*, vol. 15, pp. 23-45, 1992.

[2] D. Brzakovic, N. Vujovic, M. Neskovic, P. Brzakovic, and K. Fogarty, "Mammogram Analysis by Comparison with Previous Screenings," Proc. of the 2nd International Workshop on Digital Mammography, York, England, 1994.

[3] N. Vujovic, D. Brzakovic, and K. Fogarty: "Detection of Cancerous Changes in Mammograms Using Intensity and Texture Measures," Proc. of SPIE's Medical Imaging 1995, San Diego, California, pp. 37-47, 1995.

[4] R. Kories and G. Zimmerman, "A Versatile Method for the Estimation of Displacement Vector Fields from Image Sequences," Proc. of Workshop on Motion: Representation and Analysis, 1986.

[5] D. Skea, I. Barrodale, R. Kuwahara, and R. Poeckert, "A Control Point Matching Algorithm," *Pattern Recognition*, vol. 26, no. 2, pp. 269-276, 1993.

[6] M. Unser, "Texture Classification and Segmentation Using Wavelet Frames," *IEEE Trans. on Image Proc.*, vol. 4, no. 11, pp. 1549-1560, 1995.

Acknowledgment
This work has been supported in part by NSF Grant IRI-9504363. The mammograms were supplied by St. Luke's Hospital in Bethlehem, PA.

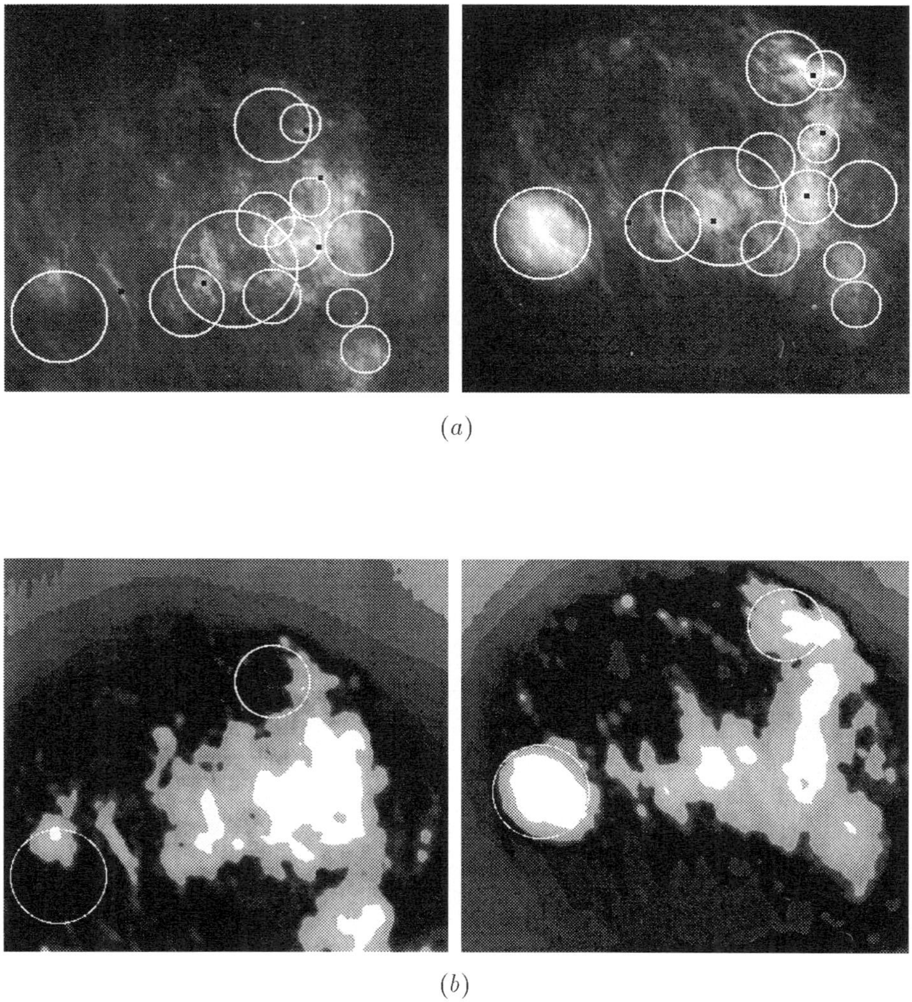

Figure 2: (a) A mammogram pair with superimposed control points and circular regions. (b) Suspicious regions detected after processing.

Computer Based Tracking System for Mammography Compliance

Pankaj J. Mowji, M.D., Mahfuz Ahmed, M.D., Ph.D., Curtis Anderson, R.T., Charles Stuewe, B.S. and Carol Ahmed, D.O.
Kaiser Permanente Medical Center, Anaheim, California

INTRODUCTION

In order to reduce cost, in this era of cost containment, there is an increase emphasis on preventive care. Breast cancers is the most frequently diagnosed malignancy in women. It is well established that the use of screening mammography in asymptomatic women can detect breast cancer at an early stage and reduce mortality. For an optimal screening program, patients need to be tracked to insure that they are receiving their mammograms in a timely fashion.

We describe a computer program that evaluates patient's risk factors, and in conjunction with mammography screening guidelines developed by the physicians in the medical group, reminds physicians when to appropriately request the examination. When the risk factor changes the program automatically adjusts to the appropriate guideline. This program, although developed in a managed care setting, has wide application, and may be utilized to evaluate patient and physician compliance in any health delivery system.

During the last four years we have developed a database of all the patients in our HMO service area. Recently the data base has been used to monitor the National Committee for Quality Assurance (NCQA) indicators on all patients, by utilizing a "Preventive Health Screen (PHS)". The PHS is used to alert physicians as well as any health care provider with whom the patient has an interaction, when one or more of the indicators are not met. This paper emphasizes the use of the PHS specifically for mammography screening.

SYSTEM CONFIGURATION

The complete computer system is described elsewhere in this issue[1] and will not be dealt with here.

SYSTEM PROCESS

When the patient visits the health care provider and the patient's medical record number is entered into the computer, the PHS appears on the computer screen (Fig:1). The PHS lists the date of the last mammogram. If the patient is compliant there is a notation as to when the next mammogram is due in months. If the patient is overdue for a mammogram, a flashing reminder, "overdue" is noted in the first column, along with the number of days the examination is overdue in the last column. There is also a date to evaluate compliance for "Self Breast Exam Education".

KPMC, O.C.	**MEMBER PREVENTIVE SCREEN**			
Patient: Jane Doe	**DOB: 04/15/35**		**Age: 60 Sex: F**	
Personal Physician:	**A. Jones, MD.**			
VITALS	> WT: HT:	TEMP:	B/P:	PULSE:
ALLERGIES	> DARVON-Nausea,	ASA-Profuse Bleeding		Valium-Hives
	PREVENTIVE SERVICES			
***OVERDUE**	**Mammography**	**Last >**	**03/15/94**	**Overdue 24 months**
Compliant	**Breast Self Ex Educ.**	**Last >**	**03/29/95**	
*OVERDUE	Tetanus - Diphtheria	Last >	03/15/84	Overdue 24 months
No Info On	Chlamydia	Please Inquire		
No Info On	Safe Sex Education	Please Inquire		
No Info On	Syphilis Test	Please Inquire		
Compliant	Blood Pressure Record	Last >	03/29/96	
Compliant	Cholestrol	Last >	03/20/96	Next Due 59 Months
Compliant	Influenza	Last >	10/09/95	Next Due 6 Months
**Refused	Pneumococcus	Last Asked> 03/15/96		
	ACTIVE RISK FACTORS			
HIGH - Breast Cancer		HI - Diabetes (Pers/Family/Hi alcohol use)		
		SLT - Asbestos Exposure		

Fig:1 Preventive Health Screen. Screen shows patient to be overdue for a mammogram by 24 months. Patients last mammogram was on 3/15/1994.

Under the heading of "Active Risk Factors", the patient is assigned to a high or low risk group based on the clinical guidelines which is used to determine patients follow up mammogram. At the time of the mammogram or patients visit to the health care provider, if there is a change in the patients risk factor status, the "Problem and Risk Factor Screen" (PRFS) (Fig:2) maybe manually changed to reflect the new risk factors. A change in the risk factors may change the follow-up interval in accordance with established guidelines, and the PHS will be updated.

The PRFS can be viewed by any health care provider the patient may come in contact with, as well as the physician.

KPMC-CHAMPS **PATIENT CARE NETWORK**

MEMBER PREVENTIVE SCREEN SYSTEM

Patient: Jane Doe **DOB:** 04/15/35 **Age:** 60 **Sex:** F

Personal Physician : A. Jones, MD

TYPE	LVL	DESCRIPTION	X	RISK FACTOR	ONSET	STS	LVL
Prob		Anticoag-Warf	X	**Breast CA (Pers)**	**06/88**	**(A)**	**5**
Prob		Diabetes					
Prob		Cancer-Brain					
Prob		Cancer-GI		1. Normal			
Prob		Cataract		2. Family history of breast CA			
Prob		Chemotherapy		Onset above age 40			
Prob		Depression		3. Family history of breast CA			
Prob		DVT		Onset below age 40			
Risk	High	Alcohol use		4. Biopsy with hyperplasia			
Risk	**High**	**Breast Cancer**		5. Personal history of breast CA			
Risk	Low	Asbestos Exposure					
Risk	Low	Sex Trans Ds					
Risk	High	Diabetes					

Function (A) A-Add, D-Delete, M-Modify, R-Risk, P-Problem Code #(B)

Fig:2 Problem and Risk Factor Screen. This screen shows the patient to have a high risk factor for breast cancer. Patient has a personal history of breast cancer. Patients risk level (LVL) is 5.

Following review of the screen the provider may take the appropriate action for mammography compliance based on the information provided. If the patient is past due or due for a mammogram, the provider orders the examination on the Order Entry System (OES)[2]. The patient is tracked on the OES until a mammogram report is transcribed on the computer system. During transcription the PHS screen is also updated and the patient is removed from the tracking system on the OES.

At our institution each physician is assigned a panel of patients and the physicians are grouped into "Primary Care Units" (PCU) at the various clinics. The PHS is used to track and follow-up on noncompliant mammogram patients. A list of noncompliant patients assigned to a particular physician is generated by age group and can be seen on the "Member Health Analysis" screen.(Fig:3). The list shows the patient's address and telephone number. The list maybe personalized for individual physician panel or for a particular PCU. This list is then utilized by the PCU to call patients individually to remind them of the necessity and value of the mammographic study. The computer is also used to generate letters from the physicians to the noncompliant patients in their panel. This is a form letter which is personalized for the patient, and is signed by the physician. These methods are initially being used to increase mammography compliance and results of the mass mailers as well as personal phone calls are being monitored.

PERSONAL PHYSICIAN MEMBER HEALTH ANALYSIS

MEMBER DATA DESCRIPTION DESCRIPTION	MEMBER DATA
(X) Women 50-74 years w/ mammogram	( )
( ) Member 55+ who have had pneumovax	( )
( ) Member 65+ with current influenza vacc	( )
( ) Member with current tetanus vaccine	( )
( ) Member 18+ w/ current PAP smear	( )
( ) Peds DOB 05/94 to 06/94 w/current immun	( )
( )	**( ) Print patient address label**
( )	**( ) Remove non-member from panel**
( )	**( ) Remove deceased pt. from panel**
( )	**( ) Analyze panel composition**
( )	**( ) Print current patient panel**

********************************RESULTS***************************

 # With current mammogram = 315 Without = 96 % With = 76%

This sample analyzed 100% of your patients.

Sample size > (100)% **For list of noncompliant pts; enter printer # ( )**

Dr. ID # (35597) **Place "X" next to analysis you wish and enter sample size (1-100)%**

Fig:3 Member Health Analysis Screen. Screen shows the data for physician ID # 35597. The sample size analyzed was 100%. Physicians panel shows 315 patients compliant as regards their mammogram and 96 patients who are not. Physician patient panel compliance is 76%.

The PHS is used to compare mammography compliance in each PCU as well as compliance of each physician panel. These results are reviewed on a regular basis by the physicians and the PCU managers at their department meetings. Individual physicians have access only to review their own panel.

RESULTS

At the introduction of the "Preventive Health Screen" for mammography, patient compliance was 55%. With the full implementation of the program recently, the mammography compliance has increased from 58% to 60% during the first three months of this year, with no significant change in the patient panel size during this time.

Physician panel compliance has also improved in the first three months of the year (Fig:4) Compliance has increased at an average of 2.8% though it has varied from minus 4% to positive 9% for individual physicians.

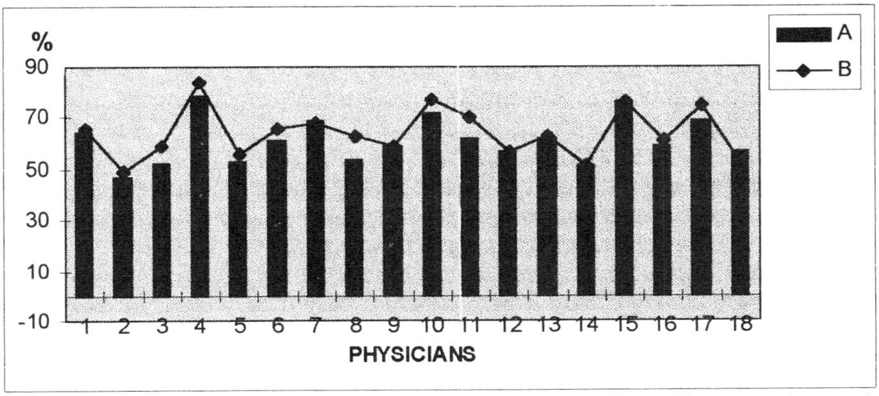

Fig:4 Physician Panel Patient Mammography Compliance. Above chart demonstrates the change in physician panel at a three month interval for a PCU. (A) is the percent of initial compliance and (B) compliance after three months.

The results of the personal letters as well as personal phone calls to the patients with a selected sample of physicians was evaluated. Increase in patient compliance is noted with personalized phone calls where three selected physicians showed an increase in compliance of 2 to 12% with an average of 6.6%. Similarly for three different physicians the mass mailers resulted in an average of 2 % with a range of 1 to 3% (Fig: 5)

CONCLUSION

In the short period of six months that the mammography compliance tracking system has been instituted we have seen an increase in the mammography compliance rate of 5% overall. We have also seen an increase in patient compliance with personalized phone calls. Among the three sample physicians, the physician with a smaller initial patient compliance showed marked improvement. Physicians with an initial higher patient compliance showed a smaller gain. Personalized phone calls are more effective when compared to the mass mailers. The computer provides information regarding the compliance rate of each physician relative to his/her colleagues. With the results provided to the Primary Care Units for discussion in their meetings, we believe that the comparative results will kindle a competitive spirit in the physicians to increase patient compliance and the patients will be the final winners.

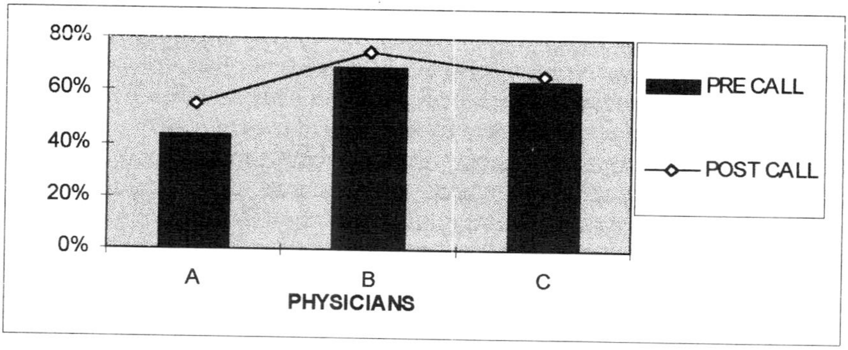

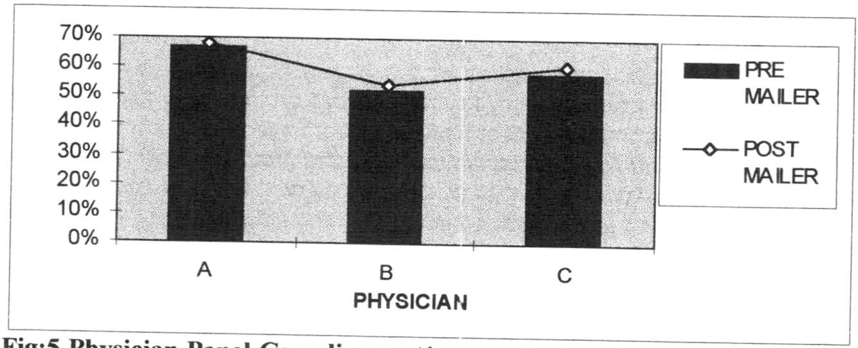

Fig:5 Physician Panel Compliance. Above graphs show the patient panel compliance of three randomly selected physicians. The results show the change in a three month period for mass mailing as well as personalized phone calls.

NOTE: The computer screens shown in Figures 1,2 and 3 are not the true screens seen on the monitor. The screens shown here contain the information necessary for this presentation. The true screens contain addition information.

REFERENCES

1. Ahmed M, Mowji PJ, Anderson C, Stuewe C, Ahmed CA. A Computer System for Improving the Score on the NCQA Health Care Report Card. **In Proceedings of S/CAR 96.**
2. Ahmed M, Anderson C, Stuewe C. A Computer System for Requesting and Reporting Radiologic Examinations, Verifying Receipt of the Reports by Referring Physicians, and Tracking Patients with Significant Abnormal Findings. **In Proceedings of the International Symposium CAR'93**, H.U.Lumpke Editor, p. 179-184.

SESSION 5

DICOM/HIS/RIS

Co-Chairs:

Ethan F. Fener
Debra Stenner

Implementing the Digital Image and Communication in Medicine (DICOM) Protocol for a Hospital Information System

Peter M. Kuzmak, MSBME and Ruth E. Dayhoff, M.D.
Department of Veterans Affairs, Technology Service, Silver Spring, Maryland

The Decentralized Hospital Computer Program (DHCP) is the standard hospital/radiology information system (HIS/RIS) of the U.S. Department of Veterans Affairs, and is installed nationwide at all 172 VA medical centers (VAMCs). DHCP includes an Imaging System that provides a full diagnostic quality (2k x 2k) image management infrastructure as part of the HIS/RIS.

The VA has developed a set of DICOM interfaces as part of the DHCP Imaging System. Currently, DICOM interfaces allow DHCP to communicate directly with commercial medical image equipment to download patient study information and to obtain digitized images. Other interfaces allow DICOM images to be retrieved from DHCP image storage. The VA is beginning to use DICOM for TeleMedicine applications. Additional capabilities are forthcoming. A bidirectional DICOM interface connecting the DHCP HIS/RIS to Picture Archiving and Communication Systems (PACS) is being developed for handling text and image data transfer. The VA is implementing the DICOM Worklist Management service.

It is the intent of the VA to make DHCP a fully compliant provider or user of many of the DICOM Service Classes. The VA will use DICOM to support image acquisition, storage management, and diagnostic quality display capabilities as part of the DHCP Imaging System.

INTRODUCTION

The DHCP Imaging System is an integral extension to the VA's HIS/RIS that is designed to provide a wide-range of image capture, retrieval, and display capabilities. The DHCP Imaging System integrates clinical images with the associated report text in the patient medical record, and provides a full diagnostic quality (2k x 2k) image management infrastructure as part of the HIS/RIS.[1, 2]

The VA began working with ACR-NEMA Version 2.0, the predecessor to DICOM, in early 1992. The VA developed a bidirectional text and image interface to the Loral PACS at the Baltimore VAMC. Since October 1993, all admission, discharge, and transfer transactions, patient demographic changes, radiology orders, reports (over 500,000 text messages) and images (over 800,000) have been sent between DHCP and the PACS.[3, 4] The text-only portion of the interface was subsequently installed at six additional VA and DOD sites.

DICOM is the Digital Imaging and Communication in Medicine standard that brings open systems technology to medical imaging.[5, 6, 7] The VA began development of the DHCP DICOM interface capability in December 1994. The VA has several different uses for the DHCP DICOM interface:

1) Image Server -- allow DHCP to store and retrieve images from commercial image servers and allow DHCP to act as an image server.

2) Image Capture Modality Interfacing -- allow DHCP to send patient study information to commercial modalities, such as CT and MRI scanners and Computed Radiography, and acquire images from these sources.

3) PACS Interfacing -- bi-directional communications between commercial PACS systems and DHCP.

4) Image Display Interfacing -- allow DHCP to send image data to a commercial display system for viewing or display DICOM images on its own workstations.

5) TeleMedicine -- allow a remote examination site to have images read at a central site; provide transfer of patient, study, result, and image data between sites. The goal is to provide seamless integration of image and text data at both sites (peer-to-peer system communications).

DHCP DICOM INTERFACE ARCHITECTURE

The DICOM standard includes various components and messaging paradigms. For example, DICOM includes both an event notification approach("Push Model") and a query based one ("Pull Model"). DICOM is object-oriented and defines the class semantics (services) and the corresponding information objects (service-object pairs or SOP classes). Institutions must select appropriate components and approaches and tailor the DICOM SOP classes to meet their needs. The VA has applied its experience with ACR-NEMA Version 2.0 in developing the design and implementation of its DICOM interfaces.

The DHCP DICOM architecture consists of a generic interface for text transfer, and separate image storage and retrieval interfaces. The generic interface is separated into an upper DICOM message handler layer and a lower DICOM TCP/IP communications layer. In order to provide prompt notification of time-critical events, the generic interface uses a set of prioritized first-in-first-out queues to process incoming and outgoing DICOM messages.

With the exception of the lower communications portions of the image transfer interfaces, which are written in C for performance reasons, all the rest of the interface is written in MUMPS, the same programming language that was used to implement the DHCP HIS/RIS.[8]

DICOM APPLICATIONS

Standard Storage Service Provider & User

DICOM defines the behavior of standard image storage devices. This Storage Service SOP Class is supported by DHCP both as a provider and as a user.

To date, the DHCP Storage Service provider and user software has been tested with Mallinckrodt "send_image" and "simple_storage" routines.[9]

Modality Interfaces

The VA has three active modality interface projects.

Remote Patient/Visit/Study Interface. The first DHCP DICOM modality interface to use DICOM Upper Layer Protocol for TCP/IP was with DeJarnette and Fuji, and became operational March 1996. The DICOM messages are sent over a T1 line from the Baltimore VAMC DHCP HIS/RIS to a DeJarnette modality interface at the Perry Point VAMC, about 50 miles away. For each radiology order, the Baltimore DHCP sends three separate DICOM N-EVENT-REPORT requests to the Perry Point DeJarnette system, one each for the Patient, Visit, and Study Management SOP Classes. DeJarnette creates a local database with the patient, visit, and study event data, and provides a worklist facility for the Fuji Computed Radiography modality.

Picker PQ-2000 CT Scanner Interface. The second project is to demonstrate that DHCP is able to acquire images directly from modalities via DICOM. The DHCP Storage Service provider was successfully tested with a Picker PQ-2000 CT scanner in March 1996.

Modality Worklist SOP Class Interface. The third interface project is to implement the new DICOM Modality Worklist SOP Class. DHCP Patient demographics and study information will be downloaded to the modality and images will be acquired. Vendors participating in this project include DeJarnette, Fuji, and Picker.

Several different functions will be performed. The DHCP Modality Interface will obtain patient demographics and ordering information from the DHCP HIS/RIS. The interface will dynamically maintain the schedule of imaging procedures to be performed. The interface will act as a Modality Worklist Service Provider to pass information about the scheduled imaging procedures to the modality.

The DHCP Modality Interface will include the Storage Service SOP Class Provider that allows the modality to send DICOM images (i.e., composite objects) to DHCP. Images will be incorporated into the DHCP Image Database and will be stored permanently. Images will be able to be retrieved using the DHCP Query Retrieve Service Provider. The modality may interrogate the DHCP Storage Commitment Push Model Provider to determine whether or not DHCP has successfully stored an image.

The DHCP Modality Interface also contains a Study Component Management Service Provider that allows the modality to notify DHCP about the study's images. This procedure permits the linking of images to studies in the DHCP Image Database, and is required for proper operation of the DHCP Imaging System.

The VA has written a draft DICOM Conformance Statement describing this modality interface.

PACS Interfaces

In the coming year, the VA's operational ACR NEMA Version 2.0 PACS interfaces will be upgraded to DICOM. Four additional medical centers will be installing new PACS with DICOM interfaces. The VA's specifications for the DHCP DICOM PACS Interface are included in RFP's for all new VA PACS systems.

Data Requirements of the PACS Interface. The PACS requires several different kinds of text data from the HIS/RIS. The HIS/RIS sends current patient identification and order entry information to the PACS so that it can register patients and process orders. All patient demographic changes are sent to the PACS to prevent patient mismatch and avoid duplicate patient registration. Examination progress information is sent to the PACS to trigger event processing, such as printing labels when the patient arrives. The examination verification step is performed on the HIS/RIS, and is passed to the PACS to trigger the release of the images. Radiology reports are entered on the HIS/RIS and are passed to the PACS so that they can be displayed on the PACS in conjunction with the images. Clinical scheduling information is also needed for prefetching images from the storage archive. Patient tracking information is needed for display of patient information by ward.

The PACS must supply the HIS with information about examinations that have been performed. Notification of completion of an examination must be sent to the HIS in order to update the order status and identify which examinations have digitized images. The PACS must also send to DHCP a list of the images associated with each completed order. The PACS images may then be transferred across the interface and displayed on DHCP imaging workstations. In a similar fashion, DHCP images must also be able to be transferred, stored, retrieved, and displayed on the PACS. Master file updates of the HIS/RIS dictionaries such as provider lists must be passed to the PACS.

PACS Interface Implementation. The DHCP HIS/RIS is designed to operate on event-driven data. The DHCP DICOM Application Entity for the PACS interface is implemented using the data "Push Model" paradigm to fit this existing framework.

An interface design goal is that there be a one-to-one mapping of events to the DICOM messages. Every event maps to a single DICOM N-EVENT-REPORT request message. Each applicable data field is translated into its corresponding DICOM element VA-specific SOP Classes were created for the event transactions. All of the patient information from each event transaction is included in each DICOM request message. The redundant patient information allows the PACS to create the patient database entry, if necessary.

The Data "Pull Model" paradigm (based on the N-GET DIMSE-N service request) was not used because of the lack of a DHCP HIS/RIS query mechanism.

CONCLUSION

Providing DICOM interface capabilities to DHCP is a great advancement in a rapidly becoming all-digital medical imaging environment. DICOM capabilities, coupled with the order of magnitude improvements in network speed, storage capacity, processor performance, display capabilities, and image size, make it now possible to incorporate a full diagnostic quality (2k x 2k) image management infrastructure into the HIS/RIS.

These efforts are important for two reasons. First, by demonstrating the usefulness of DICOM HIS/RIS interfaces, the federal medical community is promoting the acceptance of the DICOM standard by the general HIS/RIS community. That these interfaces can be implemented in MUMPS is significant because of the size of the MUMPS medical information systems community. Second, because the DICOM standard provides direct access to the images, these interfaces permit integration of PACS capabilities into HIS/RIS applications. The DICOM standard also allows shared storage devices for many specialties within a hospital. These have the potential of tremendous cost savings.

Acknowledgements

The authors would like to thank Dr. Eliot Siegel and the Radiology Department at the Baltimore VAMC for the opportunity to develop the initial interface. The authors would also like to thank Col. Fred Goeringer of the MDIS Project Office for giving us the opportunity to gain experience with the interface at the Department of Defense sites. The authors would like to thank the staff of the Washington VAMC for allowing us to test the direct modality interface to the CT scanner. Finally the authors would like to acknowledge Dr. Fred Prior for his work at Pennsylvania State University in advising us about DICOM.

References

1 Dayhoff Ruth E., Kuzmak Peter M., Maloney Daniel L., and Shepard Barclay M., "Experience with an Architecture for Integrating Images into a Hospital Information System", *Proceedings of the 4th Annual IEEE Symposium on Computer-Based Medical Systems*, Baltimore, MD, 1993.

2 Dayhoff Ruth E., Kuzmak Peter M., "A Network of Fully Integrated Multispeciality Hospital Imaging Systems", *Proceedings of Medical Imaging 1994: PACS Design and Evaluation*, SPIE Vol. 2165, pp 556-562, 1994.

3 Kuzmak Peter M., Dayhoff Ruth E., "A bidirectional ACR-NEMA interface between the VA's DHCP Integrated Imaging System and the Siemens-Loral PACS", *Proceedings of Medical Imaging 1994: PACS Design and Evaluation*, SPIE Vol. 2165, pp 387-394, 1994.

4 Kuzmak Peter M., Norton Gary S., Dayhoff Ruth E., "Using Experience with Bidirectional HL7 - ACR-NEMA Interfaces between the Federal Government HIS/RIS and Commercial PACS to Plan for DICOM", *Proceedings of Medical Imaging 1995: PACS Design and Evaluation*, SPIE, 1995.

5 Digital Imaging Communication in Medicine (DICOM), *NEMA Standards Publication PS 3 (1994)*, National Electrical Manufacturers Association, 2101 L Street, N.W., Washington, DC 20037.

6 Prior Fred, Channin David S., Zaidel Mark, Kikday Judy, "DIOCM User Conformance Profile: Proof of Concept", *Medical Imaging 1994: PACS Design and Evaluation*, R. G. Jost (ed.) Proceedings SPIE, Vol. 2165, p. 348-358, The International Society for Optical Engineering, Bellingham Washington. 1994.

7 Jensch Peter, Hewett Andrew, Cordonnier Emmanuel, Mattheus Rudy, "DICOM V3.0 - The CEN trial implementation" *Medical Imaging 1994: PACS Design and Evaluation*, R. G. Jost (ed.) Proceedings SPIE, Vol. 2165, p. 368-377, The International Society for Optical Engineering, Bellingham Washington. 1994.

8 Kuzmak Peter M., Dayhoff Ruth E., "Implementing the Digital Image and Communications for Medicine (DICOM) Protocol in M", *M Computing* 3:3 (June 1995 Proceedings) p. 33-40.

9 Moore Stephen M., Beecher David E., Hoffman Sheldon A., "DICOM Shareware: A Public Implementation of the DICOM Standard," *Medical Imaging 1994: PACS Design and Evaluation*, R. G. Jost (ed.) Proceedings SPIE, Vol. 2165, p. 772-781, The International Society for Optical Engineering, Bellingham Washington. 1994.

Survey of DICOM Conformance Statements

D.A. Clunie
Mollard Consultants, New York

I. INTRODUCTION

Essential to selecting and purchasing DICOM equipment is the Conformance Statement, whose role and structure is strictly defined in ACR/NEMA DICOM PS3.2 [1]. The statement specifies which services are available in which roles to operate on what kinds of object in response to what real world activities, as well as choices of encoding and hardware connections. Feasibility of interconnectivity between devices is determined by matching Conformance Statements. Equipment cannot be considered to conform to the DICOM standard unless such a statement is made available.

This study aims to evaluate the availability of these statements, including their availability in electronic form, their compliance with the standard format, and the extent of services defined within them.

II. METHODS

Conformance Statements were solicited from various known equipment vendors by approaching local sales representatives, field engineers, key individuals in the DICOM field, variously by telephone, letter, electronic mail, as well as publically on the Usenet news service, over a period of six months.

When multiple statements for the same equipment were obtained, only the most recent version was evaluated. Where multiple statements or sections of statements pertained to different application entities operative simultaneously on the same device, these were considered as one statement and device.

Each statement was evaluated against the standard requirements specified in PS 3.2 [1]. Each statement was examined in detail to determine what Service Object Pair (SOP) Classes were specified and in what role as Service Class User (SCU) or Provider(SCP) or both, which Transfer Syntaxes were supported, and what limitations on Associations were present.

III. RESULTS

Thirty-nine (39) statements were obtained, 17 in paper form only and 22 in electronic form or both. Currently 15 of these are available publically on the World Wide Web or by anonymous FTP.

Table 1. Vendors and Organizations.

3M	Icon Medical	Philips
Agfa	Infimed	Picker
Algotec	Intech	Polaroid
ALI	ISG	Sectra-Imtec
Cemax	Mallinckrodt Institute	Siemens
Duke University	Merge	SMS
EMED	Mitra	UCDMC
GE	PBT	

Statements were obtained from 23 vendors and organizations listed in Table 1.

Table 2. Types of devices.

6	Gateways and convertors
13	Primary acquisition devices
4	Image archives
11	Workstations
3	Printing devices
2	Test software suites

The types of devices represented are displayed in Table 2.

All statements complied with the layout specified in PS 3.2 [1]. All statements contained sufficient information to determine the parameters being evaluated.

Only one statement indicate support for offline media as defined in PS 3.10,11 and 12 [2,3,4].

Table 3. Composite Image Storage SOP Class support.

SOP Class	SCU	SCP	Both	Total
CR	2	6	14	22
CT	9	6	17	32
MR	7	6	17	30
US (old)	2	5	12	19
US MF (old)	0	2	9	11
US (new)	0	0	0	0
US MF (new)	0	0	0	0
NM (old)	1	4	11	16
NM (new)	0	1	3	4
SC	7	5	16	28
XA Single	0	1	3	4
XA Biplane	0	0	2	2
RF	1	1	3	5
Overlay	2	0	7	9
Curve	0	0	7	7
Modality LUT	0	0	6	6
VOI LUT	0	0	6	6
Any	14	6	17	37

Support of various Composite Image Storage SOP Classes is displayed in Table 3.

Table 4. Query/Retrieve SOP Class support.

SOP Class	SCU	SCP	Both	Total
Patient Root	4	7	2	13
Get	0	4	1	5
Move	4	6	2	12
Both Get & Move	0	3	1	4
Study Root	5	10	3	18
Get	0	4	1	5
Move	5	9	3	17
Both Get & Move	0	3	1	4
Patient/Study Root	3	6	2	11
Get	0	4	0	4
Move	3	6	2	11
Both Get & Move	0	4	0	4
Any	5	10	4	19

Support of various Query/Retrieve SOP Classes is displayed in Table 4.

Table 5. Print Management Meta SOP Class support.

Meta-SOP Class		SCU	SCP	Both	Total
Gray					
	Basic	4	3	2	9
	Referenced	0	1	0	1
Color					
	Basic	1	1	0	2
	Referenced	1	1	0	2
Any		4	3	2	9

Support of various Print Management Meta SOP Classes is displayed in Table 5.

All statements indicated support for the default little endian byte order implicit value representation transfer syntax, for all presentation contexts, as is mandated by the standard. Fifteen (15) other devices variously supported either the little endian or big endian byte order explicit value representation or both. Three (3) devices supported some form of compression transfer syntax, one image server indicating support for all JPEG transfer syntaxes, another image server supporting JPEG lossless 8 bit non-hierarchical transfer syntax with any predictor, and one workstation supporting JPEG lossless 8 bit non-hierarchical with a predictor selection value of 1.

Two (2) devices supported negotiation of asynchronous windows on association establishment, 15 devices did not limit the number of associations accepted, for 8 devices this parameter was configurable, and for 6 this parameter was fixed at ranges from 4 to 20 in order to limit downgrading of performance with multiple simultaneous associations.

All network support utilized TCP/IP. No statement indicated support for OSI protocols.

IV. DISCUSSION

Though some vendors eagerly supplied Conformance Statements upon request, in other cases they were not as readily forthcoming. In some instances, statements were provided by competitors, customers in other marketing regions, or other interested parties. Several major vendors totally ignored repeated requests at trade shows and by electronic mail and failed to provide statements directly at all.

Despite these difficulties, reasonable coverage of a large number of both major and minor vendors was obtained. European and North American vendors are well represented. Not one statement was forthcoming from a Japanese vendor.

During the survey period a request for proposals for an acquisition device indicating that bids must be accompanied by a DICOM Conformance Statement satisfying the DICOM requirements in the proposal, resulted in not one of the 5 bidders presenting such a statement, though 4 of the 5 were known to comply with the specifications.

Towards the end of the survey there was a noticeable improvement in the availability of statements, particularly in electronic form. Despite this, the awareness of the critical importance of the Conformance Statement amongst those responsible for purchasing on the consumers side, and sales on the vendors side seems remarkably low. Continuation and expansion of the major educational effort in this regard is necessary.

All the statements that were available were complete, well presented, and compliant with the requirements of the standard, though some were more informative than others particularly with regard to which type 3 attributes were supported and in what manner.

Of those statements made available, the majority were for either acquisition devices acting as composite image Storage SOP Class Users, or workstations acting as composite image Storage SOP Class Providers or both Users and Providers.

Few acquisition devices provided Query/Retrieve SCP services, nor did all workstations act as Query/Retrieve SCUs. Of those that did, the preferred service is the C-Move rather than the C-Get. Only one workstation claimed to provide C-Get as an SCU, which leaves the one image archive server that only offers C-get as an SCP with few connection options. This presumably reflects the simplicity of implementing the C-Move service on a separate association as opposed to sharing and turning around the existing association for C-Get requested C-Store sub-operations.

Only a small number statements covering Print devices was available, and not surprisingly most of these covered devices offering the Basic Grayscale Meta SOP Class as an SCP. Notably, few workstations and primary aquisition devices supported this class as an SCU, indicating that printing from these devices is for now obtained outside the context of DICOM.

No statements indicated support for the new part PS 3.13 [5] covering point-to-point communications support for printing. Whether this reflects lack of implementation or merely the immense difficulty of obtaining recently approved parts from NEMA is uncertain.

Of the statements surveyed, very few indicated support for other than the mandatory default transfer syntax. The use of alternative transfer syntaxes that don't offer compression and hence any significant performance advantage may seem pointless to most implementors. This state of affairs may change as wider support for offline file formats as described in PS 3.10 [2] is offered, since the little endian byte order explicit value representation is mandated for the File Meta-Information Header and the DICOM Directory File.

Support for JPEG transfer syntaxes seems sporadic, and in most cases confined to the lossless form of compression also utilized in the cardiac angiographic media storage application profile[4]. The author of the one server claiming to offer all defined JPEG transfer syntaxes may not have been aware that a composite image Storage SOP Class SCU and SCP storing an image offered in a compressed syntax is required to be able to translate it to the default transfer syntax to transfer it to another SCP that does not support the compressed transfer syntax, rather than merely regurgitating the stored byte stream.

In conclusion, despite the high quality of the surveyed statements, the difficulty with which they were obtained is dismaying, and indicates a need for continued education of vendors and consumers. The DICOM conformance described in the statements is largely confined to simple TCP/IP network transfer and retrieval and printing of images with minimal support of the more advanced elements of DICOM. OSI support is non-existent. Offline media seem largely ignored by all but the cardiologists.

V. ADDENDUM

More detailed and recently updated summary information outlining the services described in each Conformance Statement is always available electronically from "http://www.rahul.net/dclunie/dicom-conformance/survey.html".

VI. REFERENCES

1. ACR/NEMA DICOM PS 3.2 - Conformance.
2. ACR/NEMA DICOM PS 3.10 - Media Storage & File Format.
3. ACR/NEMA DICOM PS 3.11 - Media Storage Application Profiles.
4. ACR/NEMA DICOM PS 3.12 - Media Formats & Physical Media.
5. ACR/NEMA DICOM PS 3.13 - Print Management Point-To-Point Communication Support.

MUMC IMACS: A Digital Image Display, Communication and Management System

D.B. Kenyon, L. Tan, D.M. Hynes, G.W. Stevenson and C. Nahmias
Department of Radiology, Chedoke-McMaster Hospitals and McMaster University
Hamilton, Ontario, Canada

INTRODUCTION

McMaster University Medical Centre (MUMC) is a 656-bed health care institution with a complete range of diagnostic imaging services encompassing plain film radiography, Computed Radiography (CR), Digital Fluoroscopy, Digital Angiography, CT, MRI, Ultrasound, Positron Tomography (PET) and other nuclear medicine techniques. The need for a well-designed image management and communication system (IMACS) has produced the MUMC IMACS, which is capable of adapting to changing technology and expanding with increasing demands on digital imaging. At the same time, MUMC IMACS is easily accessible and adaptable to the needs of the radiologists and physicians who access diagnostic images daily. This paper describes the implementation and current state of the art of the MUMC IMACS. A discussion of several key issues follows the description of the system.

MUMC IMACS

MUMC IMACS was developed to link all of the existing digital acquisition devices in the Department with workstations, printers, and storage devices in one high-speed network. Currently, the devices on the network include two fluoroscopy units (GE DRS Prestilix 1600X and 1694D), two angiography units (GE DX LUA and AFM), a Fuji AC-1 CR unit, a GE 9800Q CT scanner, a GE Signa 1.5T MR Imager, a CTI/Siemens ECAT 953/31 PET scanner, and three gamma cameras. An ALI mini-PACS serving Ultrasound will soon be linked to the MUMC IMACS network. Two 3M XL Laser Imagers, the film processor on the Fuji CR unit, and a Codonics NP 1600 (600 dpi, colour) dye sublimation paper printer serve the network's hardcopy needs. As well, there are 7 primary viewing area imaging workstations (Sun Sparcstations with MUMC software, both described below), 1 workstation in the Intensive Care Unit, and 8 other Sun workstations for imaging research and development. Analogic DASM devices provide the interface between the Sun machines and the CR unit, and between the Sun machines and the 3M Laser Imagers.

Network

MUMC IMACS runs on a 10Mb/s ethernet TCP/IP communications network spread over two floors of the Medical Centre. A fibre-optic cable between the two floors acts as a trunk to which five coaxial (thin-net) subnets (Radiography & Fluoroscopy, CT, Angiography, MRI, and Nuclear Medicine) are connected (Figure 1). Links to the Hospital Information System (VAX/VMS) and to the network server (DEC Alpha) of Radiology Department PC LAN are via Network File System (NFS) protocols.

Image acquisition

A requirement from the outset was to acquire raw image data directly from the scanners, at their original resolution and bit depth. For CT, MRI, and CR, software routines poll the acquisition devices for the presence of new exams. For CT and MRI, the software routine queries the GE consoles and transfers any new series to an intermediate database. From here, the series are converted and transferred to the MUMC IMACS, and the MUMC IMACS database is updated. With digital fluoroscopy, a transfer request is initiated at the GE console by the technologist. The study is then automatically sent to a MUMC IMACS file server via File Transfer Protocol (FTP). Transfers of studies from the gamma cameras are initiated by the radiographer at the console, and a GE proprietary software performs the file transfer to the MUMC IMACS. With the PET scanner, a MUMC IMACS program converts and transfers PET studies to the MUMC IMACS database.

Database management

Each acquired image or exam is automatically entered into the MUMC IMACS database, identified by patient name, patient ID, date and time of exam, exam type, number of images, and a status of 'filmed' or 'not filmed', 'reported' or 'unreported'. As well, the database keeps track of the network location of each study (be it on a magnetic disk, an optical disk, or a tape).

Workstations

Imaging workstations are located in every primary reporting area, eg. Chest, Fluoroscopy, CT, MRI, etc. These workstations have full capabilities for viewing and manipulating images as well as network database querying, all through software described below. A typical reporting area workstation is a Sun Sparcstation IPX (or better) running SunOS or Solaris, with a 424MB internal disk, a 2.4GB external hard disk, a minimum of 32MB RAM, two 1000-line 16" or 20" colour monitors, a keyboard and a mouse. The Chest workstation, which handles the most demanding of the digital image types, 2Kx2K CR images, is equipped with two 2000-line high luminance black and white monitors.

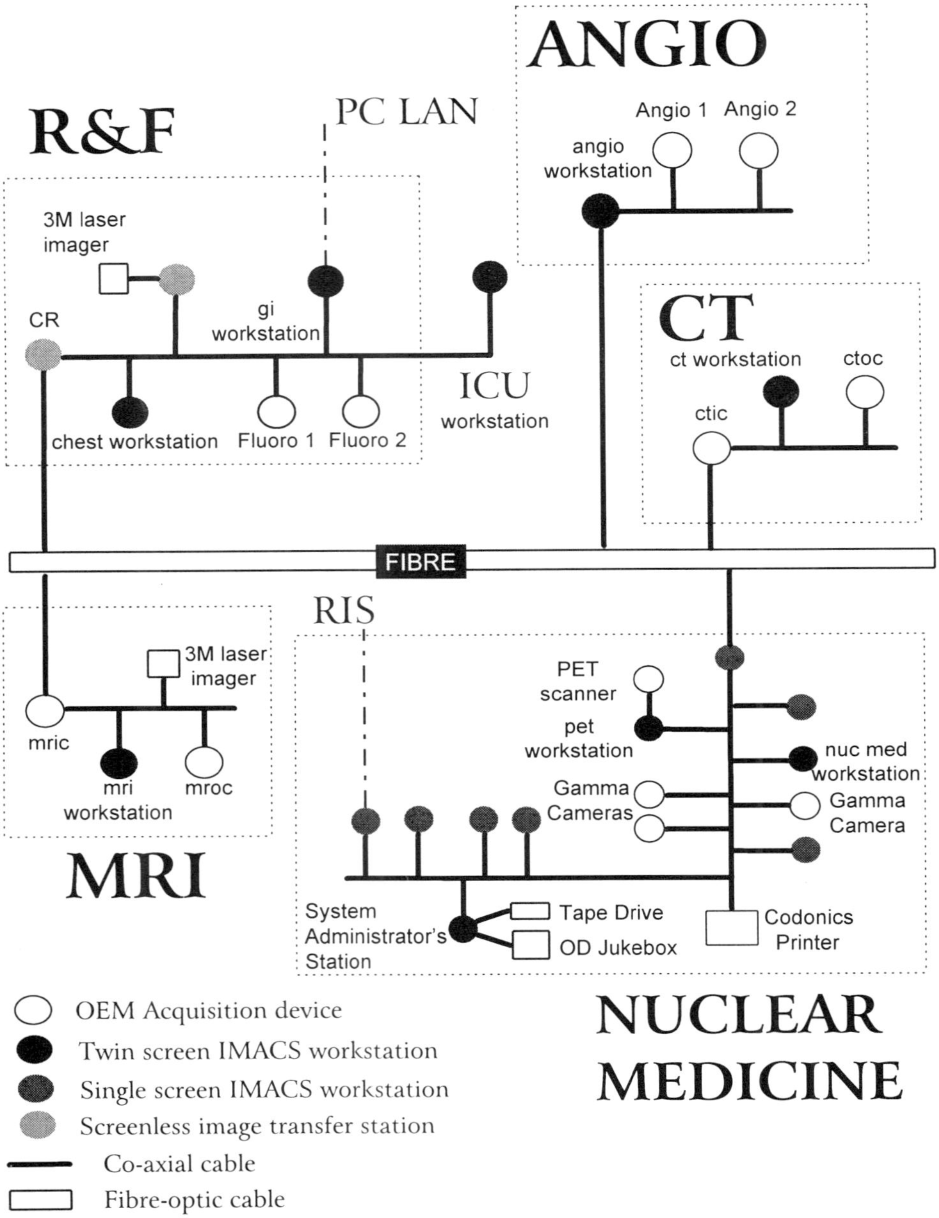

Figure 1. MUMC IMACS network diagram

Image display and manipulation

Image viewing software was designed for the imaging workstations with direct input from radiologists. Functions are taken or adapted from a comprehensive X-window based package called MUMC Display, to create simplified icon-driven Image Viewers customized to the needs of each primary reporting area. Each Viewer package has full capabilities for network database query, full resolution image display, customized film printing formats, and the generation of softcopy consultation films. Image manipulation functions which are integrated as required for each modality include real-time window and levelling, pan and zoom, image rotation and flipping, length and ROI measurements, and many sophisticated routines available from MUMC Display. All of the Viewers share a similar look and functionality, and all are accessible from an icon toolbar on every workstation.

Storage and archiving

Short-term on-line storage of images are on typically 2.4 GB magnetic disks, each dedicated to storing images from one modality only. These disks are attached to each of the seven primary imaging workstations (associated with the seven imaging modalities), which then act as file servers for images of that modality. Automatic routines carry out nightly transfers of images (1500MB/day losslessly compressed to 500MB) from these local disks to a 56-platter optical disk jukebox, and free up the necessary space on the local disks for the next day's image acquisition. Depending on image modality, each local disk stores from 3-10 days of current images. Beyond that, the optical disk jukebox archive serves online image retrieval requests for exams up to 3 months old. Backup of five optical disks to 8mm digital video tape is done manually once every 10 days. A RAID disk has been added to the network to provide fast-access high density storage, and is in the process of evaluation.

Image retrieval

Upon request, studies which have been archived to optical disk or to digital tape can be easily retrieved. A *Jukebox Retrieve* program automatically accesses the optical jukebox or tape and transfers a copy of the selected study to the IMACS workstation. A typical CT study with 30 images takes about 2.5 minutes for retrieval.

Integration with RIS

The IMACS has established an ethernet link with the Radiology Information System (RIS). Text reports are automatically copied from the RIS to a common file server. The IMACS automatically polls the file server every hour to determine the presence of new reports. New reports are matched to digital consultation films, and the RIS database is updated with a softcopy of the digital film. Both the IMACS workstations and the PC-based RIS workstations are then able to display both text report and digital consultation film on-screen, simultaneously.

DISCUSSION

MUMC IMACS has been in place for two years. The network and the image viewers have been developed to a mature and stable level of functionality. The introduction of the IMACS into the work processes of the department has been a gradual and phased process. Presently, although all reporting is still done from printed film, many of these films are being composed from the IMACS workstations.

Benefits to the work process

The IMACS provides many benefits to the work process – fast, online, one-stop database searching and retrieval of diagnostic images and online consultation films; flexibility in image manipulation; flexibility in filming; efficient retrieval of lost films, thus reducing the need for repeat examinations; and the integration of text reports with online consultation films. These benefits are achieved through a network database and distributed data storage; through keeping to the premise of storing original images without compromising the image data; and through easily customized image viewer software.

Integration and expandability

From a system design perpective, MUMC IMACS, through customized software routines built on the X-Window platform and through the use of widely available hardware, is capable of running on different platforms and integrating all types of acquisition devices. In this way, the system has circumvented the need to purchase equipment from a sole manufacturer. The network itself is easily expandable by installing the desired network cabling. Thus the network can be upgraded as higher performance networking technologies become more available and less expensive.

Storage redundancy

There is a need for more redundancy in the way IMACS stores images. Presently, for most of the modalities, the daily images reside in a minimum of two locations at any one time – the acquisition device disk, and the IMACS local disk. However, in the case of CR, the CR unit does not store data after it has been processed by the unit. If a system failure prevented immediate acquisition of CR data from the unit to the IMACS server, then the data is lost and cannot be recovered. A second storage area where redundancy is required is in both the optical disk and the tape archives. There are periods of time when images on the optical disk are the sole copies on the IMACS network. With the recent installation of the RAID, and the future installation of a tape jukebox, we plan to provide a satisfactory level of storage redundancy. This point will be especially important when hardcopy filming is eliminated.

Dicom compliance

MUMC IMACS was designed to integrate acquisition devices which were already in place in the department long before the introduction of the DICOM 3.0 standard. In recent months, we have put DICOM protocols into place, and have successfully tested their functionality in the transfer of images from the GE Signa MR Imager to the MUMC IMACS. Consequently, while many PACS systems offer the promise of compliance to the DICOM 3.0 standard, MUMC IMACS has proven its versatility in handling both old and new image transfer protocols, thereby circumventing the need to depend solely on one manufacturer in order to ensure compatibility.

Film or filmless

Presently, hardcopy films continue to be printed and filed in film bags. The issue of whether or not to go filmless is irrelevant to the development of the network, since the IMACS provides the ability to carry out filmless reporting as well as the ability to print hardcopy films.

Beyond the Radiology Department

Currently we are developing plans for expanding to other key areas of the hospital which frequently require diagnostic images, such as Emergency, ORs, Orthopedics, Neonatal, etc. Our first extension outside the Department of Radiology was the placement of a workstation and a customized Image Viewer package in the Intensive Care Unit. Benefits have already shown to be in the immediate availability of the images for timely monitoring of a patient's progress.

MUMC IMACS is successful as a totally integrated image management and communication system because it is designed for the way we work at McMaster University Medical Centre, a medium-sized facility equipped with all of the digital imaging modalities. Although the physical state of MUMC IMACS is continually changing with the addition of and adaptation to newer technologies, its fundamental design premises remain to ensure its continued integration and expansion.

Integrated PACS with HIS, RIS and Reporting System

Nabuo Okazaki, M.D.
Respiratory Division and Information Medicine, Toshiba General Hospital, Shinagawa Tokyo, Japan
Gen Kubota, M.D.
Department of Radiology, Toshiba General Hospital Shinagawa, Tokyo, Japan
Akihiro Toshimitu, M.S., Shinichi Tsubura, M.S., Eitaro Nishihara, M.S. and Toshihiko Kihara, M.S.
Toshiba Corporation, Tokyo, Japan
Osamu Hasumi, B.S. and Hiroyuki Okubo, B.S.
Toshiba Medical Engineering Company, Ltd., Tokyo, Japan

1 Introduction

Since 1993, the Toshiba General Hospital has installed the Hospital Information System(HIS) directly connected to the Pharmacy Information System(PHS), the Laboratory Information System(LIS) and the Radiological Information system(RIS) with the Picture Archiving and Communication System(PACS). Clinicians input the orders of the prescription, laboratory and radiological examination into HIS. Then, the history of the prescriptions, the laboratory data and orders can be displayed on HIS workstations in the outpatients' clinics and wards. PACS and Reporting System were only serving in the radiological department[1-3]. At this phase, clinicians refer the paper reports and the film images from the department of the radiology.

In the next phase, PACS was expanded the service of the outpatients' clinics in the end of 1995 as shown in Fig.1. It is integrated with HIS for realizing the filmless outpatients' clinics. We report our experience of using the HIS/PACS integration to help our medical decision making process and the informed contents to the patients.

2 System Requirements of Clinicians in Toshiba General Hospital

The Toshiba General Hospital has 310 beds and about 900 outpatients' visits a day. It has 20 clinics. 100% of clinicians have been routinely using the workstations of HIS in the outpatients' clinics and wards. Their works in the outpatients' clinics are to read all medical images in the purpose of the double check and the explanation of the results, the diagnosis and the treatment to the patient. They must do those works during the 7 to 10 minutes medical consultation time because of so many patients consulting.

Major requirements of systems in outpatients' clinics can

1) display the diagnosable images on PACS workstations
2) compare the previous examinations on PACS workstations
3) display radiological reports on HIS workstations
4) know the urgent information backing on HIS workstations
5) acquire every information by using one key.

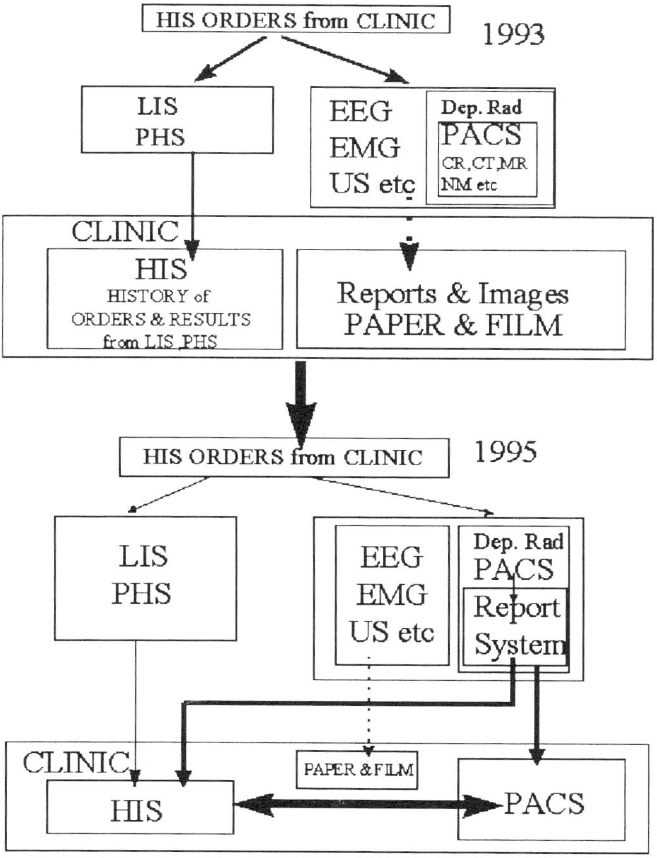

Fig.1 LIS: laboratory information system PHS: pharmacy information system
Doted line: non-digital information Solid line: digital information

3 System Issues for Clinical Requirements

3-1 Displaying Diagnostic Images

Clinicians want to display the diagnostic images on HIS workstations. However, the HIS workstations do not have enough quality to display the radiological images because of the color and low resolution monitors. Therefore the high quality monitors as shown in Fig2 were equipped in the outpatients' clinics. The diagnostic images without compression are sent from the file server in the radiological department to the clinic PACS workstations through the FDDI (data volume is CR 2kx2kx10bits, CT 512x512x8bits, MR 256x256x8bits, NM depends on images).

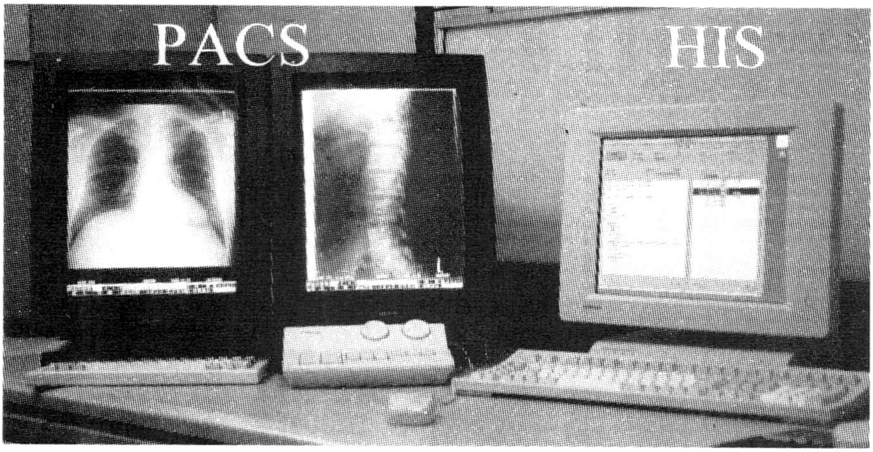

Fig. 2 Monitor of PACS and HIS at Clinic

3-2 Prefetching Algorithm for Comparing Previous Images

It is very important to compare current images with the previous images for reading the images. Many clinicians want to refer the images of the multi-modality and/or the marked images which have significant meanings. For example, the CR and CT or CR and MR images just before and after the treatment and the admission etc.

To solve these requirements, the prefetching algorithm was installed into original PACS that was running in the department of the radiology. The prefetching algorithm for clinical PACS is considered to be sent the images of high priority. However it should not to reduce the current system performance. Our newly developed algorithm has two parts as shown in fig.3. One is the images that are not yet explained to the patient at the outpatients' clinic (NYEPC). Another one is the images that are already explained to the patient at the outpatients' clinic (AEPC). PACS can recognize the difference between them by getting the date of the last and the reserved visit from HIS database.

In NYEPC, the system sends all NYECP with the previous and/or marked exams of the same modality and body position at first. Next, the images of other modality with the same body position are sent. In AEPC, the system sends the latest and marked images. When PACS get the date of the exams and the body position obtained from HIS, it can select the images of the high priority[4].

3-3 Timing of Image Prefetching and Selecting Destination

If the prefetching images of all departments are transferred from the file server to the PACS workstations at outpatients' clinics, the load of net work exceeds the performance of our system. Therefore, the system needs to limit the destination of the departments and to send the prefetching images during the night time. If PACS can get the patient's next visiting date, the system can send all prefetching data during the night time until the next visit. Our PACS have realized to send the prefetching images by getting the reserved date of next consultation from HIS database.

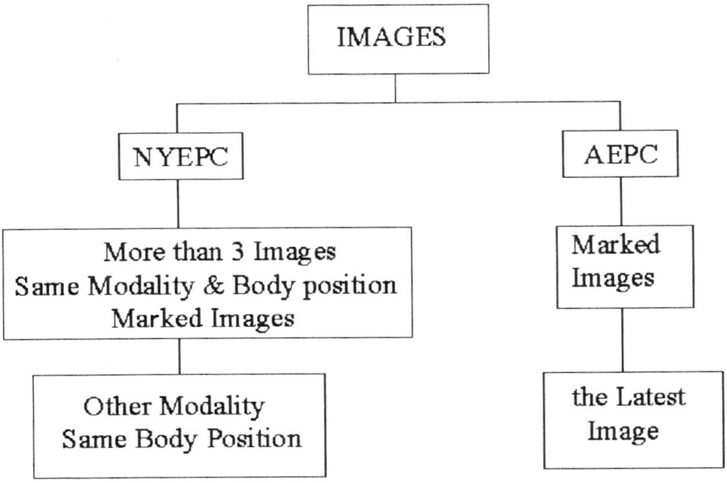

Fig. 3 Prefetching Algorithm in our System

NYEPC: not yet explain images to the patient at clinic
AEPC : already explain images to the patient at clinic

The result of the departmental characters as shown in Fig.4. It shows the rate of the reserved visit, the NYEPC, the immediately back images to the outpatients' clinic(IBIC) and the expected rate of the prefetching a day. The department of the orthopedics has the low rate of the consultation reservation and the high rate of IBIC as compared with the other department. On the other hand, the department of the respiratory division has as the high expected rate of prefetching and the middle rate of the NYEPC and the IBIC as shown in figure. If we chose these departments to expand PACS, the system's work load is exceeded to our capacity. Therefore, we chose two departments, neurosurgery and urology, for the prototype system. Because these two departments need the diagnostic images in the outpatients' clinic and have many urgent orders properly.

Department	Number of Patients' visits a day	reserved visit %	NYEPC %	IBIC %	expected prefetch rate %
Orthopedics	31	65	2	54	61
Urology	39	90	6	23	46
Neurosurgery	38	90	20	10	71
Respiratory	25	95	25	21	100

Fig.4 Departmental Characters of Images

NYEPC: not yet explained images to the patient at outpatients' clinic
IBIC: immediately back images at outpatients' clinic

3-4 Referring Images and Reports in Outpatients' Clinic

Patient ID and order number of HIS flow between PACS workstations and HIS workstations. The HIS workstations and the PACS workstations are connected in the same outpatients' clinics. Then, it is realized that clinicians can get the reports on the HIS workstations and images on the PACS workstations immediately after selecting the patient name from HIS. It can display the reports on the HIS workstations by pushing the button on the PACS workstation. Also, it can display the images on the PACS workstation by selecting the HIS workstation button.

3-5 Urgent Information

Clinicians want to know the timing of the patient call to explain the urgent images and the results. In our system, the urgent information input into HIS is transmitted to PACS. When the urgent images and reports are backed to the outpatients' clinics from the radiological department, HIS can show the special mark on the patient waiting list. Then, the clinician can see the patient of the IBIC.

4 Conclusions

Our system is realizing the integration between HIS and PACS in the outpatients' clinics. In that results, clinicians can refer many images on the PACS workstations by pushing the HIS buttons. For getting this results, we clarify that the most important information among the systems is the patient ID, the order number of HIS and the latest and the reserved date of the consultation.

After the installation of our system, our clinicians use the images on the CRT instead of the films for explaining the results to the patient. Clinicians told us the system is very convenient. We think our system is well accepted by our clinicians even though the system does not support all the clinician's work completely. This system integration work resulted our clinicians to be interested in and motivated to use the digitized information system on their clinical practice.

Reference

1. Eitaro Nishihara et all: RIS/PACS Architecture to Assist Daily Practical Reading at Toshiba Hospital. Proc SPIE; 2165,172-175,1994
2 Eitaro Nishihara et all: Integrated RIS/PACS Architecture for Daily Practical Reading (Utilization of HIS/RIS Information for Image Distribution) Proc SCAR;219-226,1994
3 Gen Kubota et all: Evaluation of time-effectiveness in RIS/PACS based radiology department Japan J. of Clinical Radiology;40,13,1585-1591,1995(Japanese)
4 Akihiro Toshimitu et all: The Toshiba General Hospital for routine in and out-patient clinics ProcSPIE 1996 ,353

A "Personal" Medical Image/Information Processing System

Jeffrey P. Leal, B.A. and Jonathan M. Links, Ph.D.
Quantitative Image Analysis Laboratory
Department of Radiology, Johns Hopkins Medical Institutions, Baltimore, Maryland

I. INTRODUCTION

The greatest challenge facing those who manage or implement computing applications in Radiology departments is the consolidation of tasks and processes currently diversified among several platforms and systems into a unified "environment". From ordering a study, through image acquisition and analysis, to the final reporting, several different, and disparate, systems are currently used, with data often transferred from one system to another by hand. While the networking of systems has facilitated the digital transfer of data, automated, seamless distribution of processes between processing systems and consolidation of user-access features through an integrated user-interface still need to be realized. We believe that, as personal computer platforms become increasingly powerful, and their operating systems become likewise more sophisticated, tasks once delegated to powerful — yet expensive — workstations, or dispersed piecemeal among many different systems, can be consolidated onto a single, economical desktop system or controlled by a "smart" network of systems via a unified user-interface.

II. VISION

Our vision of the ultimate Image/Information Processing System for a Radiology department of the future is an integrated client/server system utilizing industry standard network protocols, user-interfaces and operating systems along with industry standard data access methods. Preferably, this system would make use of economical clients which could off-load tasks to the server, or other available clients, as the need arises.

By employing the client/server paradigm, multiple systems are *integrated* to form a system that is more powerful than simply the sum of its individual parts. By using industry standard data access methods, such as SQL database queries, formats and database servers, data from multiple sources and of multiple types — possibly even stored on multiple physical servers — are *consolidated* with respect to access and queries. Finally, tasks once limited to a particular machine architecture, or machine configuration become *incorporated* into the system as a whole and accessible to clients anywhere in the system, as the server intelligently manages and distributes processing resources. Processes need not be performed on the client machine requesting the process. Instead, they can be performed on the processing system best suited for that particular task. Only the results of the process need be directed to the requesting client.

III. FIRST STEP

As a step in this direction, we have developed a 'Personal Image Processor': *Imager-3D* — a software package running under the MS-Windows operating system on a PC. *Imager-3D* allows the user to perform most of the image processing tasks which previously could only be done on a workstation-class system. These include windowed display with 8-bit palette, image resampling and co-registration, spatial and Fourier filtering, and image quantification.

Imager-3D was developed from the ground-up using Object-Oriented Programming (OOP) techniques. While the original version was a stand-alone, single-tasking application, its OOP architecture facilitated the modelling of data and functionality in the client/server model described above. The system is multi-modal, thus integrating data from a variety of modalities: PET, SPECT, CT, MRI, Ultrasound, as well as non-medical modalities such as electron microscopy and satellite imaging. In the OOP model, data became encapsulated into a data object. Multiple data objects could then be integrated by the application. An example is the integration of PET and MRI data. MRI data can be overlayed and registered with a PET dataset, allowing simultaneous region-of-interest (ROI) placement on the anatomical MRI and quantitative analysis of the functional PET image.

Functionality also becomes encapsulated in the OOP model, and distributed and shared between data instances. Functionality can also be added at run-time, by the run-time linking of user-written code modules (Dynamic Linked Libraries — DLLs — in MS-Windows). Thus, the system, at run-time, can encapsulate an unknown process and execute it with an encapsulated data object, regardless of the underlying data type — incorporating a family of processes under the management of a single system.

IV. HISTORY

Imager-3D was developed to solve a very real problem — to provide our PET investigators with a tool with which they could display and perform quantitative region-of-interest analysis of their PET data. The PC was the target platform as it represented the most accessible machine for our users at that time. Because of the multi-modal nature of PET data analysis, data type and format independence was mandated from the start of the project.

V. PRESENT STATUS

The currently-released version of *Imager-3D* employs and offers a powerful set of image/information tools to the image analyst. First, it offers a system which runs on an off-the-shelf PC system running MS-Windows 3.1 (or greater) with a 256 color display (or greater), which will load and display most image data one might encounter (excluding proprietarily formatted or encrypted data). Supported data types include 8-bit integer pixels through 64-bit floating-point pixels and even 32-bit floating point complex pixel structures. The system provides for 8-bit display of image data with user-controllable window and level with palette manipulation. It employs the Multiple-Document-Interface (MDI), which offers a consistant look and feel across applications on the desktop as well as the ability to simultaneously work with several data sets at the same time.

The feature list of the application is long and extensive, but hightlights include the following: the integration of a variety of file formats, including DICOM v3.0; quantitative region-of-interest (ROI) analysis with various ROI types (i.e., rectangular, elliptical, polygonal, auto edge-detected); image filtering (both spatial and Fourier domains);

image resampling (2-, 3- dimensional resampling as well as oblique volume resampling employing multiple user-selectable interpolation algorithms); and a user-programming API, enabling users to write their own image/information processing code and have it executed within the framework of the application and its encapsulated data objects.

VI. CURRENT DEVELOPMENT

Our current development efforts have involved extending our past efforts to more fully embrace our stated goals: *integration*, *consolidation*, and *incorporation*. To this end, our next generation system, tentatively named *Imager-95*, makes greater use of Object-Linking and Embedding (OLE), thus integrating *Imager-95* with other desktop applications and applets. Also, whereas the previous version permitted encapsulated processes, the new version extends that encapsulation by running select processes as their own separate threads of execution. Thus, at least on a multiple-processor system, processes are free to run on whichever processor the host finds most suitable. Processes are now “free” to execute with peak efficiency wherever and however the “server” (read Operating System) dictates, while remaining incorporated under the umbrella of the host application.

The most difficult, yet exciting, development taking place is the effort to consolidate data on a grand scale; that is, consolidating access to data through a single, industry standard network database. Initial efforts are limited to specific data types residing on a single server, and are also limited in functionality to primarily storing and retrieving data “blobs” through an industry standard database server.

VII. FUTURE DEVELOPMENT

The next phase of development for this system will involve the complete integration of the client software onto the desktop by turning it into both an OLE client and OLE server. This moves the image data into the position of primary focus while the application quietly sits in the background, appearing only when called.

Incorporation of remote processes and processors will be handled by an extension of the already encapsulated threaded processes to Remote-Procedure-Calls (RPCs). The processes which are currently running as individual threads on the client machine will now be free to execute on other machines. As this is handled by the operating system, the applications will be self-scaling, utilizing a single processor as efficiently as possible on a stand-alone machine, while utilizing multiple processors on a multi-processor or networked workstation without a single change in code.

The consolidation of data through network databasing will be extended through the development of more "data intelligent" objects and communication between multiple databases.

VIII. SUMMARY

We have demonstrated the usefulness of employing industry standard machines, operating systems, and tools in the clinical and research Radiology environment. It is our belief that further embracing these standards and environments will lead to more successful, efficient, and economical use of existing and future systems.

How Much Bang for the Software Buck? Guides for Choosing Productive Applications

Karl T. Dockray, MD, DABR, ABNM
Lubbock, Texas

ABSTRACT. Productivity applications suites are several programs integrated to make work better, faster and cheaper. As a Swiss knife cuts, bores, and magnifies, combined softwares should provide five solutions for a broad spectrum of jobs. These are the making of records, their messaging, storage, retrieval and finally, the analyses of results. The major solutions must address fifteen specific information management challanges as they take, hold and manipulate any concept symbolized by alphanumeric characters now put on paper.

In this presentation, institutional recommendations for the ideal electronic medical record have been reviewed and annotated with results from one early productivity suite. Its use helped one x-ray interpretor make immediate faxed reports by cutting entry typing 84% and the computed replay of old reports cut diagnostic error rates for new reports fifty percent. Automated coding of diagnoses and charges decreased billing entry costs by half.

PROPOSITIONS

Computer applications for televideo and image archiving have raced ahead (1). But, few programs help with the repetitive jobs of registrations, labeling films, transmitting reports and then satisfying the post-hoc mandates of managed care (2).

Most radiologists still tape their dictation, wait for transcripts, and lose more time with proof reading (3). Information that could help doctors be better diagnosticians remains hidden in paper journals and shelved books.

Medical softwares trying to help with these problems fail because they do not meet the three computer imperatives of faster, better and cheaper. Single-function programs run slowly because they are scattered between differing machines and even differing directories of the same computer (4).

Five elements of information processing need integration to record, message, store, retrieve and count...anything.

Business softwares are good at single projects but fail in medicine because our work requirements are radically different. We see patients in groups, lists and batches. Recent medical softwares fail because they are heavily reliant on mouse control to issue work commands. Precise eye-hand coordination is required before a button click makes something happen. And, mice are like first-day assistants that have to be told exactly what to do each time each new task comes up (5).

Gates estimates that there can be "softer software" in the sense that programmed agents will learn about us as we do our jobs. The agents will then help us with improved strategies, auto-sequencing or forms of power assistance.

One productivity suite has some of these powered features in that it automatically screens the next-logical entry fields of repetitive records-making jobs. Operators are freed from mice so eyes and brains can concentrate on the job. Touch-typed entries need only a glancing check by the operator to verify what is going on the screen.

A last difference between healthcare and business. Medical workers are now forced by government and the regulators of managed care to make regular analyses of what we do, see and decide. This is relatively easy if information programs have supporting relational databases. Some do. Most do not.

Old programs and legacy machinery allowed only focused or single solutions to patient registration, appointments and billing. New softwares need to be the electric equivalent of a Swiss knife integrating many utilities for us. In the following, fifteen institutional recommendations for ideal electronic patient records are examined in terms of the results found in processing 100,000 cases with one early productivity suite.

1. PATIENT IDENTIFICATION
As pointed out by the Medical Records Institute, stored information must be linked with a patient's computed identity (6). This can be done by putting a multi-element header at the top of each record, procedure or finding. But, thirty-eight percent of machine-registered, unchecked names contained spelling errors of one kind or another. Creation of an automated identity checker reduced these errors to eight percent.

2.ELIGIBILITY DETERMINATION
This is taken as data showing whether or not some institution will pay for a given client's care. One suite does it by recording free text or abbreviation/acronyms indicating insurance coverages. The same eligibility record can show known allergies, advance patient directives and alerts to patient-name changes from marriage or divorce.

3. ACCESSION OF ALL PATIENT INFORMATION WITHIN AN ENTERPRISE
This function is to save knowledge workers the reading of lengthy paper charts. One applications program enables a file-naming strategy that will abstract data only from specific clinical activities. It can recover 172 specially named files out of 66,000 others in 5 seconds. The complete transcript of any single record appears in three more.

4. RECORD THE HEALTH CARE PROCESS
Menued check lists and templates have been the favored methods for records creation in the past. One system showed entry speeds approaching that of dictation if operators made their own symbolisms, abbreviations, and mnemonics (2). One radiologist recorded 100,000 on-line reports averaging 130 words generated from five entered acronyms and 72 characters of free text. These entries were done in the one minute previously taken by dictation (2).

5. PROVIDE HELP FROM KNOWLEDGE BASES
For radiology, one of the most troublesome problems is that of getting old reports (1,2,3,7). One applications suite screens lists of old reports and their texts as the header of a new report is built (2). If code entry errors are made, an automatic checker presents browse lists closest approximating what the operator may be intending to enter. "Garbage" does not go in the database.

If an operator suffers memory loss, more data can be summoned with function keys. A file of "BREAST FACTS" can be reviewed as a mammogram is being read. Distant information services such as the PaperChase can be dialed (8).

Convention, conference, class and bed-side notes have been taken with the productivity suite installed in a note-book machine. These are then transferred into main systems by disk. This creates an "on-line pearl book" or electric approximation to the pencilled ward notes of Oslerian times (2).

6. DEVELOP AND SUBMIT CARE PLANS
The same case records and memo fields that hold clinical reports can be filled with care plans (9).

7. AUTOMATIC ORDER MANAGEMENT
As in care plan development, orders can be copied from memory caches or written de novo as free text in a patient's order record.

8. PATIENT EDUCATION
Here again, memoranda files can be filled with any material now given to patients as a form.

9. AUTOMATIC CODING AND CLAIM MANAGEMENT
This requirement implies that an approved number be added to every diagnosis and chargable procedure done in patient care (6). One productivity suite automated this. Then, when these numbers were modem-transmitted to a central billing system, clerical salaries dropped 50% because of reduced re-entry costs. Charge captures improved three to five percent (2).

10. REFERRALS AND POST-ENCOUNTER MANAGEMENT FUNCTIONS
Medical records authorities recommend that softwares have the ability to make referral requests and broadcast them by fax, telephone or internet to distant specialists and functionaries. This can be done by appending the patient's record with the question of the primary caregiver and faxing the document to the referrent.

Radiology managers and interpretors worry about report turn-around time (1,3,7). A prototype management survey of on-line reporting showed that 40 percent of patients having a study had their reports returned within hours on the day of examination. The percentage rose to 63 at 24 hours and another 25 percent were available by 48 hours.

11. MESSAGING
Printing a report at one's desk is not messaging, but when typescript is under the eyes of the reader, then, a message has been made. One productivity suite is rigged so that one to four typed initials dial local extensions or international telephone lines. A few more commands send one record, all the results belonging to one physician or mixed strings of reports for one destination. Vocal telephony is speed-dialed this way too (2).

12. BATCHED OR GROUPED INFORMATION MANAGEMENT
Much work can be saved if medical records can be managed in groups, lists and batches (1,2, 6 and 10). For example, several x-ray departments of one rural system run the same productivity software. Technologists register patients, print automated labels from header entries, add notes about film use and then transfer all the data to a disc. The disc and films are taken by courier to a consulting radiologist in a nearby city. Diagnoses are appended to the batched headers and the completed reports faxed back to the originating hospital immediately (2).

13. INVENTORY, COUNTING and ANALYSIS
When open software can record any concept represented by characters on paper, symbolisms can be made that go beyond patient care transactions to inventory supplies or even track errors (2). One radiologist found four percent case errors in 80,000 reports done before computer processing. Then, 30,000 more interpretations were checked to see if errors would be reduced when old reports were reviewed by computed replay. Error rates, following the American College of Radiology's classifcations, dropped to two percent (10).

14.INTERNAL SYSTEM CONTROLS
Systems with many users need controls for a worker's entry and audit trails that show what operations have been done, when and by whom. One productivity suite provides these together with batch processing and control "panels" that can be set to pre-define what the suite will do.

15. COSTS
Software costs and equipment prices vary but fortunately, trends are down. The suite reviewed above was run in standard disc operating system (DOS) machines integrating several off-the-shelf commercial softwares. Custom program-writing and equipment expenses were $262,000 over eleven years (2). Now, the two-disc records management part of the applications suite is advertised at $100. It is given to residents and students on request (11).

In closing, three imperatives of "better, faster and cheaper" usually decide if computer operations will be accepted in medical work. To satisfy these imperatives, five main principles of program design must address the demands posed by fifteen separate functions of medical information processing. One early productivity suite tracking 100,000 patients met many of the ideals specified for electronic medical records by processing information at low cost and recording new care transactions as they occurred. When used in radiology, radiographic interpretations could be done on-line with an 84% reduction in typing, a fifty percent improvement in diagnostic accuracy and a fifty percent reduction in billing salaries.

REFERENCES

1. Safran S, Rind DM, Sands DZ et al: Development of a knowledge-based electronic patient record. M.D. Computing 13:46-54 and 63, 1996
2. Dockray KT: Solo practice management: Value of a computerized Reporting System. AJR 162: 1439-1441, 1994
3. Frank MS and Rowberg AH: Authentication and management of radiologic reports: Value of a computer workstation integrated with a radiology information system. AJR 161: 1309-1311,1993
4. Taira RK, Breant CM, Chan HM et al: Architectural design and tools to supplement the transparent access to hospital information systems, radiology information systems, and picture archiving and communication systems. J Digital Imaging 9:1-10, 1996
5. Gates B: The Road Ahead. New York, NY, Penquin Group, 1995, see p. 84
6. Waegman CP: Toward an Electronic Patient Record V7 #7: p.7. The Medical Records Institute, Newton MA 1995
7. Wheeler PS: Error management and quality assurance. Applied Radiology 1986;Jan/Feb,41-45
8. Horowitz GL and Bleich HL: PaperChase: A computer program to search the medical literature. N Engl J Med 305 (16):924-930, 1981
9. Terry PB: Resuscitation and radiology. Radiol 198: 17-18, 1996
10. Cascade P (ed): American College of Radiology: Quality Improvement Manual. Reston, VA: pp. 1, 3, 5, 6 and Att.B2, p.10
11. American Health Information Management Association's Software Guide, p.4 in J of AHIMA 66:Sept 1995

SESSION 6

Workstation Design

Co-Chairs:

Janice C. Honeyman
Heinz U. Lemke

Computer-Aided Selection of Window and Level for Filmless Radiology

N.D. Sidiropoulos and J.S. Baras
Institute for Systems Research, University of Maryland, College Park, Maryland
E. Siegel, Z. Protopapas, S.M. Pomerantz and B.I. Reiner
Department of Radiology, VA Medical Center, Baltimore, Maryland and the University of Maryland Medical School

1. INTRODUCTION

Radiology is steadily moving towards a filmless environment [1, 2]. Computer workstations used in current PACS systems require radiology technologists or radiologists to modify the window/level settings to optimize the amount of clinically useful information that can be displayed using monitors which are currently limited to the display of only 8 bits of contrast data at a time [3]. This process is time consuming and can also be challenging for a technologist or radiologist and may be very difficult for clinicians utilizing the computer workstation. Additionally, certain types of CR images such as a foot CR typically have one window/level combination that is clinically best for evaluation of the toes, another window/level combination for the metatarsals, and still another for the hindfoot. The purpose of this study is to test the clinical efficacy of a computer algorithm[1] [4] designed to derive one or more optimal window/level settings based upon an analysis of image content for a computed radiography (CR) image.

The algorithm was sufficiently efficient to be able to suggest window/level combinations which correlated well with those subjectively determined independently by radiologists experienced in soft copy interpretation, and do so in about one second on a Macintosh Quadra 950 or Pentium 90 class computer workstation.

Manual optimization of window/level is time consuming, and, if performed incorrectly by a user not expert in soft-copy interpretation, it might result in a missed diagnosis or misdiagnosis. The algorithm that was tested increased the speed and accuracy of window/level optimization especially for an inexperienced user (the first author), and correlated well with the settings used by experienced

[1] This algorithm is the subject of a patent disclosure

radiologists. The routine incorporation of this algorithm as a workstation tool would increase productivity in a radiology department and would be expected to improve both image quality and time required for image review by less experienced users.

2. REQUIREMENTS ANALYSIS

Let us postulate a list of requirements for a computer-aided window/level control tool.

- The "optimal" choice of window/level strongly depends on the image itself. This implies that any reasonable decision for window/level settings should rely on image statistics.
- The "optimal" choice of window/level strongly depends on what the radiologist is looking for. This implies that, for any given image, there may not be one "best" choice of window/level, but rather *a set* of optimal choices.
- The tool should provide sufficiently many, yet not *too many* menu choices, for its purpose is to *aid* the radiologist in making proper adjustments by cutting down the search to a few optimal candidate settings.
- The tool should be available on-line and run in real-time. A radiologist experienced in soft-copy interpretation usually spends less than a minute to manually determine a proper initial window/level setting. It follows that the tool should run in the order of a few seconds in standard workstations used for image interpretation.
- The tool should be *generic* in that it should not be tied to any particular medical imaging modality and/or type(s) of study. The tool should be able to *learn* its parameters by observing the responses of a radiologist who uses it.
- The tool should *aid* the radiologist in quickly reaching a satisfactory window/level setting.

3. TECHNICAL DESCRIPTION

Most medical imaging modalities produce images of the spatial distribution of some indirectly measurable property of a projection or slice of the human body, e.g., tissue density in X-ray imaging. The very basis of X-ray imaging is that different anatomical structures, like bone and soft tissue, have very different densities, and, therefore, very different X-ray absorption patterns. This results in radically different intensity profiles for bone and soft tissue image regions. This difference also manifests itself in the histogram of the acquired X-ray, in which bone content and soft tissue content appear as distinct (albeit overlapping) lobes. In general, different kinds of anatomical structures typically manifest themselves as distinct but overlapping lobes in the histogram. However, noise as well as measurement errors and inconsistencies often make these lobes hard to distinguish and classify. As a result, the average medical image histogram is a multimodal profile, cluttered by background outliers, and noisy local extrema.

From the above, it follows that a reasonable approach would be to attempt to *segment* the given image histogram into a relatively small number of segments which correspond to features of potential interest, then for each such segment select a window/level of width equal to segment length, and centered at the midpoint of the segment.

This idea draws on earlier published work in [5] and some references therein, notably [6, 7, 8]. It differs in the following key respects: (i) In [5] and in earlier work the methods are task-specific, i.e., geared towards chest radiographs; thus (ii) in [5] the segmentation consists of a fixed pre-determined number of segments (actually, three). In addition, (iii) in [5] the segmentation rules are reasonable, yet heuristic. Finally, (iv) in [5] and [6, 7, 8] the resulting segmentation is not used to "drive" a window/level tool; instead, it is used to design look-up tables that emphasize soft or dense tissue. In contrast, our method is generic in the sense of being applicable to different modalities and exam types, and uses a variable number of segments, as needed for each application. It is rigorous and optimal [9], and uses the resulting segmentation to derive candidate optimal window/level settings. Nowadays, the window/level operation is by far the most popular interactive image enhancement technique among radiologists seasoned in soft-copy interpretation.

A radiologist typically starts by choosing window width, e.g., initially chooses a wide window to see the "big picture", then proceeds by choosing a narrower window to focus on some feature of interest. Too narrow windows are not desirable, for they lead to very coarse quantization using few grey levels, and this results in blocky, visually inferior image renditions.

Based on these observations, we may now proceed to pose histogram segmentation as a formal optimization problem, namely, one of optimally segmenting the histogram subject to a segment runlength constraint (this corresponds to a lower bound constraint on window width). This optimization has been posed and solved in a recent paper by Sidiropoulos [9], in the context of nonlinear filtering. The tool's operation can be summarized as follows:

- The user selects a region of interest (ROI). This may be the whole image, a part of the image, or a collage of several image parts. The user may also select M, the minimum width of suggested windows, or go with the system default, at her/his option.
- The computer computes the histogram of the ROI.
- The computer automatically optimally segments the computed histogram.
- For each segment of the resulting optimal segmentation (some segments may be discarded on the basis of prior knowledge), the computer suggests a corresponding choice of window/level, level being the segment's midpoint, and window width being the segment's width. In addition, the computer may also suggest window/level combinations corresponding to a union of two or more consecutive segments. The reason is that radiologists often choose multiple *overlapping* windows for viewing a given image.
- The user refines the suggested choices, as needed.

A suitable default value for M is a function of individual preferences and imaging modality, and it can be adaptively "learned" in a PACS implementation. The entire process is best understood by means of an example.

3.1. DESCRIPTION BY EXAMPLE

Figure 1 depicts a typical histogram profile of some ROI. The resulting optimal segmentation along with one suggested choice of window/level are presented in figure 2. The first and the last of the suggested window/level choices are then discarded on the basis of prior knowledge (e.g., the first option is known to correspond to clinically irrelevant black background). The overall process runs in approximately one second on a Macintosh Quadra 950 or Pentium 90 class computer workstation. The resulting menu of choices (possibly refined by an experienced radiologist) may now be stored (with minimal overhead) along with other image header information, to facilitate viewing by others.

Figure 3 is a knee X-ray. Figure 4 depicts a computer-suggested view of the knee joint. The interested reader may peruse the following link on the Web:

`http://www.glue.umd.edu/~nikos`

and follow the link to *Computer-Assisted Selection of Window and Level for Filmless Radiology*, for a short technical description of the window/level problem, along with a suite of eight knee and foot CR's with invention highlights. These have been dithered to reduce transmission time (originals are 7.5Mbytes each); however, they still convey the basic idea.

4. CORRELATION WITH EXPERT OPINION

Nineteen CR's of eight patients from the VA Medical Center have been selected to test the proposed algorithm. These include chest, hand, knee, foot, shoulder, c-spine, L/spine, and abdomen images. This set was selected by an experienced radiologist to be representative of the typical range of images (some hard and some easy to window/level) that the radiologist might encounter when reading these radiographs.

Four radiologists experienced in soft-copy interpretation were each given four or five of the above images. For each one, they were asked (i) What would be an overall "best" choice of window/level; (ii) Provided they are allowed two "best" choices of window/level, what would these be? (iii) Provided they are allowed three "best" choices of window/level, what would these be? Note that, this being a small-scale experiment, no two radiologists were presented with the same image, although this may be of interest in assessing consistency across radiologists. Each one of the nineteen images in the test set was also processed by the proposed computer-aided window/level tool for various values of M, and the resulting window/level suggestions were recorded.

The analysis of the responses reveals some interesting points. It appears that, when asked to come up with a unique overall "best" choice of window/level, the participants consistently selected a combination that essentially captured all activity in the histogram, and potentially extended a bit more to the left and to the right. This is consistent with the requirement that such a unique combination strike a balance that allows the radiologist to see as much of the "big picture" as possible. It also coincides with the unique suggestion of our proposed tool for sufficiently large M.

It was also evident that, for a given number of allowed window/level combinations, the respective subjective optimal choices may overlap substantially; this is accounted for in the proposed tool by allowing window/level combinations corresponding to a union of two or more consecutive segments.

The overall conclusion is that the computer comes up with a set of window/level suggestions containing a subset that correlates well with the subjective (empirically determined) optimal ones, and then some more that do not seem to be perceptually relevant. The latter may be quickly discarded, and the ones that do correlate well may be further fine-tuned, as needed.

5. CONCLUSIONS

The algorithm that was tested increased the speed and accuracy of window/level optimization especially for inexperienced users, and correlated well with the settings used by experienced radiologists. The routine incorporation of this algorithm as a workstation tool would increase productivity in a radiology department and would be expected to improve both image quality and time required for image review by less experienced users.

References

1. E. Siegel and E. Pickar, "The Transition to the Filmless Imaging System, Early Experience at the Baltimore VA Hospital", in *S/CAR 94*. Society of Computer Applications to Assist Radiology, 1994, p. 5.
2. E. Siegel, "Parameters Required to Evaluate a Filmless Imaging System", in *S/CAR 94*. Society of Computer Applications to Assist Radiology, 1994, p. 508.
3. Jr. J.R. Cox, E. Muka, G.J. Blaine, S.M. Moore, and R.G. Jost, "Considerations in Moving Electronic Radiography into Routine Use", *IEEE J. on Selected Areas in Communications*, vol. 10, no. 7, pp. 1108–1120, September 1992.
4. N.D. Sidiropoulos and J.S. Baras, "Computer-aided determination of window - and - level settings for filmless radiology", University of Maryland at College Park, OTL Disclosure IS-95-53, Sept. 1995.
5. M. F. McNitt-Gray, R. K. Taira, S. L. Johnson, and M. Razavi, "An automatic method for enhancing the display of different tissue densities in digital chest radiographs", *J. of Digital Imaging*, vol. 6, no. 2, pp. 95–104, May 1993.
6. P. McAdams, A. Johnson, A. Suddarth, and et al, "Histogram directed processing of digital chest images", *Invest. Radiol.*, vol. 21, pp. 253–259, 1986.
7. H. Sherrier and A. Johnson, "Regionally adaptive histogram equalization of the chest", *IEEE Trans. Medical Imaging*, vol. 6, pp. 1–7, 1987.
8. I. Sezan, M. Tekalp, and R. Schaetzing, "Automatic anatomically selective image enhancement in digital chest radiography", *IEEE Trans. Medical Imaging*, vol. 8, pp. 154–162, 1989.
9. N.D. Sidiropoulos, "The Viterbi Optimal Runlength-Constrained Approximation Nonlinear Filter", *IEEE Trans. Signal Processing*, vol. 44, no. 3, March 1996.

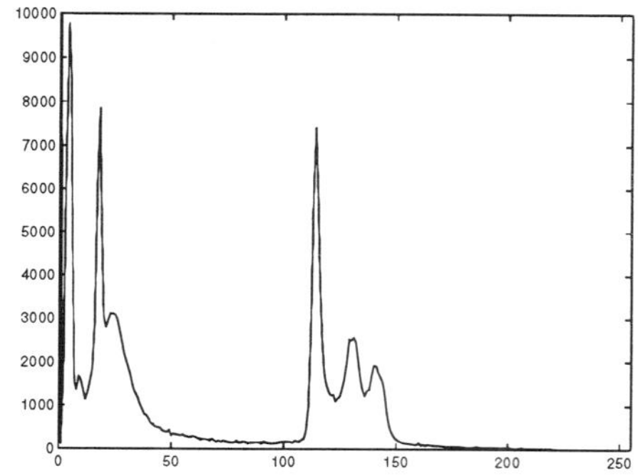

Fig. 1. Image histogram

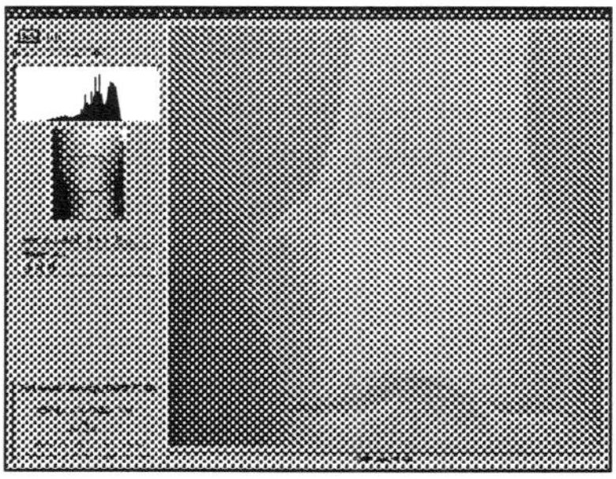

Fig. 3. A knee X-ray

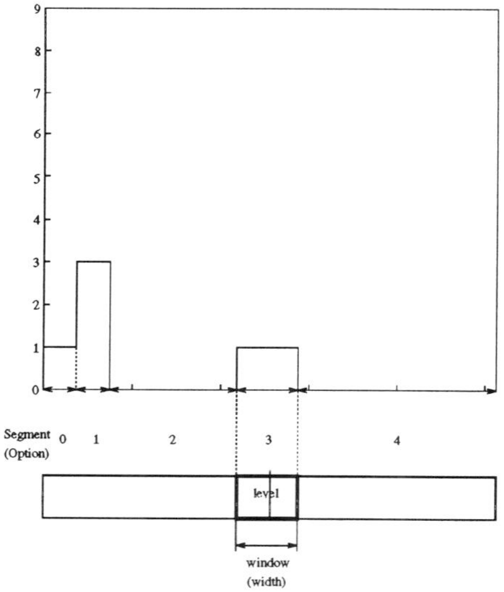

Fig. 2. Optimal segmentation, and one of suggested choices of window/level

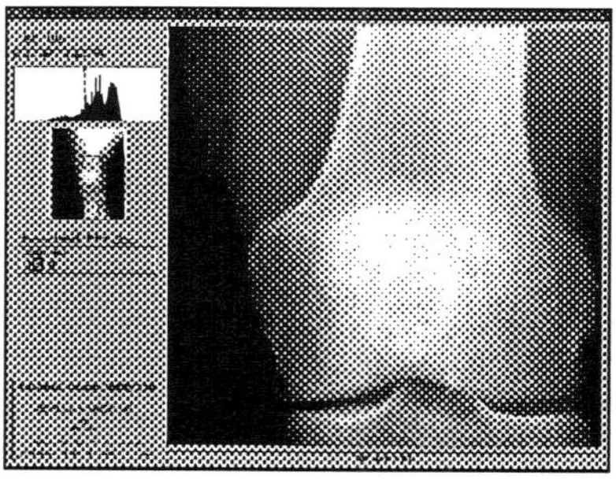

Fig. 4. Computer-suggested view of knee joint

Multi-Tasking Network Communications and the User Interface in a Macintosh Diagnostic Workstation

David E. Avrin, M.D., Ph.D., Katherine P. Andriole, Ph.D. and Ronald L. Arenson, M.D.
Laboratory for Radiological Informatics
Department of Radiology, University of California at San Francisco

I. INTRODUCTION

Macintosh PC-based diagnostic workstations for digital modalities have been demonstrated by several groups (1-3,8). Such workstations have the advantages of the friendly Macintosh graphical user interface (GUI) and lower cost compared to UNIX based workstations. However, the Macintosh is not a truly multi-tasking platform at this time. This results in contention between activities of the user-interface and data communications for incoming image studies.

We have developed methods for creating two-level cooperative multi-tasking that preserves the integrity of data communications (TCP/IP in our case), and results in minimal impact at the user interface. The underlying problem, the algorithm for resolving the conflict, and performance results will be described in detail.

The management of this problem enables development of integrated diagnostic workstations and academic tools such as computer-based interesting case teaching files in this popular and user-friendly Macintosh environment. It is anticipated that the next generation Macintosh operating system (Copland) will have true *pre-emptive* multi-tasking. The temporary solution described here will then no longer be necessary. Until such time, the algorithms presented allow full functionality of Macintosh workstations in a diagnostic environment.

The Problem

A diagnostic workstation in a clinical environment must process two major categories of events: user interaction via mouse or keyboard; and network events for transmission of incoming image data. One of the criticisms of the use of the Macintosh platform for diagnostic workstations is that although it is multitasking, it is not *pre-emptive:* (i.e. it cannot automatically interrupt processing of one event to service a second event). From the application and systems programming perspective, it does not have priority interrupt capability.

To make the Mac workstation clinically functional, the following requirements must be met:

1. Network communication of image data must be completed without loss or interruption that would terminate the process prior to completion.
2. The user or human interface should not experience noticeable delay in responding to mouse actions while such communication of data is ongoing.

At the core of a Macintosh application is an *event loop* which continuously checks for event status. In the prototype workstation application described here, the only events of significance are mouse clicks or movements in the GUI, or network activity (e.g., receiving buffer full). If one of these events occurs while processing of another event is underway, the new event will have to wait until processing of the other event is completed.

An example of two particularly troublesome scenarios are: (a) no response to mouse clicks/movements until received data is moved to memory; (b) delayed processing of network data transmission while the GUI is active, leading to interruption of that process. For example, a worst case scenario for (a) is transmission of a 60 image CT data set in 30 Mbytes, at effective Ethernet rates of 200 Kbytes/sec, yielding a 150 second transmission, locking out the GUI for that period of time. This is a clearly unacceptable circumstance for a clinical diagnostic workstation.

Network activity events occur for one of two reasons: a "file get" has been initiated by the workstation; or a "file send" has been initiated by the PACS controller for pre-routing. The first event could result in an unacceptable GUI lockout while receiving the requested image data, while the second event can usually wait for GUI "quiet time."
This technical shortcoming (lack of pre-emptive multitasking) of the Macintosh platform forced exploration of this contention, and an attempt to manage it, and measure the performance of the algorithm solution to such contention. This algorithm is described below.

II. MATERIALS AND METHODS

A prototype Macintosh 1K three monitor workstation served as the test bed (4,9). It has an Ethernet connection to the UCSF PACS Controller, running TCP/IP communication protocol. The PACS Controller pushes CT and MR studies to the workstation. The workstation software is implemented in Think C (5), Macintosh Toolbox (6) and the DOME (7) support library.

The algorithm developed to manage network/GUI contention executes the following rules:

1. If the GUI has been active in the last T seconds, notify the PACS controller to not initiate any new file transmissions; transmissions under way are allowed to be completed.
2. If the GUI is not active in the last T seconds, open TCP/IP communications.
3. Exit the communications process every megabyte of data received (approximately 5 seconds) to check for mouse activity.

This algorithm is illustrated in Figure 1.

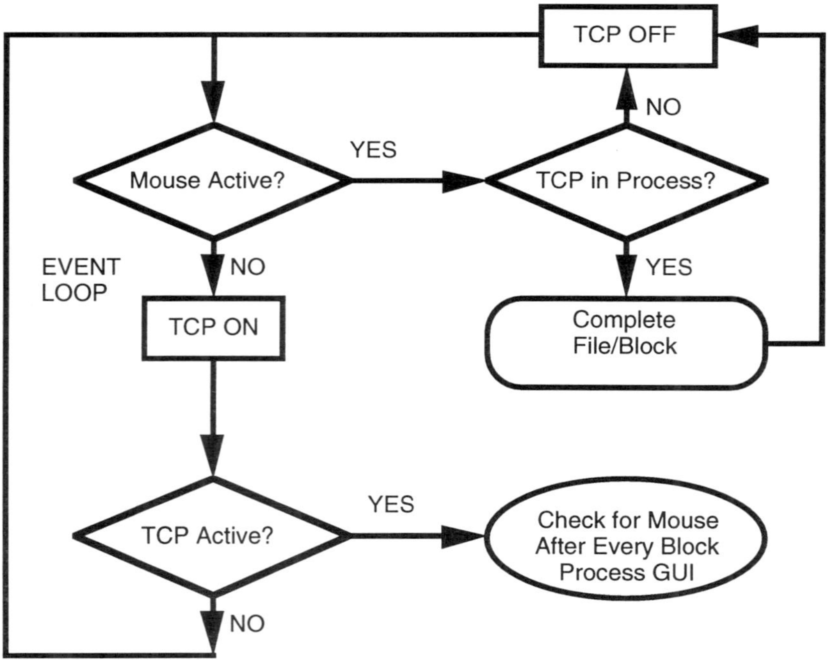

Figure 1. Algorithm for managing contention between network and user interface actions.

An event timing and logging process was installed in the workstation event loop to monitor initiation and completion of file transmission and "GUI active" periods.

The following conditions were also explored:

1. Is the event loop re-entered to check for mouse events between buffer filling by the TCP/IP process?
2. If it is checked, and there is activity, is the interruption in file transmission handled well or poorly?

III. RESULTS

At the meeting, the following data will be presented: Baseline timer data for TCP/IP communications with GUI inactive will be obtained as a benchmark. Repeat timer data for TCP/IP communications with GUI active will be presented to demonstrate the performance of the algorithm in managing the contention described above. GUI response time will be measured during TCP/IP long file transmission.

IV. DISCUSSION

A UNIX-based system can eliminate any perceived contention between GUI activity and network communications. This is not the case with the current generation Macintosh operating system.

There remains significant interest in using the Macintosh platform for clinical workstations. First, the user interface is well-known and well-liked. Second, mass-market PC's will be less expensive than UNIX workstations for the foreseeable future, while their technical differences will continue to narrow. Third, there is an interest in convergence of tasks (i.e., clinical, research and educational) to a single workstation, and that workstation will probably be a Macintosh or PC for economic reasons.

The question we have tried to answer is: Can the perceived contention be held to an acceptable and very minimal level by the techniques described above? Until the introduction of the new Macintosh operating system (Copland), which is reportedly a truly pre-emptive multitasking environment, becomes widely available, the algorithm described here facilitates the use of the current Macintosh platform in a clinical environment.

ACKNOWLEDGMENTS

Mohan Ramaswamy, M.D. provided technical insight. Albert Wong provided technical support and image data communications from the UCSF PACS Controller.

REFERENCES

1. Arenson RL, Chakraborty DP, Seshadri SB, Kundel H. The digital imaging workstation. *Radiology* 1990; 176:303-315.
2. Avrin DE, Lou A, Andriole KP, Ramaswamy M, Arenson RL. Cost effective many-monitor workstation. *European Congress of Radiology*, Vienna September, 1993.
3. Arenson RL, Avrin DE, Wong A, Gould RG, Huang HK. Second generation folder manager for PACS. *SCAR* 1994.
4. Ramaswamy M, Avrin DE, Andriole KP, Wong AWK, Bazzill TM, Arenson RL. Use of personal computer technology in supporting a radiological review workstation. *SPIE Medical Imaging Proceedings*, 1994.
5. THINK C is a trademark and product of Symantec Corp.
6. Macintosh Toolbox is a trademark and product of Apple Computer Corp.
7. Dome Hydra imaging board is a product of Dome imaging systems, Waltham, MA, USA.
8. Gillespy III T, Rowberg AH. Radiological images on personal computers: introduction and fundamental principles of digital images. *Journal of Digital Imaging* 1993; 6:81-87.
9. Avrin DE, Ramaswamy M, Andriole KP, *et al.* Preclinical Testing of a Cost-Effective Digital Modality Diagnostic Workstation. *SCAR* 1994' 496-501.

MUMC GI VIEWER: Image Display, Manipulation and Film Composition Software for GI Radiologists

D.B. Kenyon, L. Tan, G.W. Stevenson, S. Somers and C. Nahmias
Department of Radiology, Chedoke-McMaster Hospitals and McMaster University
Hamilton, Ontario, Canada

We have designed image display, manipulation and film composition software to serve the specific digital image viewing requirements of abdominal radiologists. The package, MUMC GI Viewer, provides the interface between GI radiologists and the image management and communication system, MUMC IMACS, which is in place at McMaster University Medical Centre (MUMC). MUMC GI Viewer was designed in a cooperative process between software designer and the abdominal radiologists at MUMC. It has been in routine clinical use for just over a year.

Platform

MUMC GI Viewer is developed for the X-Window graphical user environment. Thus, GI Viewer will run on any X-Windows based workstation such as DEC, Hewlett-Packard, and Silicon Graphics, regardless of operating system or system architecture. We use Sun Sparcstation computers (Sun Microsystems Inc.) to run GI Viewer. Together they form the imaging workstation for the GI viewing area. A minimum of 32MB of RAM is recommended for this platform. Two 1000-line 20" colour monitors are ideal for image display. MUMC GI Viewer is icon-based and requires a mouse or other tracking device. As well, a keyboard allows the user to enter text reports or annotations.

Layout

The two screens provide separate GI Viewer functions. The right screen provides an image canvas and an icon panel, as well as a status and information panel (Figure 1). The left screen is primarily an image display canvas (Figure 2). All functions are icon- or button-based. The left screen is normally the viewing screen, with a choice of display formats. The right screen is able to display one full-sized image. Usually, however, the right screen is used for composing a film.

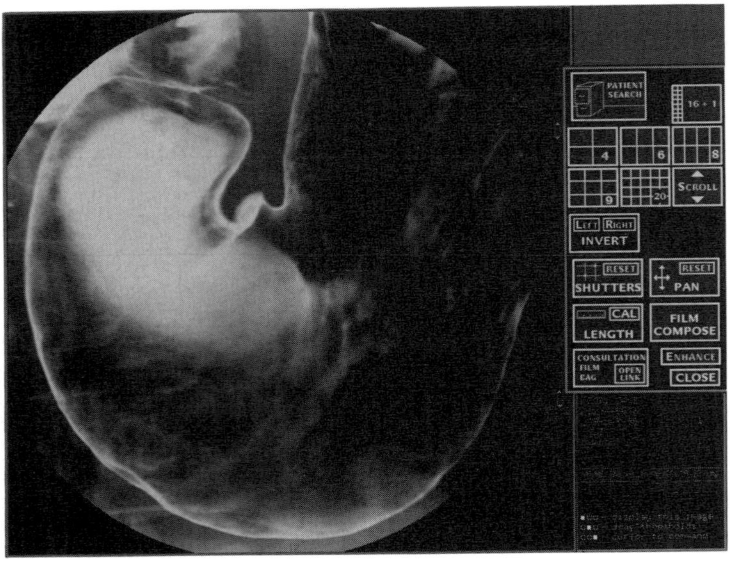

Figure 1.

Load a study

GI Viewer is programmed so that when Patient Search is selected, a list of the most recently acquired GI studies appears. The list shows the patient name, patient ID number, date and time of exam, type of exam, the number of images in the study, and the report status (filmed/not filmed). The user selects one of the listed studies (usually one that has not been filmed) and then selects one of the display formats. Alternatively, if a specific study is desired, selecting the Search button in the list dialog box opens up a powerful network database search card. The database may be searched by full or partial patient name, patient ID number, date of exam, modality type, study type, or report status. The user may also select a study from the initial list, and request a Search Same ID function. This function automatically searches the network database for all other exams undergone by that patient, not just GI exams. More than one study at a time can be selected for display.

Image display

Once a patient study has been chosen, then selecting one of the display formats (16+1, 4, 6, 8, 9, 20 images on a screen) automatically loads the selected study onto the left screen. Typically, the 16+1 display format for the left screen is preferred by the GI radiologists. This format displays 16 thumbnail preview images, leaving the rest of the canvas to display one full-resolution fluoroscopic image (Figure 2). The 16 preview images may be scrolled forwards and backwards for studies having more than 16 images. The typical time required to load an image is less than 1 second. Selecting a thumbnail image for full-resolution display is done by clicking on the thumbnail image.

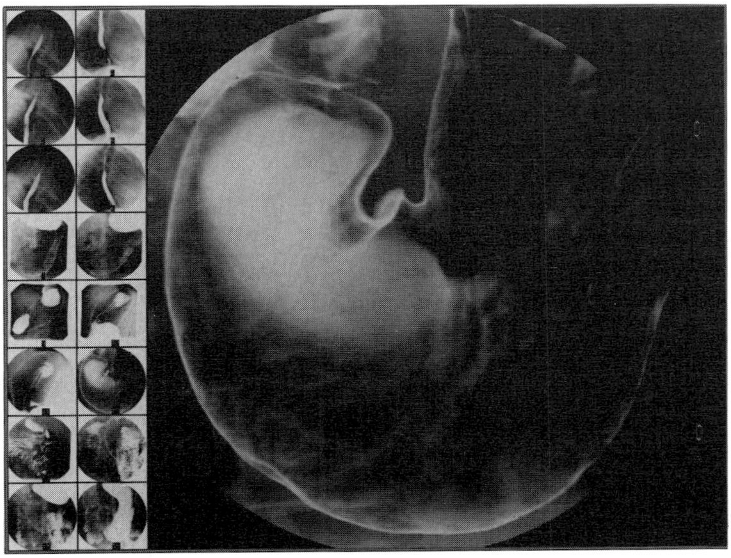

Figure 2.

If more than one study has been loaded, scrolling through the thumbnails will display the images from the subsequent studies, any of which can be selected for full-resolution display. To facilitate image comparison, an image from the left screen may be pasted onto the right screen, and then a different image may be selected for the left screen, both at the same full resolution.

Image manipulation

Various image manipulation functions are available from the icon/button panel. An Invert grey-scale button allows either the left or right, or both, screens to be inverted in grey-scale. After experimenting with various means of changing the window and level, we settled on two sliding icons on the far right side of the image canvas. The icon on top adjusts the maximum grey level, and the lower icon adjusts the minimum grey level for display. Real-time adjustments occur as the icons are dragged up and down. A reset key just below the lower icon restores the original display levels of the image. A Shutters button allows the radiologist to shutter the image on-screen, and the Pan routine moves the ends on the image into the field of view by clicking on the image and dragging the mouse. Both Shutters and Pan have reset buttons to restore the image to its original state. A length measurement routine allows the user to drag a straight line across an image and displays the length of the line in pixels and in millimetres where available. An edge enhance routine performs edge gradient filtering on the image. This function is rarely used by the GI radiologists. We have maintained the number of image manipulation functions to a minimum, although a wealth of sophisticated functions are available from our comprehensive MUMC Display software. This approach keeps the number of buttons to a minimum, keeping the GI Viewer accessible.

Film composition

The Film Compose button on the button panel opens up a sidebar of icons for film composition on the right screen. A variety of interesting formats were developed as requested by the GI radiologists. There are simple formats equally dividing the film canvas for 4, 6, 8, or 9 images; and then there are formats which mix and match different aspect ratios. One format, with 3 long and narrow positions, 6 small squares, and 2 larger squares, is ideal for displaying upper GIs with shuttered images of the esophagus during a swallow exam. All of these film formats are set to fit on an image canvas that is of the same aspect ratio as a 14"x17" film. All film formats provide locations in which the institution name, patient name, patient ID, and date of exam are automatically inserted. A text box also appears, in which the radiologist may choose to type his/her observations. As with the images, texts placed on the image canvas, either in the text box or as annotations, also appear on-screen in the same relative sizes as they would on the film, once printed. Thus, film composition with GI Viewer is done in true WYSIWYG style (Figure 3).

To compose a film, an image is selected and displayed on the left screen. Once manipulated as desired (window/levelling, shuttering), clicking on the desired image position on the film canvas on the right screen pastes that image into the film position. A new image is then selected on the left screen, manipulated, and then pasted into another film position on the right screen. Functions within Film Compose include annotations, canned text, and labelling with pointers. A particularly useful function is Film Zoom which, when selected, places a resizable zoom region on the image on the left screen. The region is set to be resizable with a fixed aspect ratio which matches that of the film position selected on the film canvas. In this way, when the desired zoom region of the image is pasted onto the selected film position, the region is resized to fill the film position entirely, leaving no black space.

As mentioned earlier, more than one study can be loaded on-screen at any time. These studies can be any of the studies in the network database, and thus can be of any modality type. The images from all loaded studies can then be pasted onto the same film canvas. One example is to have a computed radiography GI image pasted onto the same film as the images from the fluoroscopic GI study.

As it is common for radiologists to be interrupted while composing a film on the GI Viewer, a Film Bag function cleverly stores every change made to the film canvas, ie. every paste, every annotation. If the radiologist's working film canvas is no longer on the screen when he/she returns to the workstation, it is easily recreated within seconds, by selecting the appropriate time of creation from the list of films in the Film Bag.

Consultation films

Each time a film canvas is sent to be printed, a consultation film is created. In this context, a consultation film is a fully composed film canvas which can only be viewed but not changed in any way. It is essentially a softcopy film in finished form. Consultation films can be easily retrieved and reprinted. On the MUMC IMACS,

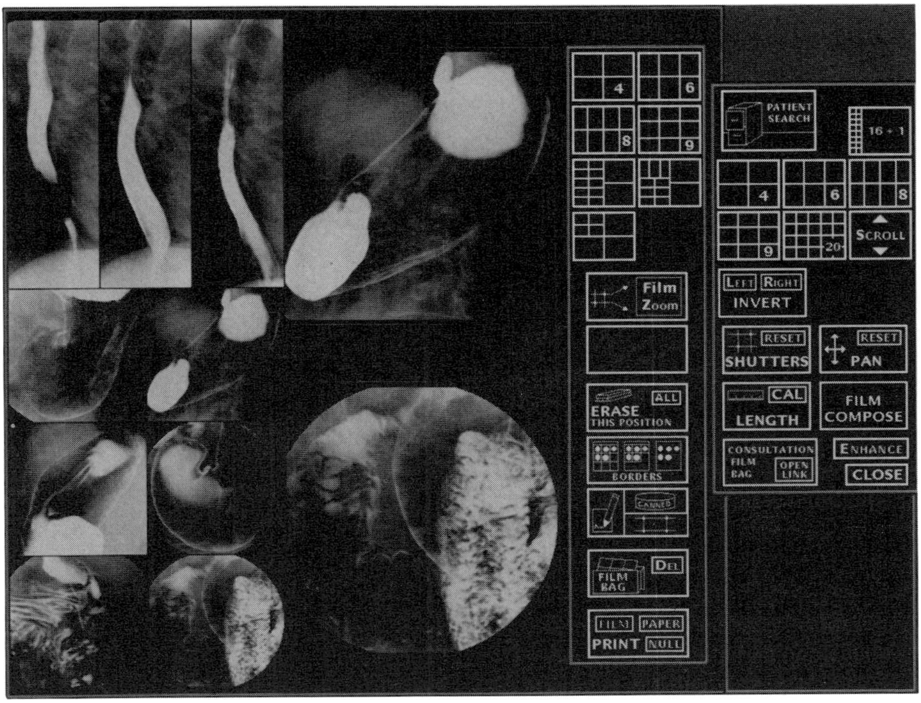

Figure 3.

consultation films are stored along with their corresponding set of original image data. In addition, any text report from the Radiology Information System is also stored alongside its corresponding consultation film(s) and original image data. Thus, on retrieving an online consultation film for viewing on the workstation, the text report is also displayed (Figure 4).

Remote online consultation

Although there is not yet a practical context in place for remote online consultation, MUMC GI Viewer does provide what it calls the Open Link function. Open Link allows a radiologist at one workstation to view and discuss (over the telephone) an onscreen consultation film that both the radiologist and his/her colleague have simultaneously displayed on their respective imaging workstations. Open Link places two arrow cursors on the image canvas, one in red for the first workstation, another in yellow for the second workstation. Each user takes control of their respective arrow cursors and is free to move them as pointers. As the first user moves his/her red arrow cursor on his/her screen, the red arrow cursor on the other workstation mirrors the movements in real-time. Both users may move their arrow cursors simultaneously.

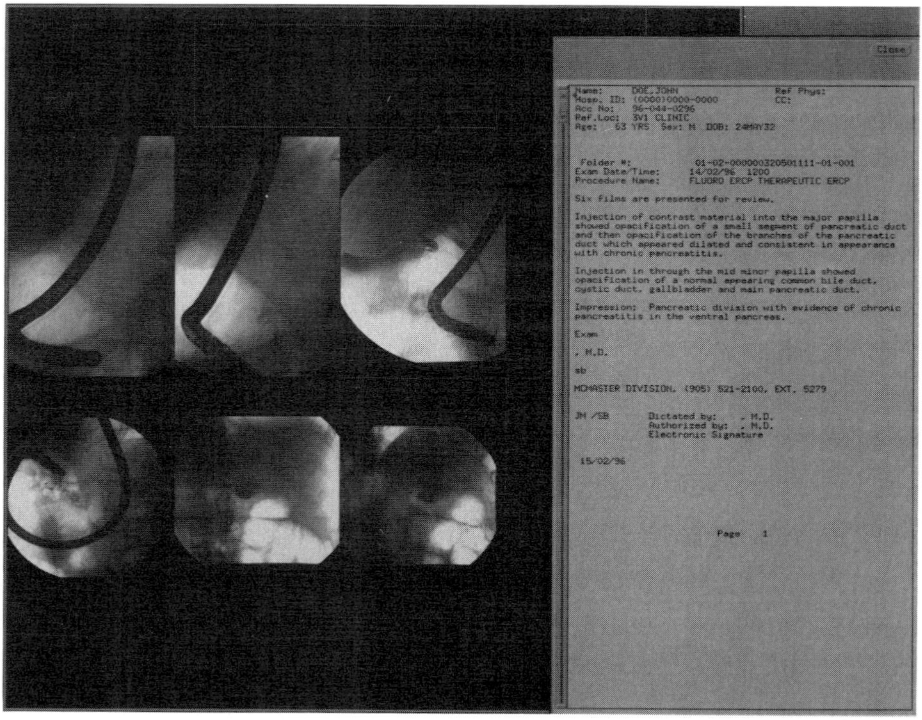

Figure 4.

MUMC GI Viewer has been well tested for over a year, in daily use by all GI radiologists, fellows, and residents in the GI reporting area. Technologists have also found ways to use GI Viewer to make their work processes more efficient. For example, CR GI images can be checked for correct patient positioning without having to wait for the hardcopy film output from the CR unit. Physicians who have ventured into the viewing area looking for film bags have found the software user-friendly enough that they were able to search for and display their desired patient studies.

Comparison of Film vs Monitor Viewing of CR Films Using Eye-Position Recording

Elizabeth A. Krupinski, Ph.D. & Pamela J. Lund, M.D.
Department of Radiology, University of Arizona, Tucson, AZ

I. INTRODUCTION

The advent of PACS and teleradiology has brought about an entirely new way of viewing radiology images. Film is still used in most situations, but viewing radiographic images on CRT monitors is being more prevalent. Some hospitals are even going completely digital. [1-3] From the standpoint of observer performance and human factors research, however, there are many questions that arise when viewing images on workstations. Compared to film viewing, there is a lot more "peripheral" information displayed on a workstation in addition to images - patient information, image processing tools etc. The question is - how does the radiologist deal with this extra information and does it influence the way they search images for lesions?

Most work in evaluating radiographic workstations still falls within the realms of hardware engineering (how to build a better, faster workstation) and software engineering (how to present images and use various image processing algorithms). [4,5] These are important areas that need to be addressed before the radiologist even gets involved, but they rarely actively involve the radiologist and address the impact of these engineering factors on observer performance. The work in observer performance evaluation also falls into two realms. The first area of interest deals with straight-forward evaluation of performance comparing standard viewing techniques (i.e., film on a viewbox or alternator) with new viewing techniques (i.e., digital images on a CRT monitor). [6-8] These studies are very important and have often yielded interesting results. In general, most studies have found that in most cases monitor viewing does not adversely affect observer performance - it just takes significantly longer to reach a diagnostic decision. In a business where time equals money and time delays can affect patient care, this increased time to use workstations in routine clinical practice is generally unacceptable.

The second area of human performance evaluation addresses this issue of time as well as many others. This area falls into the general category of ergonomics - how many monitors are needed, how should patient and image information be displayed, are there display factors that influence the time it takes to reach a diagnostic decision? Although some work has been done in this area, less has been done compared to strict evaluation of observer performance. [9]

The goal of the present study was to utilize eye-position recording techniques to evaluate how radiologists search or navigate around film images displayed on a viewbox compared to the same images displayed digitally on a CRT monitor. Overall observer performance was assessed as well, but the main concern was to determine if certain aspects of the search process can be identified which either affect diagnostic accuracy or which contribute to the amount of time it takes to reach a diagnostic decision using a CRT monitor.

II. METHODS & MATERIALS

3 radiologists and 3 orthopedic surgeons who typically read bone cases were presented with a series of 29 bone trauma cases while their eye-position was recorded. The 29 cases were displayed once on computer radiography (CR) film and once on standard screen-film (SF). The CR cases were also presented on a 1K x 1.5K CRT monitor. All the cases were from the same patients who volunteered to be x-rayed in both conventional and digital modalities. Views were the same for all cases and attempts were made to obtain the same positioning with both modalities. Ten of the cases were "normal" (i.e., no abnormalities present). 19 cases had subtle swelling. Of these 19 cases with swelling, 12 also had a single subtle fracture, 4 had some degree of displacement or subluxation, 10 had ligamentous injury, and 8 had joint effusion. Eye-position was recorded using an infra-read based system (ASL 4000SU) with < 1 degree of accuracy. Readers had the following pre-set image processing functions available : window/level set for normal, bone and soft tissue; and edge enhancement. All setting are those which are currently used on the display workstation for

emergency room radiographic reading. Also available were video reverse, zoom and pan functions.

The readers participated in 3 one hour sessions. In one session only the CRT images were displayed. In the other two sessions, CR and SF film images were randomly mixed and displayed to the observers, with the restriction that a given case could be seen only once during a session. Display modality order was randomized for each reader. The readers were given unlimited time to search each case (on average each case had 3 views on two films). Eye-position was recorded. For each case readers were asked to use a 6-level scale (where 1 = definitely present and 6 = definitely absent) to report on the presence or absence of each of the following : fracture, dislocation/subluxation, ligamentous injury, swelling, joint effusion. They were also asked to rate image contrast, sharpness and quality as excellent, good, fair or poor.

III. RESULTS

Overall, the radiologists had a higher percentage of true positives than the orthopedic surgeons ($F = 2.66$, $df = 5,70$, $p = 0.03$); while there were no statistically significant differences in false positives ($F = 1.88$, $df = 5,70$, $p = 0.11$). There were no statistically significant differences in the true-positive rates for detection of any of the five lesion types between SF, CR and CRT viewing. There were also no statistically significant differences in the types of false-positives reported for the three modalities. Overall most false positives were in the swelling, ligamentous injury and joint effusion categories, rather than the fracture or dislocation/subluxation categories.

The false negatives could be classified as either search, recognition or decision errors based on the dwell times associated with them. [10-11] Search errors are lesions which are not fixated during search and are not reported. Recognition and decision errors also go unreported, but both are fixated - recognition errors are fixated for less than 1000 msec, while decision errors are fixated for more than 1000 msec. For CRT viewing there were 21.7% search errors, for SF 17.1% and for CR 20.6%. Recognition errors were 32.6%, 28.6% and 26.5% respectively for CRT, SF and CR viewing. Decision errors were

45.7%, 54.3% and 52.9% respectively for CRT, SF and CR viewing.

Although all images were on average rated as having good contrast, sharpness and quality, there were some statistically significant differences depending on modality. Image contrast ($F = 3.21$, $df = 2,346$, $p = 0.001$), sharpness ($F = 5.23$, $df = 2,346$, $p = 0.006$) and quality ($F = 7.22$, $df = 2,346$, $p = 0.001$) were rated significantly better for CR than for SF or CRT viewing . There were no significant differences between SF and CRT ratings.

The types of image processing functions and how often they were used was recorded. Overall the normal setting was used on 68% of the cases, the bone setting on 67%, edge enhancement on 29%, soft tissue setting on 26%, zoom on 24%, pan on 13%, and video reverse on 13% on the cases. No relationships could be found between type of lesion reported and type of processing used.

Overall viewing time between the three modalities was significantly different ($F = 118.65$, $df = 2,346$, $p = 0.001$), with CRT time (mean = 91.15 sec, sd = 47.56) being significantly longer than SF (mean = 44.24 sec, sd = 21.91) and CR (mean = 46.45 sec, sd = 24.68). CR and SF viewing time did not differ significantly. Time to first fixate the lesion of interest was also determined. For all cases that had more than one lesion (e.g., dislocation with swelling), the lesions themselves all fell somewhere within a 5 degree diameter circle (i.e., in all cases the lesions were interrelated - e.g., a fracture with swelling at the same location). Thus, a first hit fixation for single and multiple lesions had to fall within this 5 degree area around the lesion(s). The time to first fixate the lesion on the CRT monitor occurred significantly ($F = 20.34$, $df = 2,266$, $p = 0.0001$) later during search (mean = 4.67 sec, sd = 4.29) than for SF (mean = 2.54 sec, sd = 2.21) and CR (mean = 2.35 sec, sd = 2.16) viewing. For all three modalities, the time to first fixate the lesion(s) was shorter for the radiologists than for the orthopedists, although this difference was not statistically significant.

With respect to general scanning patterns, the general form of patterns generated on the two types of film images were very similar. There were a number of pattern types generated, but the main thing is that all fixations were confined to the image area. On the CRT monitor, about 20% of the clusters generated during search were in the area of the image processing menu. This scanning of the menu functions was generally in the early portion of search, although excursions to the menu did occur if the reader needed to change a setting later in search.

IV. CONCLUSIONS

Viewing radiologic images on a monitor does influence the way images are scanned. It appears that readers conduct a very brief initial scan of the image to obtain a global impression of image quality (3 fixations on average), then use the image processing functions to adjust the image to their liking (accounting for about 20% of all scanning). This use of the image processing menu influences the time it takes to first fixate the lesion area of interest - almost 2.5 sec longer on the CRT monitor than on film. After this "calibration" period takes place, a scanning pattern very similar to that which occurs for film viewing takes place. In general it was observed that most of the readers tended to use only two of the image processing functions - the normal image setting and the bone setting. Most often these functions were used in the first excursion(s) to the image processing menu, while other functions such as edge enhancement or zoom were used later in search - generally after the lesion area had been fixated. These results suggest that the readers are first setting the image display parameters (i.e., window and level) to some sort of aesthetically pleasing image (normal setting) or to one appropriate for bone (bone setting) since they knew all the images were bone cases. These settings seemed to be independent of lesion identification since there was generally no extensive fixating on the lesion area prior to scanning and initial use of the image processing menu.

One possible conclusion to draw from this finding is that it might be useful for workstations to be designed so that an individual radiologist can determine their own preferred settings for the general appearance of images, enter these settings, then every time they log on for a review sessions the images would always come up initially the way they prefer. This would allow them to begin search of the image directly without having to go through this initial calibration period on practically every image. This would cut down on overall viewing time. It might also impact on performance as well. There is good evidence that a lot of diagnostic information is obtained in the global impression of the image that the reader obtains in their first glance at the image. If the reader has to stop scanning the image after this global impression to attend to the image processing menu, the information gained from this global impression may very well be lost. If this is the case, detection performance might be affected, which is what was observed in this study although the difference between CRT and film viewing was not statistically different.

V. REFERENCES

[1] Siegel EL, Diaconis Jn, et al.. (1995). Making filmless radiology work. J of Digital Imaging, 8, 151-155.
[2] Mosser HM, Partan G, Hruby W. (1995). Clinical routine operation of a filmless radiology department : three years experience. SPIE Proc, 2435, 321-327.
[3] Kim Y, Cabral JE, et al. (1995). Seahawk : telemedicine project in the Pacific Northwest. SPIE Proc, 2435, 232-238.
[4] PACS Design and Evaluation : Engineering and Clinical Issues. (1995). SPIE Proc, 2435.
[5] Gillepsy T, Rowberg AH. (1994). Displaying radiologic images on personal computers : image processing and analysis. J of Digital Imaging, 7, 51-60.
[6] Krupinski EA, Maloney K, et al. (1994). Receiver operating characteristic evaluation of computer display of adult portable chest radiographs. Invest radiol, 29, 141-146.
[7] Slasky BS, Gur D, et al. (1990). Receiver operating characteristic analysis of chest image interpretation with conventional, laser-printed, and high-resolution workstation images. Radiol, 179,775-780.
[8] Elam EA, Rehm K, et al. (1992). Efficacy of digital radiography for the detection of pneumothorax : comparison with conventional chest radiography. AJR, 158, 509-514.
[9] Beard DV, Hemminger BM, et al. (1994). How many screens does a CT workstation need? J of Digital Imaging, 7, 69-76.
[10] Kundel HL, LaFollette PS. (1972). Visual search patterns and experience with radiological images. Radiol, 103,523-528.
[11] Kundel HL, Nodine CF, Carmody DP. (1978). Visual scanning, pattern recognition and decision-making in pulmonary nodule search. Invest Radiol, 13,175-181.

Modification of Conventional Quality Assurance Procedures to Accommodate Computed Radiography

Charles E. Willis, Ph.D.
Department of Radiology, University of Texas Houston Health Science Center, Houston, Texas

John Mercier and Mahendra Patel
Tripler Army Medical Center, Honolulu, Hawaii

I. INTRODUCTION

Computed Radiography (CR, Storage Phosphor Radiography) is a relatively new imaging method for projection radiography.[1] More hospitals are introducing CR into routine service, fielding multiple CR units, and extending practice beyond portable examinations. When CR is introduced into general radiology, Quality Assurance procedures must evolve to accommodate the characteristics of this new technology. While CR affords a greater degree of control over the appearance of the plain x-ray image, it presents a challenge to the Technologist, who must substantially change his practice, to the Radiologist, who must adapt to images with a substantially different appearance, and to the Physicist, who must provide guidance on adjustment of practice to preclude and correct non-diagnostic exams. Because seventy percent of the department's workload is ordinary radiography, mastery of CR technology is a prerequisite for establishing a totally digital radiology department.

II. QUALITY ASSURANCE PHILOSOPHY

Quality Assurance (QA), *a.k.a.* Quality Improvement, *a.k.a.* Performance Improvement, includes all those activities that seek to answer the question "Are we operating our medical devices properly?" As such, QA includes all Quality Control (QC) activities (are the devices operating properly?) and a large portion of Medical Maintenance activities (are the devices properly supported?). QA provides a systematic approach to ensure consistent, maximum performance from the physician and the imaging facilities.[2] Unless devices are reliably maintained, and performance is reliably controlled, QA indicators will provide ambiguous data.

Comprehensive QA is labor-intensive and expensive. Modern QA often relies on automation to gather data. QA monitors are usually focused on sensitive indicators of performance decrement. These indicators have been developed from long-term experience and experience drawn from many institutions. The experience base needed to correctly identify sensitive indicators, to establish action limits, and to take appropriate corrective action does not yet exist for CR.[3]

A reasonable approach to dealing with new imaging technology like CR would be to conduct thorough Acceptance Testing (AT) to establish a performance baseline, conduct a periodic subset of AT to determine deviation from baseline, and try to adapt QA methods from conventional technology to CR.[4] A limitation to this approach is that CR technology is constantly changing, and the performance baseline must be frequently re-established.[5] Performance characteristics of CR also vary between different equipment vendors.

CR is not just a detector. CR affects every step of the imaging chain from acquisition of the radiographic projection to interpretation of the image. Comprehensive QA needs to address how changes at each step affect the efficient production and utilization of diagnostic information.

III. CHANGES INTRODUCED BY CR

Acquisition of the Radiographic Projection

The challenges brought on by the introduction of CR are superimposed on the usual QA problems experienced in a conventional radiology setting, that is, inappropriate technique selection, improper positioning, inadequate or incorrect patient identification can still adversely affect the ultimate quality of the CR image, but the impact of these errors can be more or less significant than with screen/film (SF) radiography.

Unlike SF, smaller format CR cassettes provide better spatial resolution because of reduced pixel dimensions at the same matrix size. Multiple images on one plate, a good conventional practice, is counterproductive because it requires a larger format cassette and the single digital image file cannot be independently manipulated by view. Different views sometimes require individualized processing. The position of the radiation field on the cassette affects the image, so collimation, and light field convergence are more critical to image quality than SF. Association of patient demographics with the image can be a source of error. When this occurs, it is important to aggressively correct the data or purge the digital image to preclude proliferation of incorrectly identified digital copies.

Development of the Image

A new set of errors arises from incorrect image pre-acquisition processing, post-acquisition processing, and management of processing parameters.[6] Selection of the wrong exam type or view can have dramatic effects on the image. When this mistake involves post-acquisition processing, the effects are reversible. When the mistake involves pre-acquisition processing, such as pattern recognition and histogram analysis, the effects are often unrecoverable. There are 5040 total processing parameter entries for 3 views of 240 exam types in the standard Fuji CR software. Subtle differences in parameter values can have enormous effects on the resulting image, but still are difficult for a human observer to recognize. This argues for automated management of parameter values.

Correction of Suboptimal Images

Technologists have an expectation that the first image should be acceptable. Corrections tend to be by "trial-and-error". Modifications that make good sense with SF do not work the same way with CR. Increasing mAs improves only noise, not density or contrast. Changing kVp affects contrast, penetration, scatter, and plate efficiency, all of which interact to affect the processing that determines the ultimate image. Where we have full-functionality post-processing workstations, QC technologists depend only on speed shift and contrast shifts when trying to recover suboptimal images.

In a setting where primary diagnosis is made from the laser-printed CR image, wasted film is a key QA indicator. The sources of wasted film can be repeated examinations, or reprinted examinations, that require no additional radiation exposure to the patient to correct a non-diagnostic image. Exams that are repeatedly reprinted are candidates for modification of processing parameters. Collimation errors are a new source of positioning repeats (see Table 1).

New artifacts are observed with CR, some of which have correspondence with SF artifacts.[6] These include dust particles on the imaging plates, scratches or cracks in the plate, and dust on light collection optics. Aliasing and *moiré* patterns have been reported because of interactions of fixed grid lines and the sampling matrix. This effect can also be accentuated by inopportune selection of magnification factor during display of the digital image. We have also observed accentuation of the edges of photocells caused by unsharp masking, clipping of data in the Hilar regions of the lung by inappropriate gradation processing, and clipping of data in the Clavicular region because of overexposure.

Control of Exposure Factor Selection

In conventional radiography, the primary indicator of incorrect technique is a film that is too dark or too light. This indicator is not useful with CR, because of the density equalization that CR provides.[7] Routine QA must monitor a digital indicator of exposure to the imaging plate (see Fig. 1).[8] There are many factors that affect the absolute accuracy of this exposure indicator. Thus, the numerical indication of improper exposure is a derived quantity subject to interpretation (see Table 2.)

The wide exposure latitude of CR has been credited with substantial reductions in repeats, especially in portable exams which lack automatic exposure control.[9] This feature also means that CR is more tolerant of overexposure than SF, which is an alternative explanation for the reduced repeat rate.[10] Other factors that can cause a decreased repeat rate include systematic under-reporting and reluctance to repeat an examination without confidence that the repeated exam will yield substantially improved quality.

The literature is equivocal about the radiographic speed of CR relative to SF. [11] The absorption of energy by the imaging plate is very different from most conventional screens, therefore the technique chart may be quite different from that used in conventional radiology. Adjustment of phototimers is also problematic, because there is no widely accepted method for setting phototimers for use with CR.

Interpretation of the Image

Reduced display formats of the 26cm x 36cm hardcopy output and "two-up" format complicate measurements and comparison to historical SF images and other views. Different magnification can cause confusion. Conventional alternators need masking to accommodate the smaller format films. Manufacturers are moving to 14"x17" hard copy output, but the complication remains in soft-copy display of CR.

There is often uncertainty among radiologists whether a difference in appearance is a clinical feature or the result of image processing. No single rendering seems appropriate for low contrast and high frequency features. The technical literature reflects concern about the detectability of cortical bone lesions[11], pleural effusions, obstructive disease, pneumothorax, interstitial disease, parenchymal masses by CR. [12] Basically, most radiologists have not yet established a "comfort level" with CR.

Maintenance

Operator maintenance tasks that have a dramatic impact on CR image quality include cleaning of the laser printer, processor, and imaging plates. It is important to use the cleaning solvent recommended by the manufacturer, because screen cleaners or aqueous alcohol solutions may damage the screen's protective layer. Cleanliness needs to extend beyond the darkroom to address the condition of cassettes, cassette storage, and the vicinity of the scanner. In our experience, cassettes are not as sturdy as SF cassettes and a new cassette design is being evaluated. Scanner jams are more complex than both automatic film processor and daylight loader jams, and require service intervention.

Organizational maintenance tasks that affect CR image quality include convergence of light and x-ray fields, scanner sensitivity calibration, scanner periodic maintenance, and software upgrades. It is essential to maintain a comprehensive log of downtime for each scanner. Unlike film processors, the capital investment in each scanner is such that redundancy is not always possible, so the impact of downtime is critical to the department's function.

Quality Control

Standardization of tests and criteria for abnormal performance are sorely needed. Because of automatic image processing, test objects that worked well with SF may not adequately simulate the human anatomy with CR, leading to erroneous interpretations.[13] Definitive physical measurements of imaging performance are too complex for routine clinical use.[14] The practical value of new test objects developed specifically for CR remains to be established in clinical practice.[15,16] Although laser output devices incorporate self-adjustment mechanisms, these are not without problems[17], and tend to mask chemistry problems until catastrophic.

IV. CONCLUSIONS

The inherent complexity of CR demands additional training for technologists, radiologists, and physicists. Existing QA resources must be redirected and additional QA resources are required. Detailed backup planning is required in the event of system downtime. Redundancy should be considered via duplicate hardware or networking. Realization of the anticipated economic benefit of CR may be adversely affected.

CR is the only credible technology available that will support large-scale Image Management and Communications Systems (IMACS) or high volume teleradiology. CR solves the image contention problem by enabling electronic distribution of images and providing unlimited reprint capability. CR provides more consistent quality of portable examinations. CR allows post-acquisition image manipulation. CR affords lost image recovery by reprinting. CR allows daylight processing of plain radiographic images. Only through conscientious, comprehensive QA efforts can we realize the full benefits of CR technology.

REFERENCES

1. Kato, H: Photostimulable Phosphor Radiography Design Considerations. in Specification, Acceptance Testing and Quality Control of Diagnostic X-ray Imaging Equipment. AAPM Monograph No. 20. 731-770, 1994.

2. Quality assurance for diagnostic imaging. NCRP Report No 99. 252pp, 1988.

3. Willis, CE, Weiser, JC, Leckie, RG, et al: Optimization and quality control of computed radiography. SPIE 2164: 178-185, 1994.

4. Seibert, JA: Photostimulable phosphor system acceptance testing. in Specification, Acceptance Testing and Quality Control of Diagnostic X-ray Imaging Equipment. AAPM Monograph No. 20. 771-800, 1994.

5. Dobbins, JT III, Ergun, DL, Rutz, L, et al: DQE(f) of four generations of computed radiography acquisition devices. Med Phys 22(10): 1581-1593, 1995.

6. Oestmann, JW, Prokop, M, Shefer, CM, et al: Hardware and software artifacts in storage phosphor radiography. Radiographics 11: 795-805, 1991.

7. Freedman, M, Pe, E, Mun, SK, et al: The potential for unnecessary patient exposure from the use of storage phosphor imaging systems. SPIE 1897:472-479, 1993.

8. Willis, CE, Leckie, RG, Carter, J, et al: Objective measures of quality assurance in a computed radiography-based radiology department. SPIE 2432: 588-599, 1995.

9. Sagel, SS, Jost, RG, Glazer, HS, et al: Digital mobile radiography. J. Thorac Imag 5(1) 36-48, 1990.

10. Schaefer, CM, Greene, RE, Oestmann, JW, et al: Improved control of image optical density with low-dose digital and conventional radiography in bedside imaging. Radiology 173: 713-714, 1989.

11. Prokop, M, Galanski, M, Oestmann, JW, et al: Storage phosphor versus screen-film radiography: effect of varying exposure parameters and unsharp mask filtering on the detectability of cortical bone defects. Radiology 177: 109-113, 1990.

12. Dobbins, JT III, Rice, JJ, Beam, CA, et al: Threshold perception performance with computed and screen-film radiography: implications for chest radiography. Radiology 183: 179-187, 1992.

13. Chotas, HG and Ravin, CE: Digital chest radiography with storage phosphor systems: potential masking of bilateral pleural effusions. J. Digital Imaging 5(1) 14-19, 1992.

14. Metz, CE, Wagner, RF, Doi, K, et al: Toward consensus on quantitative assessment of medical imaging systems. Med Phys 22(7): 1057-1061, 1995.

15. Cowen, AR, Workman, A, and Price, JS: Physical aspects of photostimulable phosphor computed radiography. Brit J of Radiol 66: 322-345, 1993.

16. Workman, A and Cowen, AR: Signal, noise, and SNR transfer properties of computed radiography. Phys Med Biol 38: 1789-1808, 1993.

17. Huda, W, Jing, Z, and Hoyle, BA: Film density calibration for computed radiography systems: is the standard three-point procedure accurate? Radiology 188: 875-877, 1993.

Table 1. Reasons for repeated examinations.

Reason	#	%
positioning	167	57.19%
underexposed	28	9.59%
motion	24	8.22%
no exposure	21	7.19%
overexposed	17	5.82%
reprint	12	4.11%
no marker	7	2.40%
artifact	5	1.71%
double exposed	4	1.37%
wrong menu selec	4	1.37%
grid lines	2	0.68%
over collimated	1	0.34%
	292	

Table 2. QA guidance based on Sensitivity (S) numbers.

S Number	Guidance
>1000	Underexposed-repeat view
>600-1000	Underexposed-QC exception required
>300-600	Underexposed-QC approval required
150-300	Acceptable range
<150-75	Overexposed-QC approval required
<75-50	Overexposed-QC exception required
<50	Overexposed-repeat view

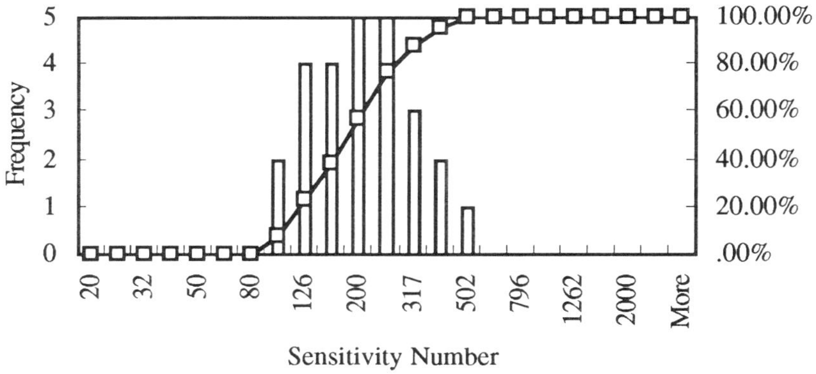

Figure 1. Distribution of Sensitivity Numbers for AP Chest Portable Examinations before QA guidance.

A Common Platform for Planning of Radiation and Hyperthermia Therapy

J. Beier
Strahlen- und Poliklinik, VIrchow Klinikum, Humboldt University Berlin
Deutsches Herzzentrum Berlin, Virchow Klinikum, Germany

J. Gellermann, O. Huth, M. Wolf and R. Felix
Strahlen- und Poliklinik, VIrchow Klinikum, Humboldt University Berlin

D. Stalling, M. Seebass, J. Nadobny and P. Deuflhard
Konrad Zuse Zentrum Berlin, Germany

1. Introduction

We present our developed multi-system, multi-architecture software for the virtual planning and simulation of radiation and hyperthermia treatment. The planning is based on complete 3D data from CT and MRI and is applied in conformal radiation therapy, regional hyperthermia, and interstitial therapies. Hyperthermia represents a new, non-invasive cancer therapy which employs radiofrequency waves to heat tumorous tissues [3, 5, 10, 11, 12]. Simulation of an efficient therapy predicts a set-up which achieves temperatures within the tumor of more than 41° C without damaging undiseased tissue. The therapy planning and simulation software HyperPlan developed at the Zuse Institute was created for applications in hyperthermia and has now been extended for planning of conformal radiation therapy.

By providing the physician with high-quality three-dimensional reconstructions of the present anatomical status, dose distributions and device adjustments the treatment is interactively planned and optimum techniques and field parameters can be selected.

2. System Design

Hyperplan is provided with a flexible, graphical, object-oriented user-interface, which allows easy handling and manipulation of the data objects. These objects are represented by icons in a working area (Fig. 1). Data objects are associated with specific visualization resp. editing objects. Thus, the user creates a graphical data flow network in the working area. Data objects, for instance, tomographic slices, contours, or a catheter array can be manipulated interactively by invoking of an editor object. The third object class are computational modules. These parametrized objects perform some computation and generate new output data. In comparison to editing modules, computational objects do not change the input data. The graphical outcome of this network is visualized by one (or more) 3D viewer(s) in a separate window. For this 3D visualization, a viewer based on SGI Open Inventor and SGI OpenGL was implemented for the display of the anatomical, physical, and technical data.

The standard set of functions can easily be extended by new, self-developed modules without the need for re-compilation. The list of available modules and their configuration is archived in a resource file. The loading and activation of a new module is synchronized by a run-time-loader. Modules which are currently not in use do not consume any system resources [13].

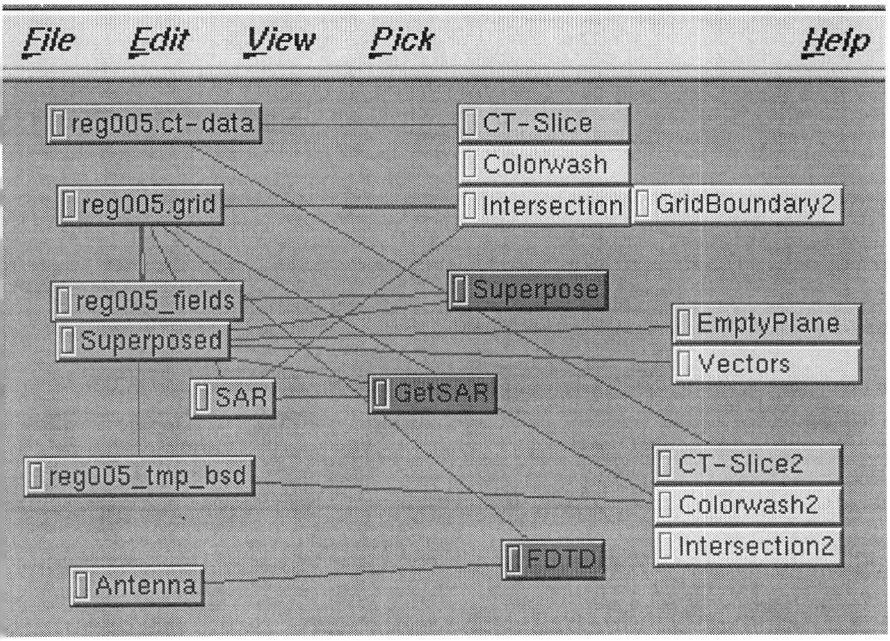

Fig. 1: Graphical user interface for object management

In the working area, the data objects (depicted in green) and their display objects (yellow) can easily be managed by the point-and-click technique. In this example, the object 'reg005.ct-data' represents a stack of CT slices which is connected to two multiplanar reformation objects ('CT-slice') in a 'colorwash' mode. Each object owns a set of parameters which are selected and adjusted separately. These features allow the fast and comfortable handling of the different data objects within the Hyperplan 3D viewer.

The HyperPlan software itself is operating in a clinic-wide (LAN within the radiological/oncological department) and inter-center (MAN, ATM-based connection to Zuse Institute and other Berlin clinics) environment.

3. Integration of Heterogeneous Information

A composite visualization of various 3D objects of different data types in one common 3D space was realized using different display techniques: objects triangulated from 2D contours, isosurfaces from thresholding, volume rendering, integration of original CT/MRI data (cut planes, data cubes), and technical structures. The data to be displayed can be divided into four classes: technical data of the treatment devices, anatomical data from CT and MRI, and physical data from radiation resp. hyperthermia (Fig 2).

Treatment Devices

The visualization of the device positions (radiation device, hyperthermia applicator / antennaes) relative to the patient and relative to the treatment room within the observer's eye view give a realistic impression of the entire set-up. For planning of interstitial radiation therapy [2, 3, 4, 5, 14], special functions for interactive generation and manipulation of catheter arrays were added [8]. After the planning phase, these catheters are surgically implanted into the tumor-bearing tissue for insertion of radioactive afterloading seeds and/or hyperthermia antennaes.

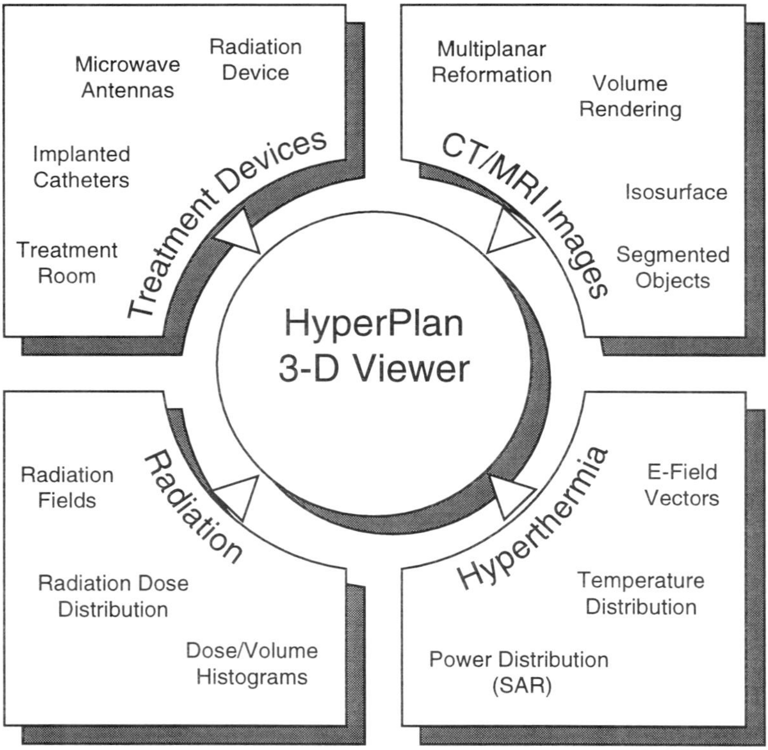

Fig. 2: Different types of anatomical, technical and physical 3D data

CT/MRI Images

The tomographic images are segmented by a self-developed software called 'Medical Image Editor' [6, 7] which provides functions for image archiving, automatic contour detection, editing and triangulation. Hence, different manual and automatic procedures were implemented:

- manual drawing of contours using the mouse,
- manual demarcation of Bezier and cubic spline base points,

- automatic region growing: seed point, two thresholds, minimal region area,
- automatic cost matrix contour tracing.

The contours can easily be manipulated by basic functions (move, add, delete base point, region editor) or by morphological functions (erosion, dilation). The resulting contours are assigned to specific objects. Several menus help the user to create and manipulate objects and contours. The contours of all or individual objects are displayed within the image. A pictorial image browser helps to navigate through the image stack. After completion of the contour detection, all 2D contours of an object are triangulated to form a three-dimensional surface.

The original and segmented CT/MRI data represent the base for visualization of image data and for calculation of radiation resp. hyperthermia field parameters.

Radiation Data

For the planning of the radiation therapy, one commercial and one scientific system (HELAX - Siemens AG, Germany; VoxelPlan - DKFZ, Germany) were successfully connected to the HyperPlan software, although these systems run on several different hardware architectures (SGI, SUN, HP, DEC) resp. different operating systems (UNIX derivates, OpenVMS). The resulting radiation dose distributions, field parameters, and statistical data are imported into the Hyperplan system and can be visualized here together with further patient data.

Hyperthermia Data

The calculation and simulation of heat treatment is directly performed within the Hyperplan software. The computation of distributions is based on tetrahedral and regular grids estimating electrical field (E-field) distributions, power deposition patterns, specific absorption rates (SAR), and temperature distributions within the tissue. Methods in practical use are the VSIE (volume surface integral equation) and FDTD (finite difference time domain) method. Furthermore, statistical analyses (volume/dose histogram, index and mean values) as well as optimization procedures are performed.

4. Results

Fig. 3 shows an example for the visualization of a patient model during hyperthermia. The circular arranged bars demonstrate the positions of the radiowave dipole antennas. Two cut planes are used for image reformation (axial and sagittal) of the CT examination. A further cut plane depicts the calculated vectors of the resulting E-field. When interactively moving these planes, its contents is updated immediately. Several anatomical objects (bone, aorta) are displayed as solid surfaces as a result of contour triangulation. For an increased speed in computation time of the hyperthermia simulation, the spatial resolution of these objects is set to a reduced value.

In particular, for the treatment of lung and prostata carcinoma the benefit of this automated approach in image segmentation, dose calculation, 3D display and therapy simulation was demonstrated. For the optimization process, variables of different dose distribution as well as biological criteria (normal tissue complication probability NTCP, tumor control probability TCP) are considered.

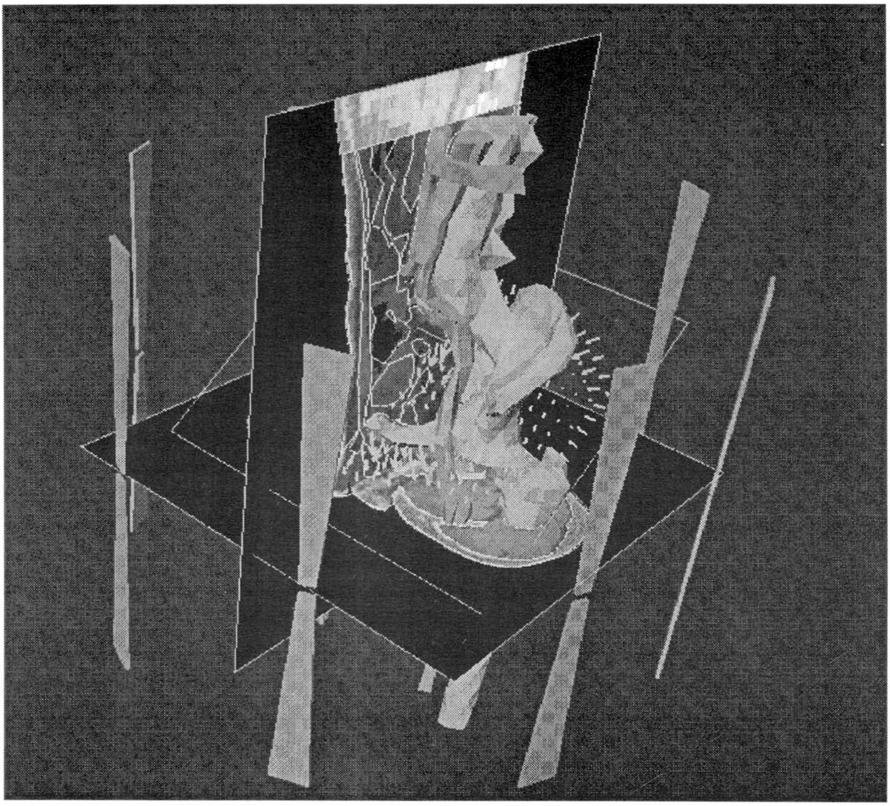

Fig. 3: Visualization of heterogeneous 3D data for hyperthermia therapy

5. Conclusions

The integration of different components for segmentation, 3D visualisation, dose distribution and therapy simulation resulted in a flexible, high-end system for planning of both radiation and hyperthermia therapy. The developed software platform allows for the calculation and optimization of radiation and hyperthermia planning in a faster and more efficient manner than conventional procedures.

The 3D reconstructions of the present anatomy in relation to treatment devices and calculated dose distributions help the treating physician to interactively plan the therapy. Based on this knowledge, the feasibility of a certain radiation plan can be assessed and compared to other strategies. By providing the physician with high-quality 3D reconstructions of the anatomical, technical and physical data the therapy can be planned in a highly interactive and comfortable manner.

References

[1] Bronen-RA; Lee-GL; Son-YH; Healy-G; Meli-JA; Sasaki-CT: CT-guided percutaneous insertion of interstitial radiotherapy catheters in head and neck tumors, J-Comput-Assist-Tomogr. 1994 Jan-Feb; 18(1): 163-165

[2] Black-PM; Tarbell-NJ; Alexander-E 3d; Rockoff-M; Zhan-MS; Loeffler-J: Stereotactic techniques in managing pediatric brain tumors, Childs-Nerv-Syst. 1993 Sep; 9(6): 343 - 347

[3] Hynynen-K: The feasibility of interstitial ultrasound hyperthermia, Med-Phys. 1992 Jul-Aug; 19(4): 979-987

[4] Brosman-SA; Tokita-K: Transrectal ultrasound-guided interstitial radiation therapy for localized prostate cancer, Urology. 1991 Oct; 38(4): 372-376

[5] Stucklschweiger-G; Schad-KA; Handl-Zeller-L; Leitner-H; Poier-E; Hackl-A: Interstitial Ir-192 afterloading therapy with sequential warm-water hyperthermia, Strahlenther-Onkol. 1991 Feb; 167(2), pp. 98-104

[6] Beier J, Bittner RC, Wust P, Fleck E, Felix R: Three-dimensional reconstruction of lung tumors based on MRI, Röfo, Thieme Verlag, 164.1, Jan. 1996, pp. 75 - 78

[7] Beier J, Bittner RC, Fleck E,Felix R: Three-Dimensional Visualization and Animation of Thoracic Tumors from MRI Images, European Respiratory Journal, ERS, 333, 1995

[8] Beier J, Wust P, Huth O, Wolf M, Stalling D, Seebass M, Bier J, Felix R: Planning of Catheter Implantation for Interstitial Radiation and Hyperthermia Therapy, CAR 96, in press

[9] Wust P, Seebass M, Nadobny J, Deuflhard P, Mönich G, Felix R: Simulation studies promote technological development of radiofrequency phased array hyperthermia, Int J Hyperthermia, 1996 in press

[10] Seebass M, Wust P, Gellermann J, Stalling D, Nadobny J, Felix R: Three-Dimensional Simulation of Non-Invasive Radiofrequency Hyperthermia, Minimal Invasise Medizin, 6(1) 1995, pp. 29 - 35

[11] Wust P, Seebass M, Nadobny J, Felix R: Electromagnetic Deep Heating Technology, in: Thermo-Radiotherapy and Thermo-Chemotherapy, Seegenschmiedt MH, Fessenden P, Vernon CC, Springer Verlag, 1995, pp. 219 - 248

[12] Gellermann J, Wust P, Wiener A, Stalling D, Stahl H, Felix R: Optimization Strategies in Hyperthermia Planning compared with those used in Radiotherapy Planning, CAR 95, 1995, pp. 1083 - 1087

[13] Stalling D, Hege HC, Höllerer T: Visualization and 3D Interaction for Hyperthermia Treatment Planning, CAR 95, 1995, pp. 1216 - 1222

[14] Stahl H, Maier-Hauff K, Wust P, Felix R: Planning and placement of catheter arrays for intracranial brachtherapy, International Brachtherapy-Program & Abstracts, 8th International Brachtherapy Conference, Nice, France, 1995, pp. 303 - 304

SESSION 7

Expert Systems/ Artificial Intelligence/ Speech Recognition

Co-Chairs:

Robert M. Allman
Jonathan Bower

Decision Support Model for Determining Appropriateness of Imaging Tests

David Piraino, M.D., Nancy Obuchowski, Ph.D., Michael Recht, M.D. and Bradford Richmond, M.D.
Cleveland Clinic Foundation, Cleveland, Ohio

INTRODUCTION

In the era of managed care doing appropriate imaging tests is increasingly important. This paper presents a general model which can be used to determine when patients should be tested and a method to choose the most appropriate test.

METHODS

A generalized model for determining appropriateness of imaging exams was developed using decision support theory and relative measures of utility. Figure 1 is a schematic of the decision tree. The square nodes indicate that a decision must be made, i.e., to test or not to test or to treat or not to treat and the circular node represent chance nodes i.e. disease present or disease absent.

Figure 1 Decision Tree

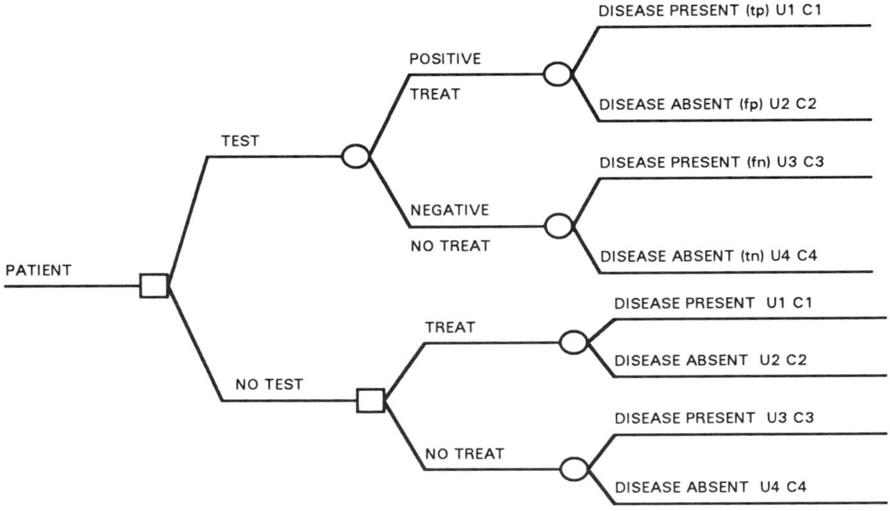

Patients present with a pretest probability of disease. The first decision is to test for the disease or not test for the disease. On the test arm the test maybe positive or negative. If the test is positive the patient will receive treatment and if the test is negative the patient will not receive treatment. For a positive test with the patient being treated, the disease may either be present (true positive) or the disease may be absent (false positive). On the negative arm of the testing tree, again the disease may be present a (false negative) or the disease may be absent (true negative).

The other decision arm involves the decision not to test. The patient is either treated or not treated. Again, there are four possible outcomes: treatment with the disease present, treatment with the disease absent, no treatment with the disease present, and no treatment with the disease absent.

The four possible outcomes with relative utilities U1 through U4 are shown in Table 1. U1 represents the utility of treating the patient with the disease, U2 represents utility of treating the patient without disease, U3 represents utility of not treating the patient with disease, U4 represents utility of not treating the patient without the disease.

Table 1 Utility	**Disease**	**No Disease**
Treatment	U1	U2
No Treatment	U3	U4

A utility or effectiveness of 1 represents completely normal health for 1 year and a utility of 0 represents death. If a treatment would provide 3 additional years of normal life as opposed to death than the utility gained by treating a sick person would be 3. Other utilities can be estimated by relative measures between 0 and 1 using data from the Beaver Dam Health Outcomes Study using the Quality of well being index (QWB) [1].

Given the above decision model the following formula can be used for calculating threshold pre-test probabilities. Two pre-test probabilities are needed: P lower and P upper. The following rule (Rule 1) applies:

Rule 1

1) If the pre-test probability of disease is less than or equal to P lower then do not test and do not treat.
2) If the pre-test probability of disease is greater than or equal P upper then do not test and begin treatment.
3) If the pre-test probability of disease is between P lower and P upper then test.

P lower and P upper are given by the following formula:

Se = sensitivity of test

Sp = specificity of test

$$Plower = \frac{-(U2 - U4)(1 - SP)}{Se(U1 - U3) - (U2 - U4)(1 - Sp)}$$

$$Pupper = \frac{Sp(U2 - U4)}{Sp(U2 - U4) - (U1 - U3)(1 - Se)}$$

Modification of the above decision tree along the lines of Phelps and Muslin with inclusion of monetary costs can be seen below[2]. Table 2 demonstrates the monetary costs of treatment: C1 costs of treating sick person, C2 cost of treating healthy person, C3 costs of not treating sick person, C4 costs of not treating healthy person. A conversion factor between costs and utility is needed so a utility to cost ratio must be defined. Also the cost of the diagnostic tests must be known.

Table 2 Cost	**Disease**	**No Disease**
Treatment	C1	C2
No Treatment	C3	C4

The formula for calculating threshold pre-test probabilities which include contribution of cost is presented below. Two pre-test probabilities are needed: P lower and P upper, the above rule (Rule 1) applies:

P lower and P upper are given by the following formula:

Ct = cost of diagnostic test
g = utility / cost ratio

$$Plower = \frac{-(U2 - U4)(1 - SP) + g(Ct + (C2 - C4)(1 - Sp))}{Se(U1 - U3) - (U2 - U4)(1 - SP) - g(Se(C1 - C2) - (C2 - C4)(1 - Sp))}$$

$$Pupper = \frac{Sp(U2 - U4) + g(Ct - Sp(C2 - C4))}{Sp(U2 - U4) - (U1 - U3)(1 - Se) - g(Sp(C2 - C4) - (C1 - C3)(1 - Se))}$$

These formulas demonstrate that the actual values of the four utilities and costs are not needed. Rather, the difference between U2 and U4 (utility gained by not treating a healthy person) , the difference between U1 and U3 (utility gained by treating a sick person) , the difference between C2 and C4 (change in cost by not treating healthy person) and the difference between C1 and C3 (change in cost by treating sick person) are needed. As can been seen from the above equation the pre-test probability range also depends on sensitivity, specificity, test cost and utility to cost ratio.

Another way to look at the decision to test or not to test is to determine the added value the test provides. The added or clinical value of the test dependents on whether or not the fallback decision is to treat or not to treat. The added value from a diagnostic test given the prior decision to treat is the gain in utility from not treating true negatives ($Sp(1-p)((U2-U4)-g(C2-C4))$) and the loss in utility from not treating false negatives ($-(1-Se)p((U1-U3)-(g(C1-C3))$). The added value from a diagnostic test given the prior decision no to treat is the gain in utility from treating true positives ($pSe((U1-U3)-g(C1-C3))$) and the loss in utility from treating false positives ($-(1-p)(1-Sp)((U2-U4)-g(C2-C4))$)[2].

The test is recommended to be performed when ever the added clinical information associated with the test is greater than the rescaled cost(test cost times utility to cost ratio). A graph of the added clinical information and the re-scaled cost provides a graphical picture of when to perform a diagnostic test. If there is more than one diagnostic test that has a value of clinical information greater than its rescaled cost then perform the one with the greatest value of clinical information. The prior probability of disease is on the X axis and the value of clinical information from the test is on the Y axis.

RESULTS

Figure 2 demonstrates the expected value of information for:

1. PERFECT test (sensitivity and specificity equal to 1) solid line and
2. GOOD test with intermediate specificity (0.85) and sensitivity (0.85) dotted line.

The cost of the test is \$2000 and utilities are held constant. The effectiveness to cost ratio is 1 to \$5000

Figure 2

PERFECT TEST	GOOD TEST
Plower = 0.04	Plower = 0.20
Pupper = 0.96	Pupper = 0.82

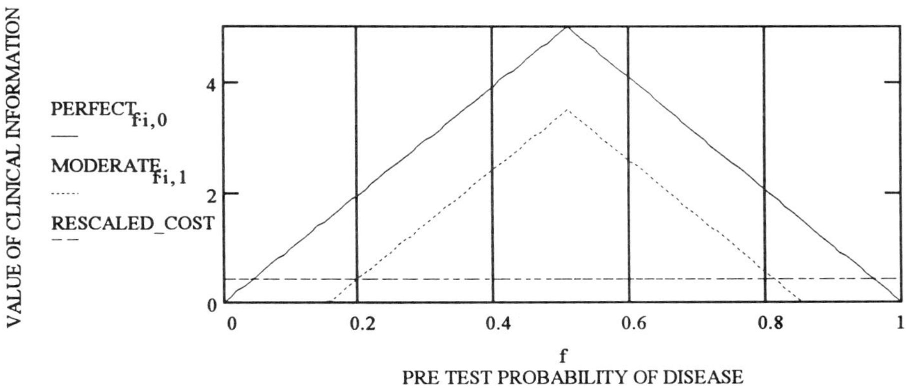

As can be seen as the sensitivity and specificity of a diagnostic test decreases the expected value of clinical information decreases and the range of pretest probability for testing decreases. With a perfect test the pre test probabilities to perform the test depend mostly on the rescaled cost of the test.

Figure 3 also demonstrates how sensitivity and sensitivity change clinical information and P lower and P upper:

1. Sensitivity = 0.80, Specificity = 0.70, solid line
2. Sensitivity = 0.60, Specificity = 0.90, dotted line

Figure 3

TEST ONE	**TEST TWO**
Plower = 0.30	**Plower = 0.21**
Pupper = 0.78	**Pupper = 0.67**

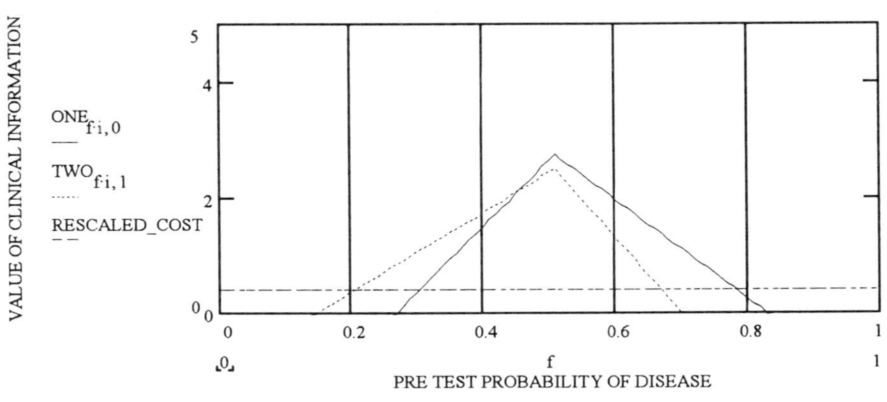

Test TWO should be performed between 0.21 and 0.45 pre test probabilities while test ONE should be performed between 0.45 and 0.78 pre test probabilities.

Figure 4 demonstrates how utility changes clinical information and P lower and P upper:

1. Utility gained from treating a sick person = 5, Utility gained from not treating a healthy person = 10, solid line
2. Utility gained from treating a sick person = 10, Utility gained from not treating a healthy person = 5, dotted line

Figure 4

TEST ONE
Plower = 0.34
Pupper = 0.88

TEST TWO
Plower = 0.13
Pupper = 0.68

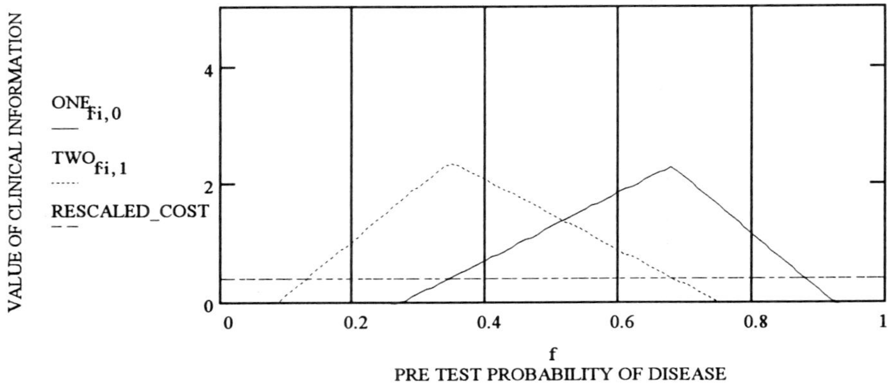

Figure 4 shows how changes in utilities can shift the added value of clinical information along the probability axis and shift the range of pretest probabilities for testing.

Figure 5 applies this model to mammography in 40-49 year old women. The following values are used in this model[3]:

Sensitivity = 0.90, Specificity = 0.80;
Utility gain by treating patent with breast cancer = 6 (20% reduction in mortality times life expectancy (30 years))
Utility gained by not treating health person = 1
Change in cost of treating breast cancer = $6100
Change in cost of not treating healthy person = $6100 [3]

Figure 5
Mammography
Plower = 0.05 **Pupper = 0.63**

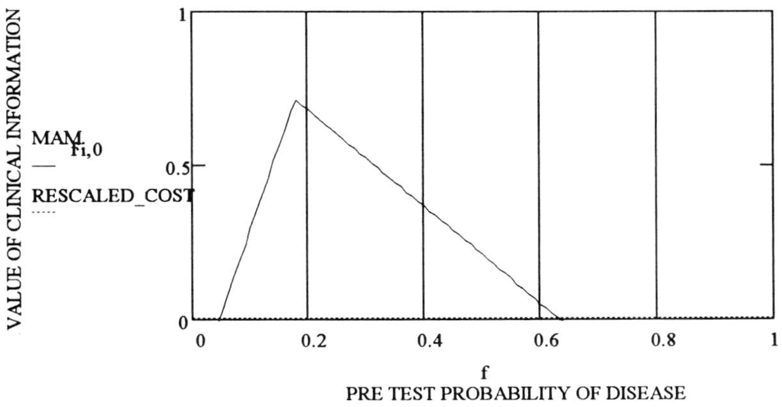

Figure 5 shows that the pretest probability range for testing starts at a very low pretest probability (0.05) as is appropriate for a screening test.

DISCUSSION

This paper presents a decision theory model which can be used to determine the range of pretest probabilities to perform a diagnostic imaging test. This model can be used to study how costs, sensitivities, specificity's and utilities change the appropriate pretest probability range of diagnostic imaging tests. Further study is needed to determine if this model can be a useful clinical tool.

Difficulties with this decision support model are obtaining accurate or reproducible information concerning relative utilities and determining appropriate utility to cost ratios.

REFERENCES

1. Fryback DG, Dasbach EJ, Klein R, et all, *The Beaver Dam health outcomes study: initial catalog of health-state quality factors.* Med Decis Making 1993;13:89-102.

2. Phelps CE, Mushlin AI, *Focusing technology assessment using medical decision theory*, Med Decis Making 1988;8:279-289.

3. Rosenquist CJ, Lindfors KK, *Screening mammography in women aged 40-49 years: analysis of Cost-effectiveness*, Radiology 1994;191:647-650.

Abdominal Organ Segmentation Using a Hopfield Neural Netwo

John E. Koss, Francis D. Newman, Timothy K. Johnson and Dennis Kirch
University of Colorado Health Sciences Center, Denver, Colorado

Segmenting images into component organs or tissue types is a necessary process to adequately calculate doses in monoclonal antibody therapy as well as in 3D treatment planning in radiation oncology. It is however, a time intensive procedure. To facilitate the segmentation process, we developed a computerized algorithm to segment abdominal organs in digital images (CT, MRI).

The segmentation algorithm separates images into component organs on a pixel by pixel basis. Pixels are represented by n-dimensional vectors where n is the number of registered images used to classify the pixels. The input data consist of abdominal digital images and images generated by calculating textural values for each pixel from the original images. The combination of textural and original grey-scale values allows proper segmentation of the images.

Classifying pixels based on textural and grey-scale values is formulated as an optimization problem and described by an energy function. A Hopfield Neural Network minimizes the energy function. Pixels are arbitrarily assigned to classes and the network evolves toward a state of lower energy by reassigning the pixels. The best solutions minimize the energy function by decreasing a metric term, along with other terms ensuring that each pixel is assigned to only one class. The metric is based on differences between each pixel vector and the centroid of the organ to which the pixel is assigned.

The neural network performed well in distinguishing organs. Textural differences in organs allowed segmentation of organs with overlapping grey-tone values. This technique shows considerable promise in automated segmentation of abdominal images.

Introduction

Segmentation of images into individual organs and/or tissue types is an important step in the visualization of tissues in the body. In radiation treatment planning, the shape, size and location of target and nearby organs needs to be known for accurate dose distribution calculations. Similarly, in absorbed-dose calculations in the application of radiopharmaceuticals, the organs ideally should be based on the patient's own organs rather than on a model organ shape and size. Manual segmentation is however, a labor intensive procedure.

Automating segmentation is a difficult problem since CT numbers overlap for most organs. Since the grey-scale values are directly (linearly) related to the CT numbers, the grey-scale image cannot be used by itself. This is similarly true for MRI images. Computing textural values from the grey-scale image(s) helps differentiate organs with overlapping grey-scale numbers. We propose computing additional images based on extracting textural features from the grey-scale images. This results in d registered images where there are d-1 textural features extracted. These d images are then segmented on a pixel by pixel basis using information from all images. Previous workers[1] have done similar segmentation on different brain tissues but by using multi-spectral MRI images rather than CT and extracted texture images.

II Texture Mapping

Texture describes the surface characteristics of grey-scale images. Textural features contain information about the spatial distribution of tonal variations within a neighborhood. Properties extracted from the image by the texture transformation include information such as homogeneity, grey-scale linear dependencies (linear structure), contrast and image complexity[2]. However, it is usually not possible to directly tie a computed textural transformation to a specific textural characteristic. The distribution of grey-scale levels can be described in terms of first, second or higher order statistics. Textures based on first order statistics include mean, standard deviation, third moment, and entropy. These first order statistics are computed without regard to where in the image the pixels are located relative to one another[3]. Second order statistics take into consideration the spatial distribution of the grey-tone levels. As originally described by Haralick et al.[2], fourteen different textural features can be described from a co-occurrence matrix. The co-occurrence matrix method, while powerful, is an extremely memory and computationally intensive algorithm. Unser[4] and Sridhar et. al[5] showed that most of Haralick's textural features could be derived from sum and difference histograms for textural analysis. The sum and difference histograms are found by adding or subtracting every horizontal and vertical pixel pair grey-scale value. Table 1 shows the textural features derived from the sum and difference histograms we found to be useful in segmenting. We also used the original grey-scale image and the mean and standard deviation computed over the entire image (first order statistics).

Textural Feature	Formula Using Sum and Difference Histograms
Mean	f1 = $\sum_i i \cdot P_{sum}(i)$
Variance	f2 = $\frac{1}{2}\{\sum_i (i-2f1)^2 \cdot P_{sum}(i) + \sum_j j^2 \cdot P_{diff}(j)\}$
Energy	f3 = $\sum_i P_{sum}(i)^2 \cdot \sum_j P_{diff}(j)^2$
Correlation	f4 = $\frac{1}{2}\{\sum_i (i-2f1)^2 \cdot P_{sum}(i) - \sum_j j^2 \cdot P_{diff}(j)\}$
Entropy	f5 = $-\sum_i P_{sum}(i) \cdot LOG(P_{sum}(i)) - \sum_j P_{diff}(j) \cdot LOG(P_{diff}(j))$
Contrast	f6 = $\sum_j j^2 \cdot P_{diff}(j)$
Homogeneity	f7 = $\sum_j \frac{1}{1+j^2} \cdot P_{diff}(j)$
Cluster Shade	f8 = $\sum_i (i-2F1)^3 \cdot P_{sum}(i)$
Cluster Prominence	f9 = $\sum_i (i-2F1)^4 \cdot P_{sum}(i)$

Table 1. Listing of second order textural features and formulas.[4,5]

Texture is a neighborhood property in that it is calculated over a contiguous block of pixels. At every pixel in the image, the textural features are calculated using a surrounding window. The textural values computed for that window are then assigned to the central pixel. In segmentation, one wants the textural feature to be calculated only within the organ being segmented and not across boundaries. Thus if the block of pixels being used to calculate the textural features is too large, it is likely that the window will cross over organ edges and the texture calculated be contaminated since it is a combination of multiple organs. But if the window over which the textural features are computed is too small, then grey-scale level tends to be the dominant property of that area since there is likely to be little variation over a small area. Thus a quandary exists in determining the size of the block over which to calculate the textural features - i.e. the area needs to be large enough to adequately represent the organ, but small enough not to cross over organ boundaries. Solving this problem involves calculating the textural features over a window that is allowed to move about the pixel of interest instead of forcing the window to be centered about the pixel[3]. As long as the organ boundaries are not too angular, at least one quadrant will lie entirely within the organ as shown in figure 1. This quadrant is used to calculate the textural features.

At the end of computing the textural features, there are twelve images (one original, two first order and nine Haralick), which are used a segmenters in a neural network. Since these images are all calculated from a single original image, they are all perfectly registered.

Pixels	1	2	3	. . .	K	Classes
1	0	1	0		0	
2	1	0	0		0	
3	0	0	1		0	
⋮						
N	0	0	1		0	

Fig. 2. Neural architecture consists of N * K neurons (N = # of pixels, K = # of classes). In this example, pixel 1 belongs to class 2, pixel 2 belongs to class 1 and pixels 3 and N belong to class 3.

III Hopfield Neural Network

Once the textural feature images have been created, the segmentation problem can be expressed as an optimization problem where there are N pixels to be partitioned into K sets where each pixel in a particular set is more similar to other pixels in that set than to pixels in other sets. Each pixel is a d-dimensional vector, where each of the d components of the vector is taken from a textural feature image. For a 512 by 512 pixel image (262,144 pixels), there are $K^N/K! = K^{262144}/K!$ possible ways to partition the

image. This number is prohibitively large and finding the one best solution may not be possible. Finding a good solution where only a few pixels are misclassified is a reasonable approach to this partitioning problem, followed by a post-partitioning filter. The Hopfield Neural Network (HNN) is well suited for this type of optimization problem[7,8]. In an HNN, all the neurons are fully connected, with no specific input or output neurons. Starting values are given to each neuron and the net iterates to a solution. The property of an HNN that makes it attractive is that the problem can by formulated in terms of an energy function or landscape where the 'lows' represent good solutions. The neural architecture consists of N columns by K rows, resulting in N * K neurons (N = number of pixels, K = number of classes) (figure 2). The energy function is constructed such that it has three terms which collectively reach a minimum when three conditions are met: 1) When only one neuron in each column is on (has a non-zero value), this prevents a pixel from being assigned to more than one class; 2) When the sum of each column equals 1, this ensures that each pixel is fully assigned to a class; and 3) A cost term that decreases in value based on a distance measured from the pixel to the class centroid to which the pixel is assigned[6].
An energy equation that meets these constraints is:

$$E = A \sum_{i=1}^{N} \sum_{p=1}^{K} \sum_{q \neq p}^{K} V_{pi} V_{qi} + B \sum_{i=1}^{N} \left(\sum_{p=1}^{K} V_{pi} - 1 \right)^2 + C \sum_{p=1}^{K} \sum_{i=1}^{N} R_{pi} V_{pi}^2$$

Where V_{pi} is the output from the neuron in class column p, pixel row I, and R is the error term. A, B and C are constants.

Initially, each pixel in the network is randomly assigned to a class. Following each iteration, the class centroid is calculated followed by an error term (R in the energy equation). This error term is calculated by doing the summation of the Euclidean distances between the class centroids and each pixel assigned to that class.

There is no training associated with a Hopfield Neural Network as there is in perceptron based neural networks. It is considered unsupervised learning. However, one must know a priori the number of classes the data is to be segmented into.

IV Implementation

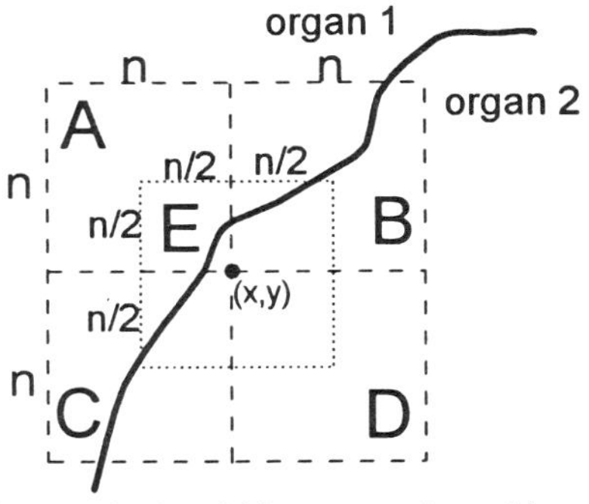

Fig. 1. Quadrant D lies entirely within organ 2 and is used to calculate the textural features for pt (x,y). n is the size of the window in pixels.

To test the algorithm we have been using a CT data set obtained from Yale University (Yaleman). Unfortunately, during the transmission and subsequent integer conversions, the data set became partially corrupted. In particular, bones have random values and cannot be segmented with our current data set. We have had some success segmenting liver, spleen and skeletal muscle - three tissue types with nearly the same grey-scale levels. Figure 3 shows the original data along with the above mentioned organs or tissues segmented out. The original data was 512 by 512 pixels. In order to speed up the segmentation process, a box was drawn around the body to reduce the number of pixels to 360 by 290. No loss of resolution resulted from this step as only background was deleted. Next, the image was rebinned to 180 by 145 - losing some resolution.

Images were formed for the two first order and nine second order textural features, resulting in pixels having 12 values associated with them. A sliding window of 5 by 5 pixels was used. This window size worked well for small organs but a larger window is preferable for large organs such as the liver.

The neural network randomly assigned each pixel to a class and was then allowed to iterate 150 times. Depending upon the random starting point, only small differences were noted between after 100 to 150 iterations. An Euclidean distance metric was used to determine differences between class centroids and pixels within a class.

Finally, a post-classifying median filter was run on the segmented data to get rid of 'salt and pepper' noise caused by local misclassified pixels. As can be seen on figure 3, most of the liver, spleen and skeletal muscle pixels have been correctly separated - although areas within each organ remain misclassified. We feel that by having a variable window size, allowing a larger window over large organs and a small window near edges and over small organs, will help reduce the number of these misclassified pixels.

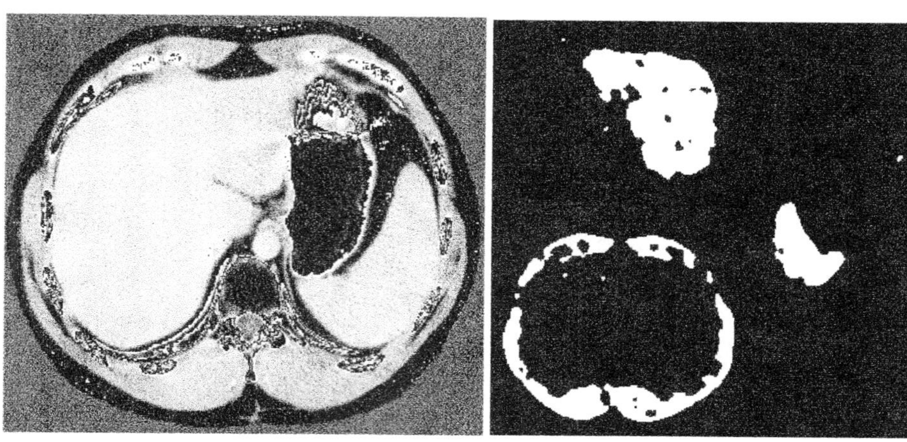

Fig. 3. CT slice used for segmentation and segmented organs. (Note that segmented organs were resized and rotated to fit on page.)

V Conclusions

This segmentation algorithm has promise in distinguishing between organs with overlapping grey-scale levels. Areas of future work include: 1) Allowing variable window sizes for texture calculations. The statistics should improve when using large windows for large organs, but still want to keep a small window for small organs and near organ boundaries. 2) Modify the algorithm so that no a priori knowledge is required. Preliminary tests suggest that, after the same number of iterations, the normalized total error as measured by the distances between class centroids and pixels is a minimum when the correct number of classes is used. 3) Test the algorithm for a variety of artifacts commonly found in CT or MRI images. 4) Distance metrics other than Euclidean may be more powerful in segmenting the image.

References

[1] S.C. Amartur, D. Piraino, and Y. Takefuji, "Optimization Neural Networks for the Segmentation of Magnetic Resonance Images", *IEEE Trans. on Medical Imaging*, vol. 11, no. 2, pp. 215-220, 1992.

[2] R.M. Haralick, K. Shanmugam, and I. Dinstein, "Textural Features for Image Classification", *IEEE Trans. on Systems, Man, and Cybernetics*, vol. SMC-3, no. 6, pp. 610-621, 1973.

[3] F. Tomita and S. Tsuji, “Computer Analysis of Visual Textures”, Kluwer Academic Publishers, Boston, 173 p., 1990.

[4] M. Unser, "Sum and Difference Histograms for Texture Classification", *IEEE Trans. on Pattern Analysis and Machine Intelligence*, vol. PAMI-8, no. 1, pp. 118-125, 1986.

[5] B. Sridhar, A. Phatak, and G. Chatterji, "Scene Segmentation of Natural Images Using Texture Measures and Back-Propagation", *NASA TM-104003*, 24 p., 1993.

[6] J.J. Hopfield and D.W. Tank, "Neural Computation of Decisions in Optimization Problems", *Biol. Cybern.*, vol. 52, pp. 141-152, 1985.

[7] B. Kamagar-Parsi, J.A. Gualtieri, J.E. Devaney, and B. Kamgar-Parsi, "Clustering with Neural Networks", *Biol. Cybern.*, vol. 63, pp. 201-208, 1990.

Detection of Malignant Regions in 3D MR Breast Images Using a Boolean Neural Network

Essam A. El-Kwae, Maria J. Bianchi and Mansur R. Kabuka

Center for Medical Imaging and Medical Informatics, Miami, Florida

Abstract

In this paper, a Boolean Neural Network (BNN) is used for the detection of malignant regions in breast MR images. The network was trained with a set of malignant, benign, and false positive patterns, from selected MR studies, using an incremental learning algorithm. After training, the network was tested using the jackknife method and using patterns from MR breast images. Results show that the BNN has a great aptitude to extract malignant regions. This saves the radiologist a great deal of time searching for suspected patterns for diagnosis.

1. Introduction

Breast cancer, a major cause of death among women, is estimated to affect 9% of American women at some point in their lives[1]. Considerable attention is given to breast cancer because of the potential to reduce the mortality rate by participating in screening programs. Even though mammography is the most common technique for cancer diagnosis, 10% to 30% of women who undergo mammography and who have breast cancer have negative mammograms[2]. Magnetic resonance of the breast is one of the most promising areas of MRI today. Two major achievements of breast MRI are improved specificity and sensitivity. Sensitivity for breast cancer detection using MRI has been reported to be as high as 98.4% [4]. Specificity, while lower still exceeds that of mammography. The use of bolus injection of Gd-DTPA is now being used to improve breast cancer detection through identification of the rapid enhancement patterns of malignancies.

In addition, some studies have shown that dynamic enhanced MR images are more accurate than mammography or ultrasound in detecting some types of cancer[5].

The images used for this study were T1 weighted, fat suppressed gradient echo images over the whole region of the breast, obtained immediately after the administration of 0.1 mmol/kg Gd-DTPA.

A Boolean Neural Network (BNN) was used for the detection of malignant regions in MR breast images. The network was trained with a set of malignant, benign and false positive patterns, from selected MR studies, using an incremental learning algorithm. After training, the network was tested using the jackknife method and using patterns from MR breast images.

An overview of the BNN is given in section 2. In sections 3 and 4, the BNN incremental training algorithm is explained, followed by the pattern recognition algorithm. In section 5, the training patterns extraction is explained. Section 6 states the results obtained using the consistency test, the jackknife test and using patterns from MR slices. Conclusions are given in section 7 followed by the set of references used.

2. Overview of the BNN

The BNN developed in [6,8] can be used to synthesize any boolean function and also performs efficient

* Corresponding Author,
Email: kabuka@cmiami.med.miami.edu

classification. It features fast learning and classification, guaranteed convergence, and simple, integer weight calculations. The BNN was also used to solve optimization problems [11]. A feature recognition BNN has been developed in [8]. It recognizes patterns after significant noise, deformation, translation, and scaling. It can be trained to recognize even rotated patterns. The BNN was also used for the design of classifiers [9] such as the NTE (Nearest-to-Examplar) classifier and the BKNN (Binary K-Nearest Neighbor) classifier.

In the medical field, the BNN was used for supervised and unsupervised segmentation of MR Brain images [10]. Also, in [12], the BNN was used for labeling MR Brain images. The BNN proved to be faster than traditional methods and other neural networks and was proved to be a feasible alternative for existing techniques for medical image labeling.

The BNN consists of layers of neurons connected in a feedforward structure. The neurons are fully connected between layers. The layers in the BNN have simple perceptron connections. While learning, traditional neural networks may never converge or stabilize while the BNN converges in a single iteration. Weight calculations are simple. After learning, a new training pattern can be applied without unlearning as in other architectures.

The concept of ROA (Radius of Attraction) is used to classify noisy and distorted patterns. The BNN can be either 'fixed radius', in which the ROA is fixed, or 'variable radius', in which the ROA is varied until a match is found. The choice of ROA is dependent on the application. Every examplar node is associated with a programmed threshold Θ_k and a ROA r_k. The programmed threshold is then decremented by the ROA to get the actual threshold $\Theta_k = \Sigma_i a_{ik} w_{ik} - r_k$. This leads to all patterns that differ from the stored pattern with a hamming distance of ROA to be classified as belonging to the class of that examplar. The ROA builds hyperspheres of radius r_k with the class programmed threshold as center. It was proved in [10] that the number of patterns enclosed by a ROA r defined over a certain neuron are: ${}^n\Lambda_r = \Sigma^r_{i=0} {}^nC_i$ where n is the dimensionality of the input pattern. For example, for a certain neuron, if n=256, and r=1, 257 patterns fall into the ROA of that neuron. Increasing ROA to 4 increases the number of patterns in the neuron's hyperspere to 177,589,057.

In [10], a generalization of the BNN for handling scalar weighted functions was given. In this case, input data is quantized into g gray level scales. These can be represented by m bits where $m=\log_2 g$. The EROA (Euclidean ROA) was introduced. One layer of preprocessing was added to the network whose weights can take fixed values from 2^0 to 2^{m-1}.

3. The BNN Incremental Learning Algorithm

Incremental learning is a multistage learning process which is used to increase the generalization capabilities of the network. It can also be used to incrementally train a network when the environment changes. The BNN incremental learning algorithm automatically reduces the training set and trains the network only with those examples which are estimated to be useful. In this case, the teacher need not make an effort to carefully select 'good' examples in the training set, since, the algorithm is capable of selecting the useful examples. Incremental learning also optimizes the number of neurons in the BNN. This is done by setting the ROA around the neuron immediately after an individual exemplar has been learned. If any of the subsequent training exemplars falls within the ROA of one of the existing neurons, it is automatically not learned by the learning algorithm.

Learning a new pattern will not affect those patterns already learned. Thus, the BNN can be used in applications where the environment is changing and it is desirable to continuously update the network during operation.

To test the ability of the BNN to select useful patterns from the training set and reduce the training set size, an experiment was conducted on a complete study of 36 images, each of size 256x256. Each pixel assumes a gray value from 0 to 255. Each image was divided into 256 patterns, each pattern being of size

==
The BNN incremental learning algorithm:
Input: A set of training vectors A_k, k=1, ..., K where K is the total number of training patterns.
Step 1 : Reset a counter *Vi* associated with each exemplar neuron *i* where *i=1,2,...,P*. where *P* is the number of neurons available.
Step 2 : *If* [(There are more input training patterns in the initial training set) OR (A request for incremental learning is received from the changed environment)
Accept a new input pattern for training $A_k = [a_{1k}, a_{2k}, ..., a_{nk}]$, $a_{ik} \in \{0,1\}$, where a_{ik}, i=1, 2, ..., n are parameters associated with A_k. Go to Step 4.
Step 3 : *If* (A pattern is presented for classification)
Classify it to the closest exemplar, increment *Vj* if the pattern is classified to *Cj*.
Step 4 : *If* (This pattern falls into the ROA of a pre-existing neuron)
Increment *Vj* if the pattern falls into the ROA of class *Cj* and go to Step 2.
Else go to Step 5.
Step 5 : For incremental learning, two cases arise :
i) In the case where there are excess untrained neurons, the next neuron to be trained is chosen for training with the input pattern. The counter of this neuron is reset after learning takes place.
Calculate $W_k = [w_{1k}, w_{2k}, ..., w_{nk}]$, $w_{ik} \in \{-1,1\}$, where w_{ik} is the weight vector associated with a_k. It is calculated as $w_{ik} = 2a_{ik} - 1$.
Set the kth neuron threshold as $\Theta_k = \Sigma_i a_{ik} w_{ik} - ROA$.
ii) In the case where there are no excess neurons in the network, training of the input pattern has to be done over a pre-existing neuron. The neuron for class C_l is selected for training such that $V_l < V \; \forall \; m \neq l$.
After learning, reset V_l to zero.
Step 6 : Repeat $\forall$ A_k by going back to step 2.
Output: A set of weight vectors W_K and neuron thresholds Θ_k.
==

16x16. Thus, the total number of input patterns was 9216. The purpose of the experiment was to find the number of relevant patterns for different ROAs. The ROA between features was varied from 0 to 10 and the ROA between patterns was fixed at 5. Results are summarized in the following table:

ROA	Rel.	Irr.	%Irr.
0	6913	2303	24.99%
1	6913	2303	24.99%
2	6840	2376	25.78%
3	6167	3049	33.08%
4	5454	3762	40.82%
5	4944	4272	46.35%
6	4221	4995	54.20%
7	3550	5666	61.48%
8	3051	6165	66.89%
9	2734	6482	70.33%
10	2486	6730	73.03%

These results show the effectiveness of the ROA in detecting similar patterns and decreasing the training set size.

4. The Pattern Recognition Algorithm

A new feature recognition algorithm was proposed in [8] and was applied to the character recognition problem The purpose was to recognize characters regardless of their positions in the image field (translation), sensor noise, some degree of deformation and rotation.

During the training session, the network is presented by training patterns. The pattern, originally a matrix, is transformed into a vector by cascading the rows successively. Thus, it becomes a fundamental memory point in the hamming space.

To be able to recognize translated patterns, the original pattern of size 16x16 is divided horizontally and vertically 4 times to give rise to 16 subpatterns, each of size 4x4. The 4x4 subdivision was selected because it divides the pattern symmetrically

The algorithm performs the following steps in succession to recognize any pattern:

1) Learns all the training patterns and remember their subsections.

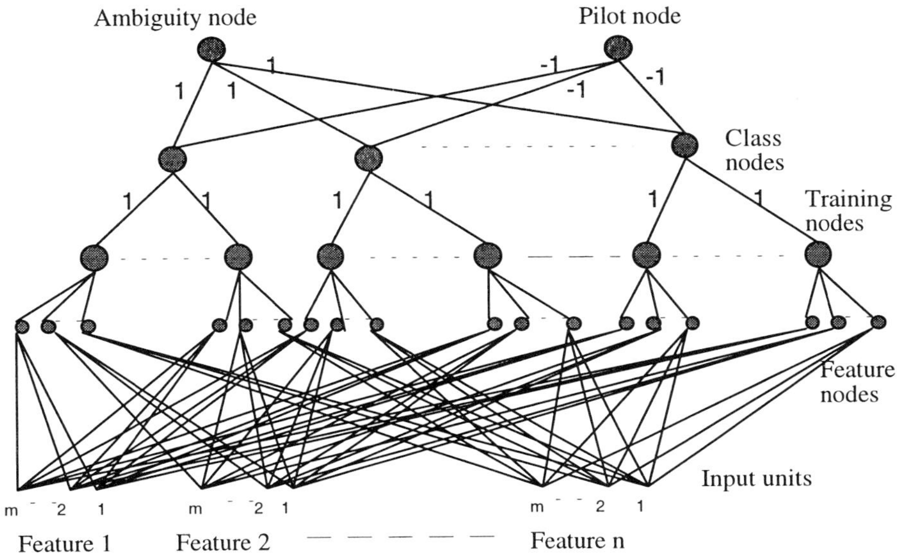

Fig. 1 : Structure of the BNN used in study

2) Divides the new input pattern into 16 segments as described above.
3) Compares each of the segments individually against the corresponding segments of the trained pattern to compute any match.
4) Finds the total number of segments that matched for any pattern and find the closest overall match. The training algorithm is the same as described in the incremental learning section. The network topology is capable of detecting any subpattern shifts that cover a displacement of ±2 in the X direction, ±2 in the Y direction. In other words, it can detect any displacement within a box of 5x5.

The network follows a 2 level detection scheme. The first level is responsible for detecting the sub-patterns and the second level is responsible for detecting the patterns themselves as well as providing the output class. The pattern grid distributes the inputs all over the first level. The neurons that detect the sub-patterns feed the single neuron in level two that fires if all sixteen sub-patterns are detected. An ROA is placed around the main pattern detection neurons in order to calculate the closest match if not all the sixteen neurons in the first level fire simultaneously.

To detect a sub-pattern whose corners are (x, y) and (x+4, y+4) and to be sure of sub-pattern detection whenever its origin lies at (x,y) or within a displacement ±2 in either or both the X and Y directions, (i.e. the origin can range anywhere from (x-2, y-2) to (x+2, y+2) or a total of 25 different points), 25 neurons are required, one for each displacement. These neurons are, connected to the neuron used for the sub-pattern detection.

5. The Training Set

The training set was collected from 8 different Breast Cancer MR studies. Three type of patterns were chosen, benign, malignant and false positive. Images having malignant regions were selected, then malignant patterns of size 16x16 were extracted. The size of the pattern (16x16 pixels) was chosen after studying tumors in many different breast cancer studies. It was found that the whole tumor fits completely in a 16x16 pattern or 32x32 pattern. The smaller size was chosen to decrease the effect of translation on pattern detection. After selecting malignant regions, an equal number of benign and false positive patterns was selected from the same image.

Each pattern was divided into 16 sub-patterns, each of size 4x4 pixels, as described above. Then the patterns were used to train the network using the incremental learning algorithm described in section 3. The number of patterns in the training set was divided as follows: 52 malignant patterns, 51 benign patterns, and 52 false-positive patterns.

6. Testing

a. Consistency Test

In order to test the ability of the network to remember the trained patterns, a consistency test was conducted. The network was first trained with all the cases in the training set and then tested with the same patterns used for training. The output values from the network were compared with the desired results. The neural network distinguished all three classes of patterns, benign, malignant, and false-positive with accuracy 100%. These results confirm the ability of the network to remember all training patterns.

b. Test by Jackknife Method

To test the ability of the neural network to generalize to patterns that were not included in the training set, a jack-knife method was employed. In this method, some of the patterns are selected at random from the training set for training the network, and the remaining patterns are used to test the trained network. The output values were compared with the expected output. Various combinations of training and testing pairs can be selected by using a random number generator.

In the first jackknife test, the network was trained using the whole set of patterns (155) except one pattern which was used for testing. The procedure was repeated for all the patterns in the database. Results are summarized in the following table.

#Patterns	155
#Correct	144
#Wrong	11
%Correct	92.9032%
%Wrong	7.0968%

Of the 144 correctly classified patterns, 33 (32%) were classified as benign instead of false positive and vice versa. This was not considered as a wrong classification because both types are negative patterns.

In the second jackknife test, the network ability to detect shifted patterns was tested. At first, a set of 25 patterns was created for each of the training patterns to cover the 5x5 window described in section 4. The total numbers of resulting patterns was 3875. The patterns were checked for relevancy by the network and the number of relevant patterns was found to be 3811 (98.348%). This shows that shifting a pattern even by one or two pixels results in a completely different pattern. For testing, half of the patterns was chosen for training and the other half was used for testing using a random number generator. The actual numbers were 1918 training patterns and 1893 for testing. Results are summarized in the following table:

#Patterns	1893
#Correct	1889
#Wrong	4
%Correct	99.7878%
%Wrong	0.2113%

These results prove the ability of the network to detect shifted patterns in the specified window with great accuracy.

c. Testing on Complete MR Studies

The jackknife tests showed that the network has good generalization, shift invariance, and training set selection capabilities. This suggested testing the network on a completely different MR study to detect malignant regions. Each image in the study is divided into 16x16 patterns and fed to the network. The patterns detected to be malignant were kept while all other benign and false positive patterns were blackened, i.e. the goal was to extract the malignant patterns in the study. Results of extracting malignant regions from a series of consecutive slices is shown in Fig. 2.

In general, the network was able to extract malignant regions efficiently but it also extracted patterns containing glandular tissues. This suggests the addition of another training class including glandular patterns to the training set. This is currently under research.

7. Conclusion and future work

A Boolean Neural Network (BNN) was used for the detection of malignant regions in breast MR images. The network was trained with a set of malignant, benign, and false positive

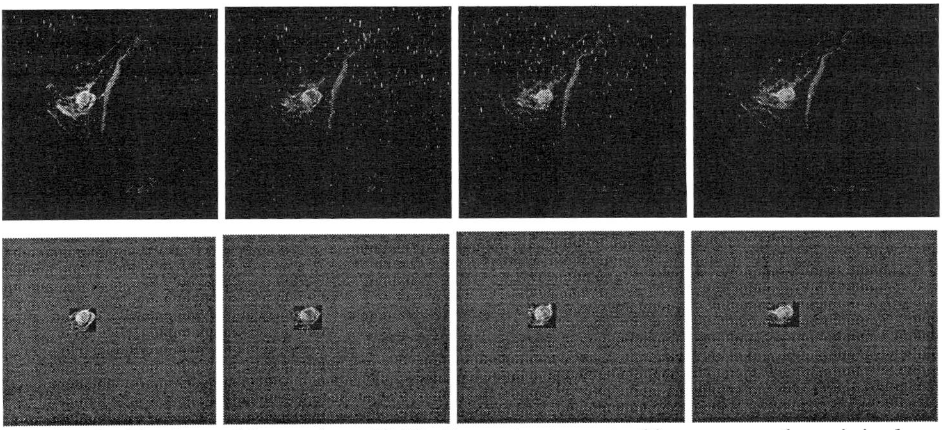

Fig. 2 . Testing with a series of MR slices, the top set of images are the original images, the bottom images are the images after extracting the malignant regions only.

patterns, from selected MR studies, using an incremental learning algorithm. A feature recognition algorithm which has immunity to shifting was used. The network ability to detect the useful training patterns and decrease the training set was shown. The generalization and shift immunity capabilities of the network were tested using the jackknife method. Then, the network was tested using complete images from MR breast studies. Results show that the BNN has good generalization, shift invariant capabilities and a great aptitude to extract malignant regions.

The adequate size of the pattern database to be used for this network is yet to be determined. One way of doing that is to test the network using MR breast images. If it fails, the network is switched to the training mode, and then taught by the malignant patterns it failed to recognize. This can be done because of the network's ability to learn during operation Also, Learning a new pattern is not done unless it is really relevant and it never unlearns currently learned patterns.

Adding a class of glandular patterns to the training set is also necessary.

References:

[1] Sun, Olsen, and Robitaille, "Design and Implementation of a Breast Coil for Magnetic Resonance Imaging," *Magnetic Resonance Imaging*, vol. 11, pp.73-80, 1993.

[2] Giger, M.L., "Computer Aided Diagnosis", *RSNA: A Categorical Course in Physics, Technical Aspects of Breast Imaging*, 1993.

[3] Harms S., Flamig D., "MR Imaging of the Breast", *JMRI*, 3:277-283, 1993.

[4] Weinreb J., and Newstead G., "Controversies in Breast MRI," *Magnetic Resonance Quarterly*, Vol. 10, No. 2, pp.67-83, 1994.

[5] Gilles R., Guinebretiere J.M., Shapeero L.G. et al., "Assessment of Breast Cancer recurrence with contrast-enhanced subtraction MR imaging: preliminary results in 26 patients," *Radiology*, 188:473-478, 1993.

[6] B. Hussain and M. R. Kabuka, "Neural Net transformation of arbitrary Boolean functions," *SPIE 1992 International Symposium on Optical and Applied Science: Neural and Stochastic methods in Image and Signal Processing* (Invited).

[7] Shirish Bhide, Nigel John and M. R. Kabuka, "A Boolean Neural Network approach for the Traveling Salesman Problem," *IEEE Transactions on Computers*, Vol. 42, No. 10, pp. 1271-1278, October 1993.

[8] B. Hussain and M. R. Kabuka, "A novel feature recognition neural network and its application to character recognition," *IEEE transactions on Pattern Analysis and Machine Intelligence,* Vol. 16, No. 1, January 1994.

[9] Srinivas Gazula and M. R. Kabuka, "Design of supervised classifiers using Boolean Neural Networks," *IEEE transactions on Pattern Analysis and Machine Intelligence*, (to appear).

[10] Shirish Bhide, "Image Segmentation with Boolean Neural Networks," *M.Sc. thesis,* University of Miami, 1994.

[11] Shirish Bhide, Nigel John, and M. R. Kabuka, "A Real-Time Solution for the Traveling Salesman Problem using a Boolean Neural Network," Proceedings of the 1993 IEEE International Conference on Neural Networks , San Fransisco, California, pp. 1096-1103.

[12] Xiahong Li, Shirish Bhide, and M. R. Kabuka, "Labeling of MR Brian Images Using a Boolean Neural Network," Proceedings of Symposium of Computer Assisted Radiology, Winston-Salem, NC, June 1994.

Iconic Reporting of Radiological Findings: A New Visual Summarization and Communication Method

Casimir A. Kulikowski, Leiguang Gong and Suzanne Stevenson
Department of Computer Science, Rutgers University, New Brunswick, New Jersey
Reuben Mezrich
Department of Radiogy, University of Pennsylvania, Philadelphia, Pennsylvania
Soraya Abad-Mota
Departamento de Computation y TI, Universidad Simon Bolivar,Venezuela
Alfred Tria and Kenneth Klein
Department of Orthopedics, RW Johnson School of Medicine, New Brunswick, New Jersey

1 INTRODUCTION

Radiological studies typically involve a large number of images, even for relatively specialized problems such as those involving the knee. While conventional dictated reports from the radiologist allow for great flexibility in describing findings, they do not provide an efficient summary to the referring physician. We have developed a new method of iconic reporting that abstracts and summarizes the findings from the radiologist's report into a compact, visually powerful representation. We have tested the ability of this method to communicate surgically significant findings about the knee to two orthopedic surgeons. In a preliminary trial taken from 100 MRI knee examinations we have found that the surgeon with most familiarity in reading the iconic reports was able to accurately identify 96.4% of the significant diagnostic findings from the text report. Iconic reporting can be seen as a new representation for *visual reporting problems.* It is based on a flexible, generic framework for describing the visual abstraction and summarization of large sets of image information [1]. The iconic report superimposes icons representing the findings onto a visual template of the knee in 3 views. The success of our preliminary trial suggests extensions to new visual indexing and retrieval techniques which will be essential in handling the flood of imaging information in clinical as well as research environments.

2 VISUAL REPORTING AS SUMMARIZATION AND COMMUNICATION: APPLICATION TO RADIOLOGICAL REPORTS

Experts in different specialties who wish to communicate their interpretations of complex image data have always been able to append schematic diagrams or sketches to their verbal or textual reports. Different fields, like medicine or geology, have also evolved their own, domain-specific sublanguages to describe commonly occurring spatial structures or contexts, and their interrelationships under both normal and abnormal (dangerous or diseased) conditions or states of nature. In direct verbal exchanges among experts these specialized natural language descriptions suffice, and are usually most effective, with transcription and textual recording commonly providing permanency [2]. In situations where rapid exchange of visual summary information is helpful or essential, with networked computers now providing the technological infrastructure [3], representations have yet to be developed for capturing *visual reports* that abstract and summarize information from large collections of image data.

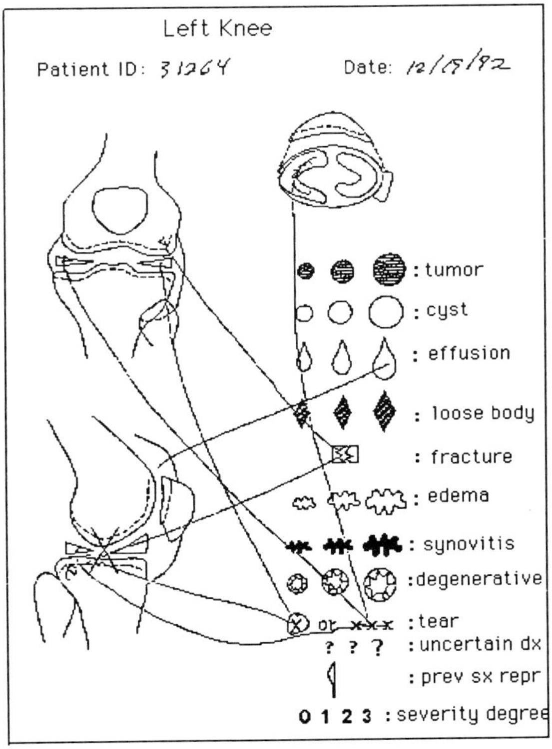

Figure 1: Prototype Iconic Report for the Knee

In our representation visual reporting is formalized as a problem of: 1) visual context template selection (views of the knee); 2) classification by selecting an icon to represent a finding, with qualifiers like size and intensity; and 3) localization of the icon within the visual context template. Experts must define the set of contextual visual templates, such as anatomical atlas renderings, geographical maps, or geological cross-sections. A standard set must be adopted for a particular reporting problem, as for, instance a set of 3 views of the knee to localize radiologically observed abnormalities in this structure, or a map of a region to localize reported cases in an epidemic, or fault-lines in earthquake reporting. In addition, the experts exchanging information must agree on a visual vocabulary of annotating symbols or *icons* to describe the abnormal states of nature being reported or tracked in the visual summary reports. Design of the icon set for a particular reporting problem must incorporate constraints of perceptual perspicuity and cognitive disambiguity among the icons themselves,

as well as similar constraints with the visual context templates on which they are to be overlaid. Validation of the representation is important, because a visual summary must be judged against the current "gold standard" of the physician generated text report. To determine a basis of comparison we have developed a common object_attribute_location descriptive database model which contains the essential visual interpretation knowledge extracted from the set of images. As illustrated in Figure 1, our prototype iconic report for the knee included ten icons to denote the various common pathological entities reported, such as tears, cysts, edema, etc, together with two modifiers to characterize the degree of severity of the finding on a scale of 1 to 3 and the degree of certainty with which the radiologist made the interpretation of the finding (with three levels). The schematic illustration of the knee was taken from the most informative examples in [4]. For this preliminary feasibility study the templates and icons were placed on a single piece of paper and the radiologist completed a report by drawing a line from the icon to the appropriate location on the template to indicate type, severity, and location of the lesion. We have designed a "drag and drop" computer-based version, but could not provide the convenient hardware (portable PCs) for the orthopedists to carry out the study rapidly and unobtrusively, so proceeded with the paper version for this study. Its results should improve with appropriately designed automatic methods that reduce the ambiguities of the paper method.
Our study was retrospective: one hundred sequential knee studies referred by two orthopedic surgeons to the Laurie Imaging Center were selected for analysis. The images and conventional text report of each case was reviewed by the radiologist experienced in orthopedic MRI (RSM) and an iconic report prepared. Patient information was hidden and reports identified only by an ID assigned to the patient by the MRI center at the time of study. The two orthopedic surgeons separately reviewed each iconic and conventional report - with sufficient time between them, and blinded so as to minimize the chances of bias - and were asked to complete a questionnaire that assessed the information transmitted by the reports. The same questionnaire (Fig 2) was used for each report to record the surgeon's determination of the location, extent, and severity of the pathology. The questionnaires were collected and compared on an item by item basis. We then determined the agreement between findings generated from the conventional vs. from the iconic report - to establish the degree to which the surgeons were able to derive or receive the same information from the two types of reports. One of the surgeons had helped develop the approach and methods of the iconic report and at the time of the study had considerable experience in reading them, while the other was only given a brief introduction to the method.

3 DATA ANALYSIS AND RESULTS:

The findings extracted by the surgeons from the iconic and conventional reports were tabulated according to the categories of finding, location and sublocation as shown in the questionnaire of Figure 2. Findings derived from the iconic report

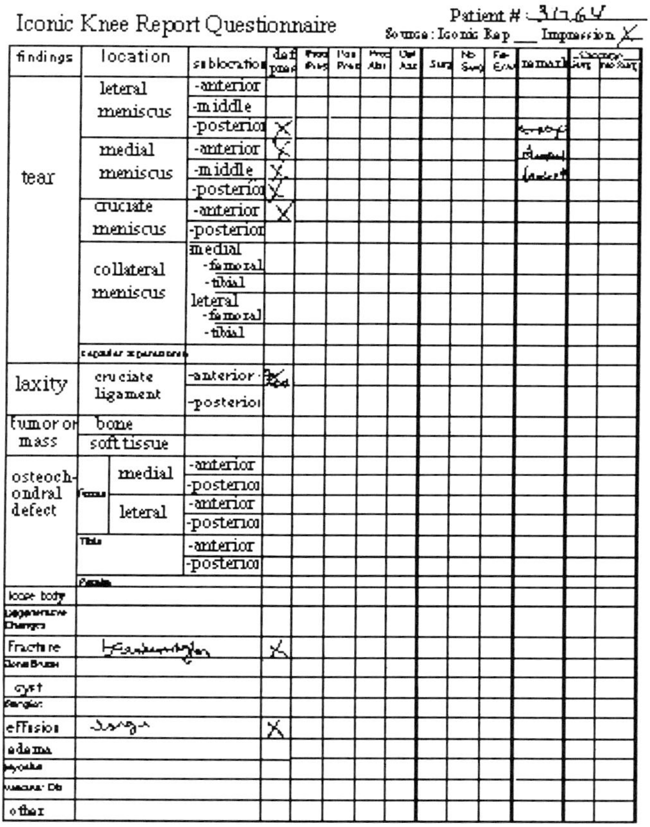

Figure 2: Questionnaire for Iconic Knee Report

were compared to those taken from the conventional report, using the latter as the reference set. For each surgeon we categorized findings according to whether they were in complete agreement in both reports, whether they were found from the conventional but not from the iconic, or whether they disagreed (difference or error from the iconic report). We applied a difference of proportions test to the number of matched findings to determine whether the two surgeon's interpretations were comparable and a chi-squared test that took into account the errors and missing findings as separate categories. After excluding data insufficiencies from report generation, reproduction, and transmission, 72 out of the 100 cases yielded comparable data from both reports and from both surgeons' questionnaires. A total of 145 findings were reported by both surgeons, of which 132 showed complete agreement between those extracted from the iconic vs conventional reports (91.1%). There is, however, a noticeable difference between the surgeons: the one who had practice with the iconic reporting system ac-

tually showed agreement in 54 out of 56 (96.4%) of the findings he extracted from the reports, whereas the surgeon less familiar with the iconic report found agreement in 78 out of 89, or only 87.6%. Findings missing in the iconic report were 6 overall, and those in error 7, but again, for the experienced surgeon these figures were 1 and 1, respectively, whereas for the less experienced surgeon they amounted to 5 and 6. We can conclude from these preliminary results that an experienced surgeon can derive substantially all findings from the iconic report that were present in the conventional one. Examining the cases that were in error or had missing findings, we see that they always involved a large number of complex findings. With the paper media and line indexing between icons and locations, this is not very surprising. The computer-based system currently under development has the ability to provide higher resolution versions of the iconic report where such complexity requires it. Comparing the results for the two surgeons, a difference of proportions z test shows that the null hypothesis that the measured differences were due to chance can be rejected at the 95% level. This is also supported by chi-squared test results, rejecting the hypothesis that the surgeons' performance is equivalent, consistent with our observation that their experience with the iconic reporting system differed considerably.
Comparing the extracted findings from the iconic report to those from the conventional report, a z test for difference of proportions showed no significant difference (at a 95% confidence level) for the experienced surgeon, though for the other surgeon it was at a lower level, again indicating that training in using the report is helpful.

4 DISCUSSION

We have designed a visual language with a deliberately limited vocabulary around a specific task: to describe the pathological changes in the anatomy of the knee as described by the radiologist. We have tested its ability to communicate the findings interpreted from a complex and large set of MR images to a surgeon. The advantages of the iconic reporting language is its precision and economy. Its disadvantage is that its flexibility (or degree to which nuances can be conveyed) is in direct proportion to the number of elements (icons) included in its vocabulary. A small vocabulary is easy to learn, which is advantageous when reports are sent to a wide audience, many of whom will not have deep or frequent experience with this format. With the limited number of icons in this study there was a measurable decrease in information transfer to the less experienced (in terms of familiarity with the iconic report) surgeon. The optimum size of the vocabulary will have to be determined by continued use to strike a balance between the detail with which small nuances can be described and the ease with which new users can interpret the report. While this study was carried out for MRI reports of the knee, the method should be generalizable to all anatomy, using all modalities with an appropriately enlarged set of icons and corresponding contextual visual templates.
We are currently designing and implementing a computer based version of our

iconic reporting method. We use drag and drop techniques in which icons are selected and dragged onto the appropriate locations on the template. Size and color of the icon is used to indicate size and severity of the lesion. Some of the icons have drop down labels attached to convey information about other attributes, such as chronicity or the differential possibilities of the lesions, and can be customized by the radiologist. In transmission by local or wide area networking, the advantage of such coded information in an iconic report is that it can be easily reconstructed in graphical format from a representation of the templates and icons, which only need be transmitted once for a given class of problems. A database of iconic reports interrogated by graphical queries provides a much richer set than textual reports, and would allow great control over search criteria and degree of match, and can also be translated into various controlled vocabularies and coding schemas. The development of computer formalisms for knowledge representation, including the contents of complex natural images, like those in radiology, raises interesting research issues in cognitive science and computer science [5,6]. In a fully developed digital radiology system it would make sense to provide the radiologist with the facilities to use icons to annotate the real images as well as serving to summarize the findings on a template. A further planned, though not yet implemented improvement would be the replacement of the three elevations of the template with a 3D view of the anatomy (using semi-transparent or wire-frame models).
In conclusion, the iconic report provides a sophisticated abstraction of the pathology and anatomy indicated in the technical aspect of a radiological study, but with a sufficient vocabulary to let the radiologist provide his or her interpretation. This preliminary study shows the feasibility of using such an iconic report to encode and communicate the findings for the radiologist to a surgeon with some experience in using the report.

5 REFERENCES

[1] Abad-Mota S, Kulikowski CA, Gong L, et al. Iconic reporting: a new way fo communicating radiological findings, Proc SCAMC-95; 915.
[2] Frank MS, Guse SL, Stern EJ, Rohrman CA. Integrating a digital dictation system with a network data base for creating and managing radiological teaching files. Invest Radiol 1994;29:652-55.
[3] Mezrich RS, DeMarco JK, Negin S, et al. Radiology on the information superhighway. Radiology 1995;195:73-81.
[4] Tria A, and Klein K. An illustrated guide to the knee, Churchill Livingstone, 1992.
[5] Sloman A. Varieties of formalisms for knowledge representation. Comp Intell 1993;9:413-23.
[6] Glasgow J. The imagery debate revisited: a computational perspective. Comp Intell 1993;9:309-33.

Clinical Impact of Speech Recognition

Paul N. Grooff, M.D., David W. Piraino, M.D., Michael P. Recht, M.D. and Bradford J. Richmond, M.D.
Cleveland Clinic Foundation, Cleveland, Ohio

Introduction:

Radiologists are under increasing pressure to render prompt printed interpretation of medical imaging exams to promote patient care. Therefore, decreasing the time from completion of the imaging exam to provision of a final printed interpretation is becoming increasingly important. This study evaluates the impact of using a commercially available speech recognition system to provide a prompt report of medical images. This method is compared to conventional exam interpretation with subsequent transcription.

Methods:

We report on the results from a single site (Cleveland Clinic Foundation) from a multi-institution study. 200 outpatient musculoskeletal exams, including plain film radiographs and bone densitometry, were reported by two radiologists over a three week period. 141 examinations (series 1) hung at one station were interpreted using a traditional digital dictation system with subsequent transcription. A similar set of 59 examinations (series 2) were interpreted using a speech recognition system (Voicerad Kurzweil AI) without the need for further review. The following data was collected for both series: 1) time (to the nearest five seconds) for dictation of the report, 2) total time (in minutes) from completion of the exam to production of a final printed report, and 3) user comments. Additionally, for the traditional method of dictation (series 1), time (in minutes) from completion of the examination to dictation, time (in minutes) from dictation to transcription of a preliminary report, and time (in minutes) for finalization of a preliminary report were gathered.

Time measurements for length of dictation were recorded by the interpreting physician immediately after dictation of each individual examination. The remaining times were calculated from electronic time signatures available within the digital dictation system and radiology information system.

Comparison between the exams interpreted in each series was performed. As the data was nonparametric, a Wilcoxon rank test was performed to compare the length of dictation time and the time needed to produce a final printed report.

Results:

59 patients were dictated using the voice recognition system and 141 patients were dictated traditionally. Median time of dictation with voice recognition software (90 seconds, range of 35-240 seconds) was significantly longer ($p < 0.001$) than standard dictation (median = 50 seconds, range of 20-120 seconds). Figure 1, "Report Dictation" depicts this difference. There is a large range of time for dictations with speech recognition, some reports taking over 200 seconds.

Figure 1

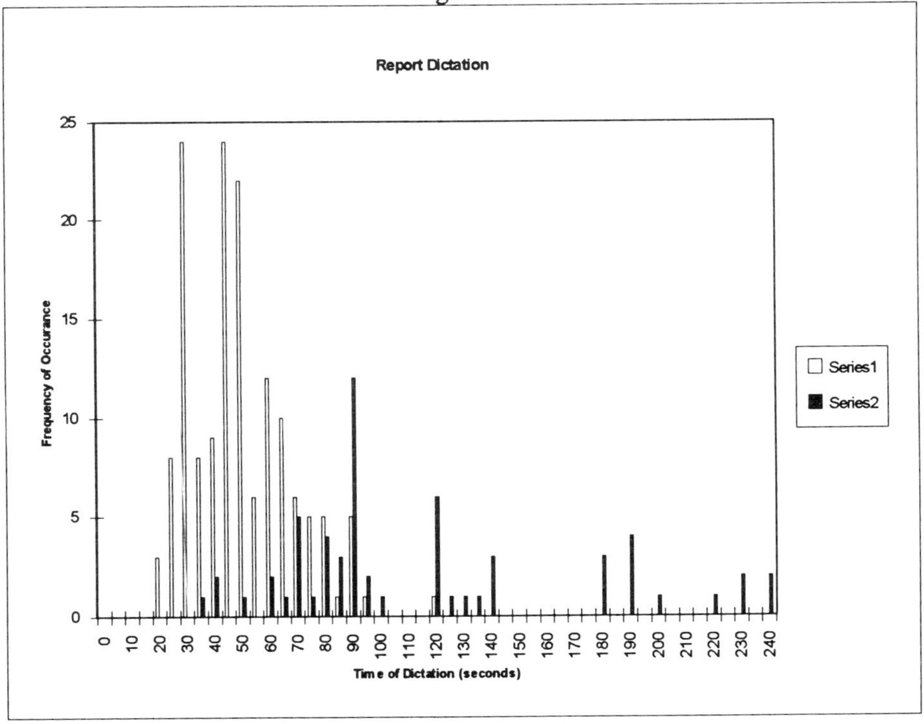

54 of 59 dictations in series 1 contained electronic time signature information, as did 125 of 141 dictations in series 2. Median time of production of a final report with speech recognition (1398 minutes, range of 22-6292) was significantly faster ($p < 0.001$) than the traditional method (median = 3071, range of 1343-17318). Figure 2, "Time from Completion of Exam to Final Report," depicts this difference. This histogram also demonstrates large ranges for both speech recognition and traditional dictation, clustered in 24 hour periods.

Figure 2

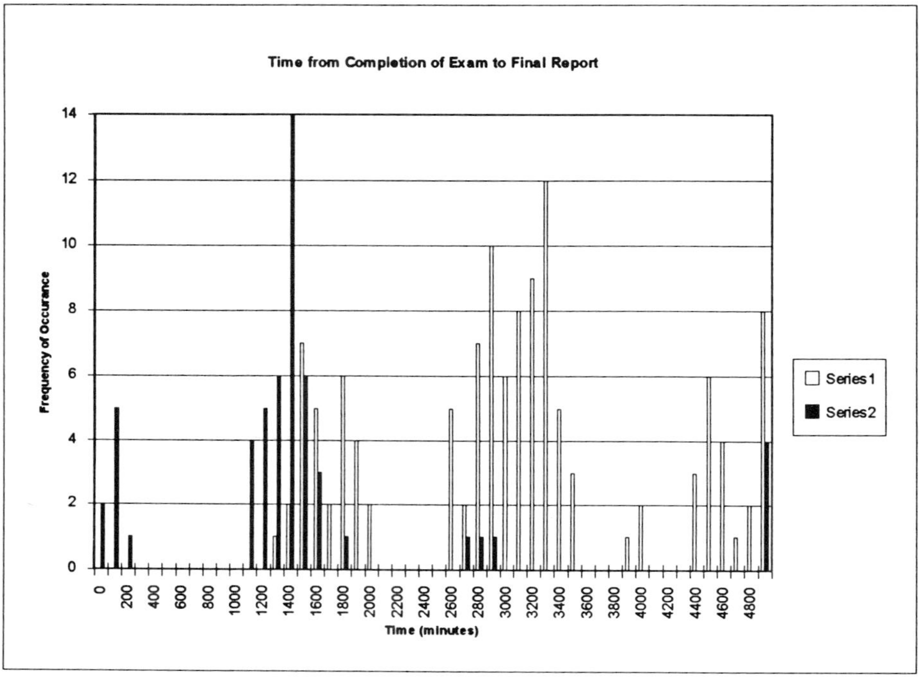

Using traditional dictation with subsequent transcription the median time from completion of the exam to dictation was 1409 minutes (range of 37-15820 minutes). Median time of transcription of these dictations was 146 minutes (range of 0-991 minutes). The median time to finalize these preliminary reports was 1629 minutes (range of 23-2346 minutes).

Discussion:

There has been much recent research in speech recognition applications in expediting medical care.[1,2,3] Radiology, with its volume of dictated material, lends itself to speech recognition research. The added time to perform tasks with speech recognition, in this case nearly doubling the length of dictation time for physicians, is a problem not easily overcome.[1] However, the benefits are substantial. Final printed exam interpretation with this new method, is rendered at our institution more than one day more quickly than with the traditional dictation system.

Other ways to expedite the production of a final interpretation need to be considered. Indeed in our study, it only took slightly more than 2 hours to transcribe the dictations in series 2. This seems expeditious, as the other 839 dictations reported by the same radiologists over the same time period took, on average, twice as long to transcribe. Nevertheless, a much larger delay in rendering a final interpretation was encountered in finalizing preliminary reports (which often took more than a day to perform). Perhaps, greater emphasis on reviewing preliminary reports would expedite the process to a greater degree. Recent work linking oral reports to digital images is another method to speed reporting.[4] However, this manner of examination reporting is not currently used in many institutions.

Eliminating the time for transcription and review of radiologic examinations greatly improves speed in reporting. We feel that our early results in this area show great promise for future application of speech recognition technology in radiology and further work is needed.

References:

1 Shiffman S, et. al. *The integration of a continuous-speech-recognition system with the QMR diagnostic program.* Proceedings - the Annual Symposium on Computer Applications in Medical Care: 767-71, 1992.

2 Nakatsu R, Suzuki Y. *What does voice-processing technology support today?* Proceedings of the National Academy of Sciences of the United States of America. 92(22): 10023-30, 1995 Oct 24.

3 Frenger P. *Inexpensive speech recognition techniques.* Biomedical Sciences Instrumentation. 30:141-6, 1994.

4 Inamoto K, Inamura K, Umeda T *Oral diagnostic reporting and synchronized image filing using magneto-optical disks.* Computer Methods & Programs in Biomedicine. 37(4):327-31, 1992 May.

Voice Recognition Utilization and Speed of Generating Radiology Reports: Two Years of Experience

David J. Curtis, Bruce Hall, Roger Shannon and Deane Marlin
Durham VA Medical Center, Radiology Service, Durham, North Carolina

INTRODUCTION:

A Kurzweil Voice Rad (KVR) (Fairfax, VA) voice recognition system is located in our outpatient reading room and is used consistently by several readers, rather than using analog dictation. One reader is no longer using it (3), one user has just begun (2), and one has used it consistently over the 4 sampling times discussed here (1). The one reader consistently using the machine was trained 1972-1975, using a digital reporter Siemen's AG SIREP (Erlangen, Germany), which is no longer made. The other two were trained using analog systems.

A much larger study, which includes the performance times of the other radiologists in our group, will not be submitted here, because analog dictation was used 20-100% of the time by them.

MATERIALS AND METHODS:

A KVR machine was utilized to report all radiographic exams in the outpatient clinic. Up to a daily 110 exams were used by 3 readers who did not utilize the backup analog dictation. A routine statistical package (Microsoft Corporation, Phoenix, AZ) was used. Time of reading was available in the Decentralized Hospital Computer Program (DHCP) master computer to which the KVR is connected by an HL7 interface. Also, the report dictated on the Kurzweil Voice Rad was immediately available after signature and printing in printed or computer format.

RESULTS:

The speed of individual reporters using the Kurzweil voice-activated machine is graphically displayed in Figure 1. Note the significantly faster speed of the individual trained on a digital system in his residency. Speed also is probably related to the number of words and phrases recorded by the computer for the individuals. Some of the three 100% KVR users have trained the KVR with additional words, phrases and complete reports. The time to do this is included in report times. Reader 1 has almost 60,000 voice profile recordings, while reader 2 has slightly over 56,000, and reader 3 is about the same as reader 2.

The KVR saves one transcriptionist ($23,000 + 20% benefits) when used, since it takes 10-30 minutes to transcribe one report. The cost may be higher in a different environment.

Also, the system saves the radiologist 1-3 minutes per report, because the reports do not need to be reviewed and corrected.

DISCUSSION:

Voice-activated technology has been available in digital form for 3-4 years. Of significance in this study was that the fastest reader used fewer phrases and mostly individual words spoken in a staccato manner to complete reports, while the others routinely used phrases and complete reports. Random phrases generated by the KVR made looking from the film to the screen a frequent necessity, and selective deletion was not available; nor were other word processing capabilities which would allow more utility and create higher accuracy. Accuracy of reading is examined quarterly, and no significant detriment in reading rapidly was noted over the two years of the study. Distinct enunciation makes the machine more receptive to the appropriate word, although the correct word may be in the alternates which can be chosen without redictating. This feature is helpful. Background noise is an intermittent problem which is partially overcome with a filter mechanism.

The third reader was frequently interrupted from reading by administrative duties which artificially inflated his time for dictation. The second reader was just learning the system through persistent use of the KVR because of the time it saved in dictation and reviewing reports on the DHCP. These alterations are noted in Table 1. The first reader used less time in looking between the screen and the film and had fewer dictation errors, presumably because of his large number of voice recognition recordings.

Overall, the administrative and radiologist time and money savings make the KVR a tool which pays for itself in one year, if used.

The major advantage of the system is that a hard copy and directly available DHCP computer reports are created immediately, whereas a report created by an analog system takes 1-7 days to be generated.

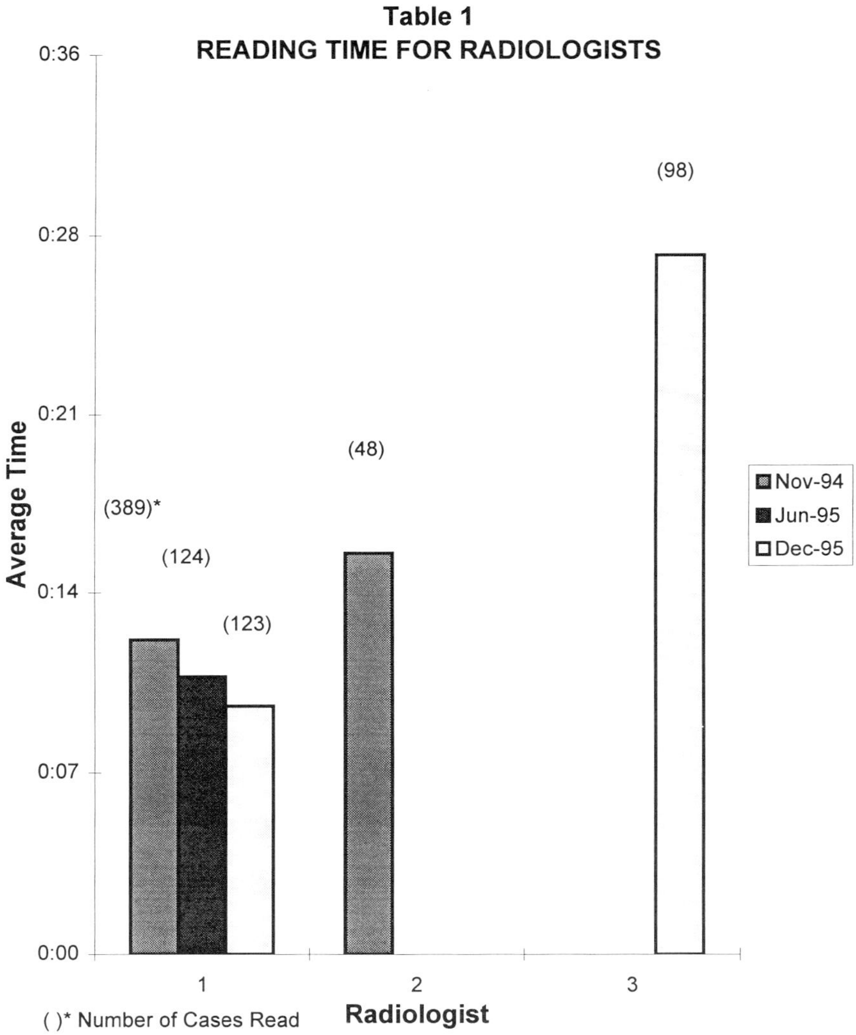
Table 1
READING TIME FOR RADIOLOGISTS
0:36
0:28
0:21
0:14
0:07
0:00
Average Time
(98)
(48)
(389)*
(124)
(123)
Nov-94
Jun-95
Dec-95
1
2
3
( )* Number of Cases Read
Radiologist

BIBLIOGRAPHY

1. Stromgren BJ. Voice recognition: a new technology for operative reporting. J Am Rec Assoc 1988;59(2):20-2.

2. Yokubaitis PR. Voice recognition: technology with a future. J Ahima 1992;63(7):93-7.

3. Williams KA. Voice-recognition/knowledge-base reporting systems for ambulatory care patient records. J Ambulatory Care Manage 1992;15(3):55-66.

4. Mrosek B, Grunupp A, Keppel E, Moese G, Mohr K, Stargardt A, and Gunter RW. Computer-assisted speech recognition and display of x-ray findings [German]. Rofo 1993;159(5):481-483.

5. Haber L. Searching for the speech recognition holy grail. MIDRANGE Systems 1992;5(11):39.

6. Voice-processing speeds communications. (The Clinic of Richlands, VA, uses Dictaphone's Digital Express voice-processing in Office Technology). 1989;34(11):26.

7. Mosser H, Urban M, and Hruby W. Filmless digital radiology--feasibility and 20-month experience in clinical routine. Medical Informatics 1994;19(2):149-59.

8. Fusi A and Vidal B. [Automatic voice recognition for radiologic reports. Experiment with a prototype in an operational environment]. [Italian]. Original title: Il riconoscimento automatico della voce per la refertazione radiologica. Esperimento di un prototipo in ambiente operativo. Radiologia Medica 1991;81(3):309-13.

9. Altman J. Hospital utilizes voice recognition. MIS Week 1988;9(28):1-2.

Integrating Automatic Retrieval of Reference Images With Report Dictation: 'Continuous Education' – A Functional Evaluation

Henry A. Swett, M.D., Pradeep G. Mutalik, M.D., Vladimir P. Neklesa, M.D., Laura Horvath, M.D., Carol Lee, M.D., Joan Richter, M.D., Irena Tocino, M.D.and Paul R. Fisher, M.D.

Yale University, School of Medicine, Department of Diagnostic Radiology, New Haven, Connecticut

INTRODUCTION

Continuing education is critical if radiologists are going to remain unchallenged as the preeminent imagers in the rapidly changing healthier landscape. Most radiologic education is quite removed from the time and place where it is needed and therefore is suboptimal. We have developed a method of integrating immediate 'continuous education' into an on-line reading environment. Our approach automatically extracts finding descriptors from a dictated report and uses these values to spawn multiple searches of an image database. As a result, the radiologist may immediately view proven reference images which have findings in common with the case being dictated. In this paper, we review the design and function of this system and present a functional evaluation of the effectiveness of this approach.

MATERIALS AND METHODS:

IMAGE DATABASE. An image database of 347 digital mammography cases was assembled and image features were coded. The distribution of pathologic entities included:

HISTOLOGY	# CASES
Carcinoma(Various histologies)	64
Malignancy (Non epithelial)	6
Inflammatory Lesions	6
Benign Entities	112
Fibroadenoma	
Lipoma	
Cysts	
Benign Calcification	
Scar	
Ruptured Implant	

Table 1.

A multidimensional database search strategy was developed so that retrieved images could be grouped in sets (axes) intended to address common questions that arise during image interpretation.

IMAGE CODING. A detailed image description lexicon was developed to allow coding of all mammographic findings. The lexicon includes descriptors for all Mammographic findings and scalar values for most findings so that similar images could be retrieved and arrayed in logical sequences. For example, a group of retrieved masses could be grouped by progressive size of masses, density of masses, sharpness of mass border, or Boolean combinations of findings. The image description scheme is cross referenced to the ACR Bi-rads lexicon and can be thought of as a superset of this convention. An excerpt of this representation is shown below:

Field Name	Field Description	Format	Possible Value
Mass Findings Table			
MASS_SIZE	mass size, qual description	Char (1)	small, intermediate, large
MASS_DIM_X	mass dimension-long axis	real number (4)	
MASS_DIM_Y	mass dimension-short axis	real number (4)	
MASS_DENS	mass density	char(1)	Radiolucent (0)* Low (-) High (+) Combined-Random Combined-Lucent Center Equal (=)

Table 2.

VOICE REPORTING. We employed a commercially available speech recognition radiology reporting system (VoiceRAD, Kurzweil Applied Intelligence, Inc., Waltham, Mass.) to prepare standard written reports and at the same time to inform the decision support system of the findings present in the case being analyzed. This system translates 'trigger phrases' into complete sentences which are concatenated into a formal radiology report. At the conclusion of the finding description phase of reporting, we asked the radiologist to provide a diagnostic hypothesis. We mapped the trigger phrases into input tupples which were then processed by meta-rules which generated multiple searches of the database. The results were arrayed in a series of 'image axes'.

USER INTERFACE/IMAGE AXES. The results of each search are displayed in sets of images intended to anticipate common clinical questions. These image sets or 'axes' include:

1. *All Images.* All retrieved images are displayed regardless of other features.

2. *Hypothesis Axis.* All images which have findings in common with the index case and are caused by the hypothesized diagnosis. The images which are most like the index case are presented first in each axis with progressive dissimilarity in proportion to distance from the first case.

3. *Differential Diagnosis Axis..* This image set contains images which share similar features to the index case but are caused by any etiology. This is intended to provide a visual differential diagnosis.

4. *Spectrum Axis.* Images arrayed on this axis are constrained only by etiology. Axis ordering strategies cluster images with similar features. This axis presents the spectrum of findings by diagnosis.

5. *Malignant Axis.* All images representing examples of any malignancy are placed on this axis.

6. *User Defined Axis.* This axis allows findings to be added or subtracted from the index finding set, or a new set of findings and hypotheses be supplied. Here, the radiologist may view reference images exhibiting any specific finding or group of findings.

7. *Best Match Axis.* All images in the database are placed on this axis in order of similarity to the index case. The first images presented are most like the index case.

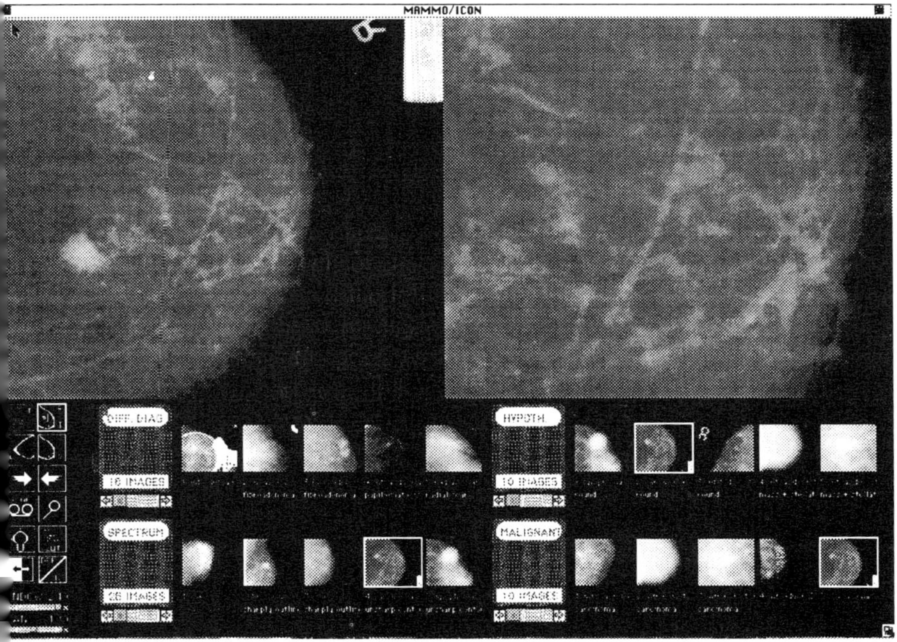

Figure 1. Mammo/Icon user interface. Four axes are displayed on the bottom half of the screen; the Differential Diagnosis Axis, the Hypothesis Axis, the Spectrum Axis, and the Malignancy Axis. Each axis is scrollable with the number of images present indicated on the axis header. Selection of an image token causes it to be displayed on the top half of the screen. Icons at the lower left provide common

image processing tools and access to descriptive information about each case.

FUNCTIONAL EVALUATION. A functional evaluation of the system was performed as a guide for subsequent system development. Eight prototypical cases were selected which demonstrate a variety of common findings. These included:

1) Stellate mass
2) High density mass
3) Low density mass
4) Combined density mass
5) Radiolucent mass
6) Multiple masses
7) Clustered calcifications
8) Scattered calcifications.

Two mammographers submitted the findings for the index cases to Mammo/Icon and graded the systems response based on:

1. Response time
2. Helpfulness of retrieved images (10 point scale)
   by image
   by axis
3. Appropriateness of image sequencing within each axis
4. Appropriateness of array placement of each individual image (10 point scale).

Their findings are summarized in the following table:

RESULTS:

VOICE RECOGNITION. Voice dictation using a controlled vocabulary of trigger phrases successfully produced written reports and initiated appropriate searches of the image database and array set up during repeated system testing after suitable period of system training. The functional evaluation of the system used menu input of findings rather than speech recognition since our goal was not to test the accuracy of speech recognition, but the qualitative value of the systems response.

SUBJECTIVE EVALUATION OF CLINICAL UTILITY.
Image Axes. Images were generally correctly retrieved and displayed in the image arrays. A small number of cases were displayed inappropriately due to inaccurate feature coding. An irregularity in the database caused 43 cases not to be displayed. Image arrays in order of clinical usefulness, (10 point scale):

User defined axis (8.4)
Best match axis (7.8)
Differential diagnosis axis (7.6)
Malignancy axis (6.8)
Hypothesis axis (5.6)
Spectrum axis (5.6)

The number of images retrieved varied based on findings present in the index case, and proposed diagnosis. Helpfulness is a subjective determination derived from a 10 point scale where 1=not helpful and 10=very helpful. 'Inappropriate images' were images that the reviewers felt should not have been displayed on the relevant axis. This also varied with index case. 'Incorrectly coded images' were inappropriately arrayed images for which we determined the findings were coded incorrectly. 'Incorrect sequencing' refers to an image which was placed in the correct array, but was out of sequence based on clinical ordering criteria.

AXIS:	Diff. Dx	Hypoth.	Spect.	Malig.	Best Match
Images retrieved	1-28	0-11	2-27	0-11	141
Helpfulness	7.6(7-9)	5.6(5-7)	5.6(5-8)	7.06(6-9)	8(4-9)
Inappropriate Images	4	1	0	0	0
Incorrectly Coded	3	0	0	0	0
Incorrect Sequen.	1	3	0	0	42

Table 3.

As illustrated in table 3, the clinical 'helpfulness' of the system was found to be greatest for the 'best match' axis, the 'differential diagnosis' axis, and the 'malignancy' axis. The 'user defined' axis is not shown in this table because the evaluators used this utility to freely explore the image database and therefore the results of these searches was variable. For certain lesions, however, other axes were considerably more or less valuable. For example, for both of the lesions shown in table 4, the 'differential diagnosis' and 'best match' axes were found to be most useful. The 'spectrum axis' was found to be more useful for high density masses than for stellate masses.

Axis:	#	Diff.Dx	#	Hypoth.	#	Spect.	#	Malig.	#	Best Match
		Val/In/Cor		Val/In/Cor		Val/In/Cor		Val/In/Cor		Val/In/Cor
Stellate Mass										
Eval. 1	18	8/3/0	9	7/0/0	27	5/9/0	10	6/0/0	141	9/0/23
Eval. 2	18	9/1/1	9	6/0/0	27	5/0/5	10	6/0/0	141	8/0/42
High Density Mass										
Eval. 1	5	8/0/0	2	7/1/1	27	7/0/0	2	8/0/0	141	8/0/>10
Eval. 2	5	8/0/0	2	5/1/1	27	7/0/0	2	9/0/0	141	9/0/>10

Table 4. Functional evaluation by lesion type (excerpt). Value (Val)=clinical helpfulness(Ten point scale. 1=Not helpful. 10=Very helpful). Inapp(In)= Number of images inappropriately placed on axis. Incor(Cor)= Number of images incorrectly sequenced on axis. #=Number of images retrieved.

DISCUSSION.

Medical education often occurs at the wrong time. Traditional learning methods provide good general background knowledge, but often are of limited use when a specific clinical problem arises because of human memory limitations. Some of the most effective and longest remembered education occurs when an immediate clinical problem evokes an emotional response and stimulates case specific research. Unfortunately the demands of radiologic practice often make it difficult to take time to research difficult cases. In this paper, we describe a method of retrieving potentially helpful context sensitive reference images as an automatic part of the diagnostic reporting process.

Computer based decision support systems have shown some value in a variety of different settings in radiology, including mammography [1,2,3,4,5,6,7] We previously demonstrated the ability to produce computer generated case discussions or 'critiques' of radiologic findings (ICON) [8] Because visual pattern recognition is central to the process of image analysis, we have developed several experimental computer systems which attempt to support radiologic decision making by using the findings reported by a radiologist as input values to an image database search engine (Image/Icon) [9] As a result, it is possible to dictate a written radiology report and simultaneously generate multiple searches of an image database. In effect, this system acts as an agent for the radiologist, automatically finding context sensitive reference images. This offers 'continuous education' as a part of every case interpretation provided 'just in time' to influence immediate clinical decision making.

In order to guide future system development and to establish a reality check on the qualitative value of this approach, we performed a functional evaluation of a mammography decision support system, Mammo/Icon. We found that the approach was generally considered moderately to very helpful by two experienced mammographers. Some of the image arrays were very helpful in specific clinical settings and not helpful in other settings. This reflects both the richly varied character of image analysis, and the composition of the database. A small subset of mammographic findings was represented in the test database. Findings in the index case might be highly evocative of a specific diagnosis, but would not trigger a meaningful response if there were no cases of the evoked diagnosis in the database. By the same token, when many examples are retrieved of a specific diagnosis causing the observed findings, one is given the impression of a strong causal relationship. Conversely, if one proposed that the observed findings are caused by a specific diagnosis and the system is unable to find examples of that diagnosis causing the specified findings, one might assume that the proposed diagnosis is unlikely. These assumptions are likely to only be valid for large databases where the distribution of findings and etiologies reflects their occurrence in the population under consideration. Large databases drawn from actual clinical experience are likely to have more meaningful implications, and may reflect local variations in disease incidence. Ultimately, conclusions based on actual practice experience may lead to previously unrecognized associations between findings and disease entities.

Accurate and detailed coding of findings, anatomy, and relationships of findings and anatomy is essential for useful image retrieval from large databases. This is soon to become essential as hospitals rapidly transition to filmless radiology. Conventional coding systems are too granular to be useful with large databases. The unified medical language system [1,2] and SNOMED [3] are two coding systems which are beginning to address these more demanding requirements, but none of the existing coding systems are sufficiently robust to allow precise image retieval and sequencing of multiple images. We developed a special coding system for mammography and linked it to the existing BiRads system[12]. While our approach provided generally useful retrieval and stratification of images, it is not a generalizable approach that can be extended to other domains in radiology. Our evaluation demonstrated that even this specially created lexicon did not adequately support the full range of retrieval and ordering required for the paradigm that we have created. The evaluation also revealed implementation errors in coding and the databases application of search strategies both at the level of individual image retrieval and at the meta level of axis ordering routines.

In addition to the need for better coding systems, a method of automating detailed image coding will be necessary if radiologists are to harvest the power of digital image databases. There are likely to be new incentives to accurately code findings and relate them to the efficiency of radiologic workup and to patient outcome provided by large purchasers of imaging services in a managed care environment. Additionally, radiologists are facing increasing pressure to provide almost instantaneous access to written consultation reports. These factors make alternatives to conventional report transcription increasingly viable including speech recognition and direct interaction with a finding coding interface. Either of these approaches can be coupled with evolving systematic coding strategies to enable the kind of flexible image retrieval described above.

In conclusion, we believe that automated access to reference images in real time during film reading is likely to provide a valuable resource and have described one method of accomplishing this. We have not yet attempted to determine whether this approach improves diagnostic accuracy. For this potential to be realized, there is an urgent need for the development of flexible new coding methods.

1. Kahn CE. Artificial Intelligence in Radiology: Decision Support Systems. *RadioGraphics* **1994**;14:849-861
2. Vyborny CJ. Can Computers Help Radiologists Read Mammograms? *Radiology* **1994**;191:315-317
3. Kegelmeyer WP et al. Computer-aided Mammographic Screening for Spiculated Lesions. *Radiology* **1994**;191:331-33
4. D'Orsi CJ et al. Reading and Decision Aids for Improved Accuracy and Standardization of Mammographic Diagnosis. *Radiology* **1992**;184:619-622
5. Getty DJ et al. Enhanced Interpretation of Diagnostic Images. *Investigative Radiology* **1988**;23:240-252
6. Swets JA et al. Enhancing and Evaluating Diagnostic Accuracy. *Medical Decision Making* **1991**;11:9-18
7. Swett HA, Miller PL. ICON: A computer-based approach to differential diagnosis in radiology. *Radiology* **1987**;163:555-558
8. Swett HA, Fisher PR, Miller PL, Mutalik PG. Expert System Controlled Image Display. *Radiology* **1989**;172:487-493
9. Lindberg DA. Humphreys BL. McCray AT. The Unified Medical Language System. Methods of Information in Medicine. 32(4):281-91, 1993 Aug.
10. Bell DS. Pattison-Gordon E. Greenes RA. Experiments in concept modeling for radiographic image reports. Journal of the American Medical Informatics Association. 1(3):249-62, 1994 May-Jun.
11. Rothwell DJ. Cote RA. Cordeau JP. Boisvert MA. Developing a standard data structure for medical language--the SNOMED proposal. Proceedings - the Annual Symposium on Computer Applications in Medical Care. :695-9, 1993
12. Kopans DB. Standardized mammography reporting. Radiologic Clinics of North America. 30(1):257-64, 1992 Jan.

SESSION 8

Telemedicine

Co-Chairs:

Glendon G. Cox

Tim B. Hunter

Evaluation of a Teleradiology System: Diagnostic Accuracy of Pneumothorax Detection at Three Matrix Sizes

Jeffrey L. Chenoweth, Carroll R. Markivee, Bhargavi K. Patel
Radiology Service, Saint Louis Department of Veterans Affairs Medical Center and Saint Louis University School of Medicine, Saint Louis, Missouri

Introduction

Teleradiology systems are increasingly being used to provide radiologic services in areas or situations where it is not feasible to have a full-time radiologist on site. It is important to understand the capabilities and limitations of these devices when placing them in service and to develop ways to overcome these limitations. Our previous work has shown that fine detail lesions in particular may be susceptible to error; increasing image matrix size may help to overcome these limitations to increase diagnostic accuracy.[1,2] We conducted a large scale study to evaluate the ability of a commercially available teleradiology system to detect pneumothorax, a clinically important fine detail pathology that may be difficult to detect even on conventional chest radiographs.

Materials and Methods

We used a commercially available image transmission system (Ektascan, Eastman Kodak Co., Rochester, NY) to digitize and transmit conventional chest radiographs. We have previously described the system in detail.[1] The system acquires image data via a vidicon camera mounted above a light box that holds up to a 14" x 17" radiograph. The image may be optically magnified up to 4 times before the image is digitized. The camera is interfaced via a frame grabber board to an IBM PC microcomputer. Standard image acquisition is a 512 x 480 matrix, with 8 bit image depth resulting in 256 gray levels. The images are displayed on a separate display/control module. This module permits numerous display features including: 1. window/level manipulation; 2. zoom; 3. area of interest; 4. histogram equalization; 5. reverse video image; 6. grid overlay; 7. image flip; and 8. image mirror.

Image data is sent via ordinary telephone lines from the image capture/transmit/receive module to a second transmit/receive module using a 9600 bps modem. The system employs 2:1 data compression without data loss.

We employed an image database of 200 chest radiographs for this project. Half the images were of a case of pneumothorax. Most were of average difficulty in detectability (on the original radiograph), a handful were fairly obvious, and a greater number were very subtle, as would be expected in routine clinical practice. An equal number of chest radiographs without pneumothorax were chosen. An effort was made to include radiographs with similar findings other than pneumothorax so that extraneous clues would not unduly influence the readers' decision. For example, cases of lung masses following needle biopsy with and without pneumothorax were included, as were cases of central line placement, again with and without pneumothorax.

In all cases the true state was determined by a truth committee (JLC, CRM) based on the findings on the original radiograph, findings on radiographs before and after the study radiograph, and on the clinical history and course. In the rare instance where the committee could not agree on a diagnosis, the radiograph was excluded from the study set. All patient identifying data was masked. Using the macro zoom lens each radiograph was digitized at 3 magnification levels (1x, 2x, 4x) corresponding to an effective matrix size of 512 x 480, 1024 x 960 , and 2048 x 1920. Each image was transmitted over ordinary telephone lines from the Jefferson Barracks division to the John Cochran division of the St. Louis Department of Veterans Affairs Medical Center, a distance of 12 miles.

The reader panel consisted of six staff radiologists all of whom interpreted chest radiographs as part of their routine clinical duties. The cases were presented in groups of ten to twenty at a time with normal and pneumothorax examples randomly dispersed throughout the groups. Each image was interpreted a total of four times by each reader: once at each matrix size (1x, 2x, 4x) as well as the original radiographs. Images were presented over the course of six months to prevent any memory effect. Because of the difficulty of scheduling reading periods for so many people over a relatively long time period, a few of the images were not interpreted by all readers, however substantially all cases were read by all readers. Readers were allowed to take as much time as they desired to make their interpretation. They were allowed to use any of the image manipulation controls available on the unit.

Readers were asked to rate each image on a five choice scale:

1. pneumothorax definitely present
2. pneumothorax probably present
3. pneumothorax possibly present
4. pneumothorax probably absent
5. pneumothorax definitely absent.

Readers were also asked to grade the technical quality of each image on a three point scale:

1. High
2. Adequate
3. Low.

They were also given an opportunity to comment on each image.

Rating data were tabulated and the area under the resulting receiver operating characteristic (ROC) curves calculated using a spreadsheet (Excel 5.0 for Macintosh, Microsoft, Redmond, WA) by the method of England.[3] The two-tailed paired t test was used to determine statistical significance (Excel 5.0, above) for comparing the average reader performance for the matrix sizes employed.

Results

Figure 1 shows the set of ROC curves generated by responses from one of the readers. The ROC curves of the other readers had similar distributions. As can be seen, there were large differences in the reader's accuracy depending on the matrix size used, particularly at the standard matrix size of 512 x 480. For all readers accuracy increased with each increase in effective matrix size; best accuracy was achieved with the conventional radiographs. Most readers' data values for conventional radiographs clustered in the "ideal region" of the upper left corner of ROC space, whereas the readers' data points for the transmitted images were spread out farther away from the "ideal region," particularly for the standard non-magnified 512x480 matrix size.

Figure 1. ROC curves for reader 1.

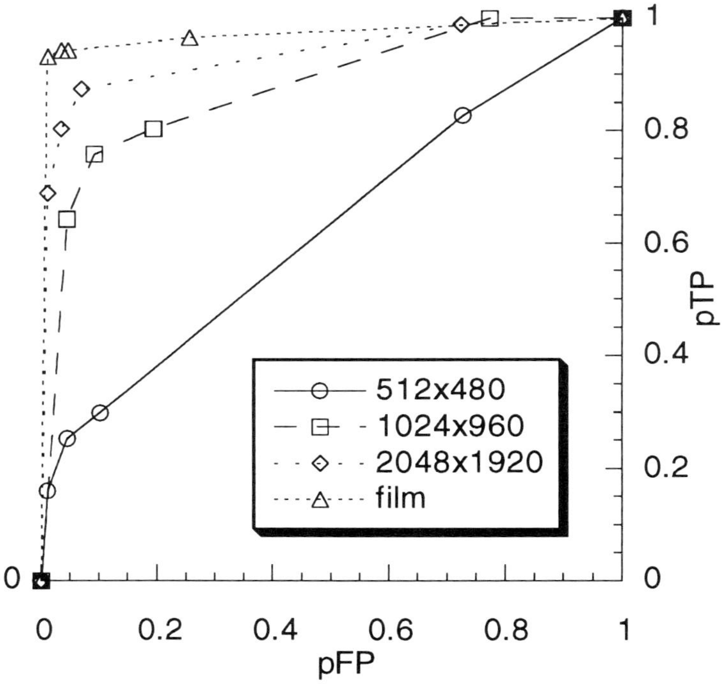

Table 1 summarizes the areas under the ROC curve for the group of six radiologists at each matrix size and for conventional chest radiographs. From this table we see a consistent trend in improvement in accuracy scores as the matrix size increased from 512 x 480 to 1024 x 960 with lesser degree of improvement as the matrix increased to 2048 x 1920. Greatest accuracy occured for conventional film radiographs.

Table 1. Accuracy index (area under ROC curve) for pneumothorax detection.

reader	Accuracy index (ROC area) matrix size 512x480	matrix size 1024x960	matrix size 2048x1920	conventional film radiograph
1	0.648	0.901	0.954	0.977
2	0.712	0.854	0.922	0.965
3	0.674	0.875	0.957	0.962
4	0.736	0.949	0.968	0.991
5	0.656	0.794	0.852	0.889
6	0.632	0.734	0.804	0.866

Table 2 gives the two-tailed t test P values for all format combinations. The improvement in accuracy was statistically significant for each increase in matrix size employed. Notably however, the accuracy in evaluating conventional plain film radiographs was significantly better than for any of the teleradiology groups. Indeed, the best accuracy ratings for all readings was with conventional films, though the 4x matrix closely approached that of film.

Table 2. p Values - comparison of modalities using paired 2-tailed t-test.

	512x480 matrix	1024x960 matrix	2048x1920 matrix
1024x960 matrix	p=0.000637		
2048x1920 matrix	p=0.000107	p=0.00123	
film radiographs	p=0.0000110	p=0.000804	p=0.0103

Discussion

We studied the ability of radiologists to diagnose pneumothorax using chest radiograph images transmitted by a commercially available teleradiology system. Pneumothoraces may be subtle and difficult to detect even on conventional film radiographs yet may have important, possibly life threatening consequences if not diagnosed. Our pilot work in evaluating this system showed that such fine detail lesions were the most difficult to diagnose and hence would provide a critical means to evaluate diagnostic accuracy of a given system.[2]

We found that the conventional chest radiographs yielded the highest diagnostic accuracy as measured by the area under the ROC curve. We also showed that increasing the effective matrix size (resolution) of the transmitted images yielded statistically significant improvements in accuracy, though still less than the original radiograph. Hammond and others using a similar image transmission system did not find a significant difference in diagnostic accuracy between transmitted images and film in evaluating intravenous urograms for hydronephrosis.[4] This is not surprising as hydronephrosis may be considered a coarse detail lesion which puts less demand on the system and reader for diagnosis. A report by Kassebaum and others also using a similar image transmission system evaluated transmitted dental radiographs for pathologic changes. They found general improvement in diagnostic accuracy with decreasing pixel size (increasing matrix size) but the differences were often not statistically significant.[5]

Using a different system, Elam and others found that readers evaluating for pneumothorax on conventional chest radiographs were significantly more sensitive than with images on a digital workstation.[6] Clearly the nature of the pathology in question will influence accuracy results. In general, subtle abnormalities and difficult negative cases are most useful in discriminating differences in diagnostic accuracy.[7]

This study demonstrated that increasing the effective matrix size of the transmitted images (effectively decreasing pixel size) could result in significant improvements in diagnostic accuracy. This improvement was not without cost, however. In order to achieve the higher matrix size, portions of the chest radiographs are optically magnified prior to the digitization. This means the entire image can no longer be seen on the monitor at the same time; multiple images are required for complete coverage. This results in increased data storage requirements (4x for the 1024 matrix, 16x for the 2048 matrix) as well as similar increases in transmission time. Probably more important however is that radiologists are used to seeing an entire image at once; viewing only portions of the original image on the screen requires effort to integrate them into a total image, resulting in uncertainty of interpertation. The increased resolution of modern scanners and displays may eliminate this drawback, though expenses will increase proportionately.

The image manipulation controls were sometimes helpful in interperation. The histogram equalization was the image manipulation control most often used by our readers. It serves to "spread out" the gray scale in a user-selectable region of the image. This increases the contrast of the range selected to achieve maximum detail and was most useful when the area in question was largely dark (such as the lung edge in pneumothorax) or bright. The window/level control was also useful to improve visualization of the overall image. The image magnification (zoom) feature was usually not helpful as it only increases pixel size without actually increasing resolution. While helpful in improving image quality in some cases, many of our readers disliked using these controls, finding them somewhat distracting and time consuming. Our readers uniformly had a preference for the original radiographs. In part this was due to familiarity, image quality, and decreased time required to read the film image. These objections need to be overcome if any teleradiology system is to be used on a routine, high volume basis. In addition, any teleradiology system employed must be evaluated for ability to achieve accurate results in the diagnosis of fine detail pathologies as opposed to coarse detail lesions. User interface issues also need to be studied to ensure acceptability issues are adequately addressed.

References

1. Markivee CR, Mahanta B, Savci S, Abbas SA, Chenoweth JL, Luther RK, Patel BK, Vas WG, Hill TG. Diagnostic accuracy of a teleradiology image transmission system. MD Computing 1989; 6: 88-93.

2. Markivee CR, Chenoweth JL. Teleradiology image transmission system: Diagnostic accuracy at three matrix sizes for various types of images. J Digital Imaging 1990; 3: 170-173.

3. England WL. An exponential model used for optimal threshold selection on ROC curves. Med. Decis Making 1988; 8: 120-131.

4. Hammond CA, Hattery RR, King BF, et.al. Quality of remotely transmitted images. In Arenson RL and Friedenberg RM, editors. S/CAR '90–Computer applications to assist radiology. Proceedings of the 10th conference on computer applications in radiology and 4th conference on computer assisted radiology of the Society for Computer Assisted Radiology; 1990 Jun 13-16; Anaheim, CA. Carlsbad, CA: Symposia Foundation; 1990. p 96-101.

5. Kassebaum DK, McDavid WD, Dove SB, Waggener RG. Spatial resolution requirements for digitizing dental radiographs. Oral Surg Oral Med Oral Pathol 1989; 67: 760-769.

6. Elam EA, Rehm K, Hillman BJ, Maloney K, Fajardo LL, McNeil K. Efficacy of digital radiography for the detection of pneumothorax: comparison with conventional chest radiography. AJR 1992; 158: 509-514.

7. Rockette HE, King JL, Medina JL, Eisen HB, Brown ML, Gur D. Imaging systems evaluation: Effect of subtle cases on the design and analysis of receiver operating characteristic studies. AJR 1995; 165: 679-683.

Acknowledgements

The authors thank Syed A. Abbas MD, Suheyla Savci MD, Robert L. Levitt MD, Lucy Morris MD, and Benett Gray MD for taking time in their busy schedules to serve on the reader panel. Eastman Kodak Co. donated use of the Ektascan Image Transmission System.

Accuracy of Diagnosis of Subtle Fractures on Digitized Teleradiology Images

A. Larson, B.S., D.A. Lynch, M.B., B. Zeligman, M.D., C. Harlow, M.D., G. Thieme, M.D. and R.F. Kilcoyne, M.D.

Department of Radiology, University of Colorado School of Medicine, Denver, Colorado

This study compared conventional skeletal radiographs with 12-bit digitized images of the same radiographs in terms of subjective image quality and accuracy of diagnosis of subtle fractures. The cases used were chosen for the subtlety of their abnormalities. They included 29 normal sets of bone images, and 26 sets of bone images with fractures normal and abnormal bone images. Each radiograph was viewed by three radiologists at a workstation with a 1K by 1K (1280 x 1024 pixel matrix) monitor equipped with an 8–bit–per pixel gray scale display. Most of the digitized images were rated as good as or slightly inferior to the original images in spatial resolution and contrast resolution. Overall sensitivity and specificity for detecting abnormality was also slightly worse for the digitized images. We conclude that digitized radiographs are adequate for clinical diagnosis of subtle abnormalities.

INTRODUCTION

Radiologists remain concerned about the possibility of missing subtle disease on digitized radiographs. Some previous studies have shown that accurate primary diagnosis can be made from digitized images (Goldberg et al). However, another study of original and digitized radiographs containing a variety of subtle abnormalities showed a significant decline in diagnostic accuracy for the digitized radiographs (Scott et al.). Bone fractures are a particular area of concern, since 2 previous studies have identified a decrease in the detection rate of subtle fractures when digitized radiographs were compared with original radiographs. Therefore, this study was performed to compare the accuracy of diagnosis of subtle fractures on digitized radiographs viewed on a teleradiology system with that of original radiographs.

METHODS

A total of 55 sets of skeletal images were chosen for evaluation- 29 were normal and 26 showed subtle fractures. Many of these abnormalities had been missed in earlier interpretations by residents or faculty radiologists. Radiographs included all commonly imaged body parts. Three independent board-certified radiologists viewed all of the images, giving a total of 165 readings. The correct diagnosis was determined by consensus of two board-certified radiologists who did not participate in the scoring of the images. The study design required the radiologist to evaluate and score the digitized image first, then the analog image, then directly compare the images.

The radiographs were laser–digitized at a spot size of 100mm and a contrast resolution of 12 bits using a Lumiscan 150 scanner (Lumisys, Inc, Sunnyvale CA). Each radiograph was viewed by the three radiologists at an AGFA RS 5000 teleradiology workstation with a 1K by 1K (1280 x 1024 pixel matrix) monitor equipped with an 8–bit–per pixel grayscale display. By adjusting the window–width and window–level settings, the radiologists were able to use all 12 bits of digitized information. The "roam" function made it possible to view all parts of each image at full resolution (2K by 2K). During the viewing the radiologists were encouraged to manipulate the images using all of these functions so that each digitized image was viewed at maximal resolution.

A score sheet asked the viewers to score each image on a scale from 1 to 5 for image quality with the following interpretations: 1=Excellent, 2=Good, 3=Borderline, 4=Nondiagnostic, 5=Terrible. When determining specific image problems the viewer chose from 1=Poor Spatial Resolution, 2=Poor Contrast Resolution, 3=Aesthetically Unpleasing, 4=Other (Specify). The score sheet then asked the radiologist to determine if a fracture was present. The confidence scale used the following values: 1=definitely normal, 2=probably normal, 3=equivocal, 4=probably abnormal, 5=definitely abnormal. Abnormalities apart from fracture were ignored. The location of the fracture was noted. After the separate evaluations of the digitized and original radiographs, the radiologists were asked to directly compare the spatial resolution and contrast resolution of the digitized and original radiographs. The contrast resolution was evaluated in high-contrast areas of the radiograph (lung or bone) and in low contrast areas (mediastinum and soft tissues). The subjective scale used was: 1=much better than original, 2=slightly better than original, 3=same as original, 4=slightly worse than original, 5=much worse than original.

For comparison of the individual sensitivities and specificities of the viewing methods for each type of abnormality, a McNemar test for paired proportions was used.

RESULTS

Sensitivity and Specificity

Table 1 shows the results of the sensitivity and specificity evaluation for detection of fractures. Teleradiology yielded a slightly higher sensitivity than conventional radiographs. The accuracy rates for all 3 observers were similar. All cases of fracture were detected by at least one observer, but 6 of 26 fractures were missed by at least one observer on the original and digitized images.

TABLE 1
SENSITIVITY AND SPECIFICITY OF DIGITIZED AND ORIGINAL RADIOGRAPHS FOR FRACTURE DETECTION

	SENSITIVITY	SPECIFICITY
FRACTURE DETECTION ON ORIGINAL RADIOGRAPHS	92%	81%
FRACTURE DETECTION ON DIGITIZED RADIOGRAPHS	94%	85%

The image quality results can be seen in Table 2. A total of 76% of the digitized images were scored as either excellent or good, compared with 88% of original images.

TABLE 2
IMAGE QUALITY

	ORIGINAL IMAGES	DIGITIZED IMAGES
EXCELLENT	87 (53%)	44 (27%)
GOOD	55 (33%)	80 (49%)
BORDERLINE	16 (10%)	12 (7%)
NONDIAGNOSTIC	5 (3%)	25 (15%)
TERRIBLE	2 (1%)	4 (2%)

The direct comparison of contrast resolution and spatial resolution is summarized in Table 3. A large majority of the digitized bone and chest radiographs, were scored as either equivalent to the original film or slightly worse. A small percentage of the images were scored as much worse than the original.

TABLE 3
DIRECT COMPARISON OF IMAGE QUALITY

	CONTRAST RES (BONES)	CONTRAST RES (SOFT TISSUE/ FAT)	SPATIAL RES
DIGITIZED MUCH BETTER THAN ORIGINAL	3 (2%)	8 (5%)	0
DIGITIZED SLIGHTLY BETTER THAN ORIGINAL	16 (10%)	26 (16%)	2 (1%)
DIGITIZED SAME AS ORIGINAL	71 (43%)	79 (48%)	90 (55%)
DIGITIZED SLIGHTLY WORSE THAN ORIGINAL	71 (43%)	50 (30%)	70 (42%)
DIGITIZED MUCH WORSE THAN ORIGINAL	4 (2%)	2 (1%)	3 (2%)

DISCUSSION

This study confirms that the inevitable loss of spatial and contrast resolution when a film is digitized is usually apparent to the radiologist as a slight decrease in image quality. However, this decrease in image quality causes only a very slight decrease in sensitivity for detection of subtle fractures. The subtlety of the fractures in this study is evident from the fact that six of 26 fractures were missed by at least one observer on both the original and digitized images. Use of subtle cases should enhance the ability of our study to detect a real difference between digitized and conventional images (Rockette).

In a series of patients with pneumonia and fractures, Ackerman and colleagues found a sensitivity of 89% for analog radiographs, compared with 78% for digitized radiographs. The lower sensitivity of digitized radiographs in their study might be due to the fact that 1280 by 1024 pixel monitors were used, and it is unclear whether all images were appropriately zoomed to maximize spatial resolution. In another study from the same group, sensitivity for subtle fractures was dramatically lower for digitized images than for original images. A study by Wilson and Hodge, using a scanner with a 175 μ spot size, and a 1200 line monitor, concluded that this system was not adequate for clinical use because of a substantial decrease in detection of fractures when reading digitized radiographs. Our study differs technically from these previous studies in that the spatial resolution of the digitized images was greater (2.87 line pairs/mm for 14 by 17 inch original radiographs and 5.03 line pairs/mm for 8 by 10 inch original films, compared with 3.5 line pairs/mm (Scott) and 2.35 line pairs/mm (Wilson and Hodge). Also, we requested the viewing radiologists to view all parts of each images at maximal resolution. Although this added to the time required for viewing the images, it did seem to overcome the disadvantage of using 1Kby 1K monitors.

The overall sensitivity of our readers for detection of fractures on bone radiographs was substantially higher than that previously found for chest radiographic abnormalities. This may have been because the fractures were less subtle than the chest radiographic abnormalities, or because the readers were able to focus on the single task of defining whether or not a fracture was present, rather than having to search for 3 separate types of abnormalities, as with the chest radiographs. Since most bone radiographs are physically smaller than chest radiographs, the spatial resolution is higher and the area for searching is smaller. It is interesting that the sensitivity of the readers for detection of fractures was slightly higher for digitized radiographs than for original radiographs. This may have been because many of the bone radiographs were physically enlarged when viewed on the teleradiology monitor, making fractures easier to see. An additional advantage of viewing bone images on a workstation is the relative ease of manipulating window and level for viewing darker areas of the image, compared to the task of using a bright light for analog images. In the near future, the use of edge-enhancing image processing algorithms, or computerized detection techniques for nodules and pneumothorax on digitized images may actually enhance the sensitivity of readers using workstations for radiographic reading.

Our study design provided a difficult test for digitized radiographs because we intentionally chose very subtle radiographic abnormalities. The fact that the original radiographs were always viewed after the digitized radiographs might have caused some of the apparent increased sensitivity of film-based reading, since abnormalities are presumably more likely to be seen on a second viewing. However, this second-look technique may also have caused the decline in specificity for analog radiographs, since it is clear that prolonged evaluation of radiographs leads to increased detection of false-positives.

Our study intentionally accentuated any potential deficiencies of the teleradiology system. The majority of our digitized images were scored as either excellent or good in terms of image quality. When the contrast resolution and spatial resolution were evaluated, the majority of the cases were scored the same as or slightly inferior to the original. In our study there were no major differences between the sensitivity and specificity of the original and digitized images. We conclude that although image digitization leads to an appreciable slight decrease in image quality in the digitized images, the resultant decline in detection sensitivity for subtle abnormalities, if present, is very small. Our study suggests that primary diagnosis from digitized images of the chest and skeleton transmitted by teleradiology is acceptable practice.

BIBLIOGRAPHY

Ackerman SJ, Gitlin JN, Gayler RW, Flagle CD, Bryan RN. Receiver operating curve analysis of fracture and pneumonia detection: Comparison of laser-digitized workstation images and conventional analog radiographs. Radioogy 1993;186:263-268.

Goldberg MA, Rosenthal DI, Chew FS, Blickman JG, Miller SW, Mueller PR. New high-resolution teleradiology system: Prospective study of diagnostic accuracy in 685 transmitted clinical cases. Radiology 1993;186:429-434

Rockette HE, King JL, Medina JL, Eisen HB, Brown ML, Gur D. Imaging systems evaluation: effect of subtle cases on the design and analysis of receiver operating characteristic studies. AJR 1995;165:679-683

Scott WW Jr, Bluemke DA, Mysko WK, Weller GE, Kelen GD, Reichle RL, Weller JC, Gitlin JN. Interpretation of emergency department radiographs by radiologists and emergency medicine physicians: teleradiology workstation versus radiograph readings. Radiology 1995;195:223-9.

Scott WW Jr, Rosenbaum JE, Ackerman SJ, Reichle RL, Magid D, Weller JC, Gitlin JN. Subtle orthopedic fractures: teleradiology workstation versus film interpretation. Radiology 1993;187:811-815.

Wilson AJ, Hodge JC. Digitized radiographs in skeletal trauma: a performance comparison between a digital workstation and the original film images. Radiology 1995;196:565-568

Assessment of Asynchronous Transfer Mode (ATM) Networks for Regional Teleradiology

André J. Duerinckx, Alex Hayrapetian, Michelle Melany and Edward G. Grant
Radiology Service, Veterans Affairs Medical Center, West Los Angeles, California and Radiology Department, UCLA Medical Center, California

Daniel J. Valentino and Sherelle L. Narin
Radiology Department, University of California, Los Angeles, California

1. INTRODUCTION

Because of the increasing availability of Asynchronous Transfer Mode (ATM) networks both hospitals and radiology groups have become very interested in their use. In some instances individual hospitals or whole regions have decided to link themselves with ATM type networks, making it easy for radiologist to use existing connections [1, 2]. In other instances radiologists have taken the lead, and have justified experimenting with ATM networks based on the very high data rates required to transfer imaging studies [3-8]. In this paper, we describe our own experiences with ATM, review the first clinical experiences with some of the ATM networks built specifically for radiology applications and speculate on the future of medical imaging networks based on ATM technology. As with PACS, the relative importance of cost considerations will dramatically change when intangible benefits such as ultrafast access to images is taken into account.

2. METHODS

In Los Angeles, California, several teaching hospitals are very closely affiliated with the UCLA medical center. Two of these even share a joint radiology residency training program (the West Los Angeles Veterans Affairs medical center and the Olive View-UCLA medical center). This cluster of three affiliated hospitals is one of the test sites for ATM networks since an ATM network was established in late 1994 and early 1995.

The ATM test described here were performed between two hospitals approximately 1 mile removed from each other but separated by a large California freeway. The alternative to ATM was to physically drive films or a radiologist from one institution to the next. In order to physically drive from one hospital to the next during busy day time traffic, one could spend up to 25 minutes driving the short distance and then spending the additional 5-10 minutes finding parking space at the UCLA Medical Center and walking to the offices. Thus a typical radiological consultation involving physical transport of films and a physician moving from one hospital to the next could take 30 minutes or more of physician time. The ATM network was set up to provide efficient interactive telemedicine and teleradiology consultation between physicians at both locations.

3. RESULTS

Initial image data transfer was successfully tested in March 1995, and initial real-time video/audio transmission in October 1995.

The initial ATM trial involved transfer of static radiographic image between two ultrasound mini-PACS: one PACS was situated at the West LA VA and the second PACS at an outpatient imaging center immediately adjacent to the main UCLA hospital (the Medical Plaza 300 Building). First the Raw Data Rate (Megabits per second) was measured. A bit generator (Hewlett Packard) was used to verify the raw data rate that could be accommodated by the ATM network (performed at GTE Laboratories in Marina Del Rey). We were able to consistently achieve a data rate of not less than 137 Mbit/sec. Second TCP/IP and DICOM Data Rates (protocol limitations) were measured. The average memory-to-memory data rate, using TCP/IP on SUN SPARCstation 10 servers, was 25 Mbit/sec. Typical variations in memory-to-memory and disk-to-memory image data transfer rates during a 30 minute session are shown in Figure 1. These changes reflect variations due to competition with other users on the same PACS. The average remote disk-to-disk image transfer, using TCP/IP on SUN SPARCstation 10 servers, was 9.6 Mbit/sec. However, using DICOM 3.0 communications protocols, the average remote disk-to-disk image transfer performance was 3 to 5 Mbit/sec [8]. The average time to retrieve up to 100 ultrasound images to a remote workstation was 60 sec. Using these capabilities, timely interactive subspecialty consultations between radiologists was successfully performed while both were at different physical locations.

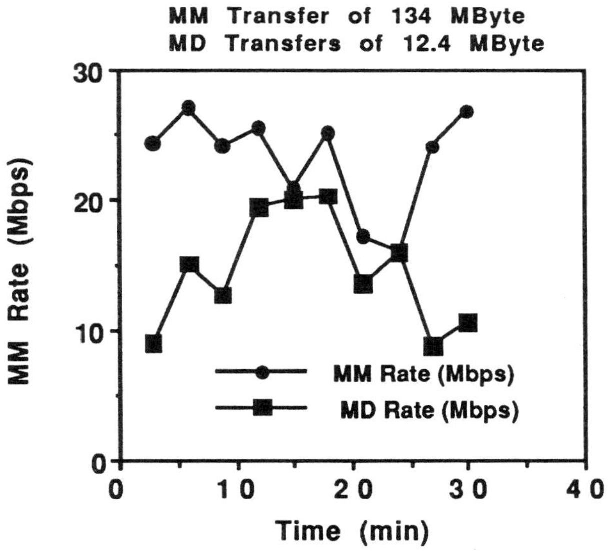

Figure 1: Typical variations in memory-to-memory and disk-to-memory image data transfer rates on the UCLA ATM network during a 30 minute session.

We also evaluated interactive audio/video communication at approximately 37 Mbit/sec band width [9, 10]. The image quality was sufficient to allow interactive teaching conferences and remote monitoring of ultrasound studies [11].

4. DISCUSSION

Ultrafast networks using Asynchronous Transfer Mode (ATM) technology can provide the bandwidth and throughput that may be sufficient to satisfy the medical imaging community. Several trials are underway to assess the effect of ATM network capabilities on the clinical practice of radiology, by providing immediate interactive radiology consultations between subspecialists and general radiologists at affiliated academic institutions. The hardware to build such networks is now commercially available and its cost is decreasing steadily, but the monthly charges for ATM bandwidth use are still high. Nevertheless, given the tremendous increase in communication capability and data transfer rates possible with ATM networks, cost alone should not be the determining factor for selecting this technology.

A similar ATM experiment among UCSF affiliated hospitals has been described by H K Huang et al. [5, 6] . Preliminary results with the ATM link between the main UCSF Medical Center and one affiliated hospital (Mount Zion Hospital) showed a data rate of 59 Mbit/sec.

Initial performance results of an ATM network at the Duke University Medical Center showed throughput rates up to 10 MByte/sec (or 80 Mbit/sec) with TCP/IP protocol [12]. These early tests of commercially available ATM hardware indicate that high throughput is achieved today using TCP/IP. The experiment was performed using switched virtual circuits (SVCs) as opposed to permanent virtual circuits. Although the standard on SVCs has not yet been set, this particular type of connection was selected because the simplicity of establishing SVC connections and the expectation that SVCs will be the typical method of connection from most PACS applications in the near future.

The discrepancy between our ATM rates and the ones reported by others is most likely explained by the fact that we had a working PACS being used for clinical operations in use at the time of our measurements.

5. CONCLUSION

The ATM networks described are in the early stages of clinical testing. Initial results and experience with these new networks are being reported as they become available.

Having such an advanced image network may create the need to discuss radiology load balancing and improved coordination of coverage of radiological services provided by a single staff physician to multiple hospitals.

6. ACKNOWLEDGMENTS

We would like to acknowledge people in several organizations who made this project possible including, GTE Telephone Operations, Bayer Corporation (Agfa division), Newbridge Networks, Inc., the UCLA medical physics and imaging group, and the Information Resource Management service at the VAMC, West LA. Richard Steckel, MD at the UCLA Medical Center and Ramesh Verma, MD at the Olive View-UCLA Medical Center also supported this project.

7. REFERENCES

1. Bruwer WA, Loop JD, Symon JA, Thompson BG. VISTAnet and MICA: medical applications leading to the NCIH. IEEE Network. 1994; 8(6): 24-31.

2. Schnepf JA, Du DHC, Ritenour ER, Fahrmann AJ. Building future medical education environments over ATM networks. Comm of the ACM 1995; 38(2): 54-69.

3. Lemke HU. Future direction in electronic image handling. Investigative Radiology 1993; 28 (Suppl 3): S79-81.

4. Dutton G. 1994- The year of the asynchronous transfer mode. IEEE Software 1994; 11(1): 102-103.

5. Huang HK, Arenson RL, Dillon WP, Lau AS, Bozzell T, Gould RG. High performance testbed network with asynchronous transfer mode technology for teleradiology (Abstract). Radiology 1994; 193(P): 141.

6. Huang HK, Arenson RL, Dillon WP, Lou SL, Bazzill T, Wong AWK. Asynchronous transfer mode technology for radiologic image communication. AJR 1995; 164: 1533-1536.

7. Duerinckx AJ, Hagan G, Valentino DJ, et al. Assessment of ATM for transmission of medical images. In: SPIE Proceedings of the EUROPT Symposium on "Advanced Image and Video Communications and Storge Technologies", SPIE Vol 2451. March 20-23, 1995; Amsterdam, The Netherlands: 1995: 345-356.

8. Duerinckx AJ, Valentino DJ, Hayrepetian A, Hagan G, El-Saden S, Grant EG. (Abstr) Assessment of Asynchronous Transfer Mode (ATM) Networks for Regional Teleradiology (Abstr.). Radiology 1995; 197(P): 377.

9. Duerinckx AJ, Hayrapetian AS, Grant EG, et al. Impact of ultrasound video transfer on the practice of ultrasound. In: SPIE Proceedings of Medical Imaging 1996. PACS: Design and Evaluation . Newport Beach, CA, Febr 10-15: SPIE Vol 2711, 1996 (In Press)

10. Duerinckx AJ, Valentino DJ, Hayrapetian A, Grant EG. Ultrafast networks (ATM): first clinical experiences (Invited Review Article). European Journal of Radiology , 1996 (In Press)

11. Grant EG, Melaney M, Duerinckx AJ, Leifer-Narin SL, Valentino DJ, Hayrapetian A. Impact of ultrafast video image transfer on the practive of US. Radiology 1995; 197 (P): 161.

12. DoVan M, Humphrey LM, Cox G, Ravin CE. Initial experience with asynchronous transfer mode for use in a medical imaging network. Journal of Digital Imaging 1995; 8 (1): 43-48.

PC-Based Access to the Multimedia Patient Record with Simultaneous Videoconferences: The Hospital Goes On-Line

Jens Ricke, M.D., Lutz Kleinhotz, Ph.D., Norbert Hosten, M.D., Holger Amthauer, M.D., Thomas Liebig, M.D., Christian Stroscszinski, M.D., Tilmann Schumacher, M.D. and Roland Felix, M.D.

Department of Radiology, Virchow-Klinikum, Medical Faculty, Humboldt University, Berlin, Germany

1. Introduction

Information management in medicine has not kept up with the pace of advances in communication technology in general. This is even more surprising since the use of communication technology designed specifically for the medical environment offers remarkable increases in quality of treatment as well as cost savings [12, 15, 17]. Optimal use of diagnostic and therapeutic resources today is restricted by time or information loss in medical data transfer. Following the BERMED project [6, 8, 16] for the development of telemedical applications, the aim of the HYPERMED project at the Virchow-Klinikum Berlin was to create a cost efficient concept for the hospital on-line. A Multimedia PC offers the basic functionalities for medical communication in daily practice:

1. access to fully integrated electronic patient records with all images and reports via hospital network or ISDN
2. teleconsultation with simultaneous access to the electronic patient record and visualization of all non digital data via document camera.

2. Technology

Multimedia PC

The Multimedia PC runs under Windows (3.1 or ´95) [9]. After authorization, a Netscape Browser [4] allows access to the electronic patient chart and offers an index of patients. For each patient, a list of examinations available is visualized on screen and single examinations can be chosen. A mouse click retrieves general examination data, the report and GIFFormated images. For visualization of original image data in ACR-NEMA or DICOM [1, 2] a proprietary viewer is implemented allowing simple functionalities of image processing like window and center modification. The software can be modified to be used on Apple Macintosh or UNIX based workstation as well. UNIX machines can be interesting due to the larger number of software tools for image processing on the market.

For videoconferencing, Intel ProShare® is used. For demonstration of patient data a „shared whiteboard“ serves to transmit data retrieved from the digital archive or scanned with a document camera. To support demonstration of findings, a telepointer can be used.

Networks
Hospitalin- and external communication base on two different networks mainly for cost reasons. At the Virchow-Klinikum, the project ARUBA served to install and test a hospitalinternal ATM-infrastructure on optical fiber with a maximal data transfer rate of 2,5 Gbit/s. This network connects the department of Radiology with the departments of Surgery, Internal Medicine, Intensive Care units, Laboratories, the German Heart Center located on the same campus, and the hospital administration [7]. In addition, copper-based Ethernet with up to 10 Mbit/s can be accessed anywhere in the hospital. Ethernet is specifically interesting for being far less expensive than ATM [13, 14].

For external communication Euro-ISDN at 2 x 64 Kbit/s is used [3]. Euro-ISDN, Integrated Services Digital Network, is a world wide standard for digital public phone and allows integration of various services (Audio, Video, Fax,...) scaleable in 64 Kbit steps.

Hospitalinfrastructure: Digital archive and electronic patient record
In Radiology, digital archiving demands integration of imaging and other information devices [5, 10]. Ideal is the integration of all sources generating medical or relevant administrative data. In HYPERMED, the concept of a Meta Patient Record has lead to establish fully integrated electronic patient records [11, 16]. Like an index card system, the central server just stores information about where the original data is stored in subsystems: storage space can be added when needed, existing devices can be integrated, and individual solutions remain scaleable. All standards can be used, focuses are HL7, EDI and DICOM 3.

3. Experiences in clinical routine

Key issue for telemedical applications is the time spent for data transfer and handling. To estimate the performance of HYPERMED in clinical routine, in 20 cases time was calculated to perform the following activities via ISDN (hospitalexternal) or Ethernet (hospitalinternal) including start up of the software program:

1. access the digital archive and visualization of an overview of all examinations of an individual patient
2. retrieval of general examination data, patient history, report and images of an average CT (58 GIFF images)
3. retrieval of a selected CT image in ACR-NEMA as original data.

In addition, 20 „whiteboards" with 6 MR images and written report (conferencing chart for a ProShare videoconference) where tested regarding time for transmission during a videoconference. In previous studies, an average of 6 images had been selected by Radiologists to demonstrate findings of MRI or CT examinations to clinicians [17].

The configuration of the PC allows 1 x 64 Kbit/s for ISDN access to the digital archive, videoconferences use 2 x 64 Kbit/s. Hospitalinternal communication is Ethernet with a maximal transmission rate of 10 Mbit/s; in practice, 4-6 Mbit/s are more realistic depending on the number of users on the network.

Time to visualize an overview of archived information of a patient was 41s with ISDN (standarddeviation SD 2s), Ethernet 19s (SD 4s). Visualization of general examination data, report and 58 CT images via ISDN took 3min 31s (SD 4s), Ethernet 37s (SD 3s). Retrieval of original ACR-NEMA data of a single CT slide took an additional 1min 20s (SD 0,9s) via ISDN and 6s (SD 2s) via Ethernet.

Transmission of a conference chart with 6 MR images and written report during a teleconsultation via ISDN took an average of 2min 20s (SD 14s).

4. Conclusion

The most important functionalities foreseen for Telemedicine in daily routine is covered by the Multimedia-PC: access to the electronic patient chart and simultaneous videoconferencing. A document camera for transmission of analogue documents is optional. It should be considered though that document cameras do not support the advantages of Telemedicine regarding speed of data transmission and unlimited access to all relevant patient data. Other aspects like integration of the hospital administration and various other software tools and services may be implemented on top of the basic PC.

For hospitalinternal communication a local area network with Ethernet features technology for rapid data transfer in seconds even for larger data volumes like CT examinations. Work flow in clinical practice can profit tremendously. Following this argument, 1000 PCs in the Virchow-Klinikum located on wards or in out patient clinics will be updated with software for access to the digital infrastructure in 1996. In critical areas like emergency or operating rooms 40 additional PCs will also feature videoconferencing hard- and software.

For external communication, the only technology available at reasonable cost is ISDN allowing access to the digital archive as well as retrieval of the complete electronic patient record within minutes. After modification of the router technology implemented, the use of 2 x 64 Kbit/s will lead to further increase of transmission speed.

Suggested readings

1. *American College of Radiology and National Electronic Manufacturers* Association *(ACR-NEMA):* Digital Image and Communications in Medicine (DICOM). Part 1: Introduction and Overview: Version 3.0. NEMA Standards Publication PS3.1 March 1993

2. *American College of Radiology and National Electronic Manufacturers Association (ACR-NEMA):* ACR-NEMA Standard V. 2.0. Standards Publication No. 300.1988

3. *Bocker, P.:* ISDN – Das dienstintegrierte digitale Nachrichtennetz. Konzept, Verfahren, Systeme. Springer, Berlin 1987

4. *Berners-Lee, T., R. Cailliau, A. Luotonen, H. Frystyk Nielsen, A. Secret:* The World-Wide-Web. Communications of the ACM 37 (8) (1994)

5. *CEN/TC 251/PT 011 EHCRA:* Electronic healthcare record architecture, first interim report. State University Gent, March 1994

6. *Felix, R., L. Kleinholz, H. Oswald, M. Ohly, N. Hosten, K. Vöge, E. Köttgen, B. Mahr, E. Fleck:* Kommunikation und Integration medizinischer Dokumente für medizinische Konferenzen. Fortschr. Röntgenstr. 161(4) (1994) 327-34

7. *Fuchs, S., L. Kleinholz, M. Ohly, R. Simon, J. Steffens, R. Felix, B. Mahr, E. Fleck:* Broadband Telemedicine Applications:

Experiences and Results of the ARUBA Project. Proc. European Symposium on Advanced Networks and Services. Amsterdam 1995

8. *Kleinholz, L., M. Ohly:* Multimedia Medical Conferencing: Design and Experience in the BERMED Project. Proc. IEEE Multimedia Computing and Systems. Boston 1994

9. *Kleinholz, L., M. Ohly, J. Ricke, J. Thomsen, D. Emmel, R. Felix:* Multimedia Medical Conferencing: Standards, Products, ATM, ISDN, and other Technical Perspectives. Proc. CAR. Berlin 1995

10. *Kleinholz, L.:* Multimedia Documents. In: E. Fleck (Hrsg) Open Systems in Medicine. IOS Press Amsterdam 1994

11. *Kleinholz, L.:* Integrated Medical Application. In: E. Fleck (Hrsg) Open Systems in Medicine. IOS Press Amsterdam 1994

12. *Langlotz, C.P., O. Even-Shoshan, S. Seshadri , I. Brikman, S. Kishore, H. Kundel, J. Schwartz:* A methodology for the economic assessment of picture archiving and communication systems. J Digit Imaging 8(2) (1995) 95-102

13. *McConnell, J.:* Internetworking Computer Systems. Interconnecting Networks and Systems. Prentice-Hall Intern. Ed., Englewood Cliffs 1988

14. *Meyer-Ebrecht, D.*: Netzwerke für die Bildkommunikation. Gegenwärtiger Stand. Radiologe 34(6) (1994) 309-16

15. *Peters, P.:* PACS oder die schleichende Revolution. Radiologe 34(6) (1994) 285

16. *Ricke, J., L. Kleinholz, N. Hosten, H. Schedel, P. Gentz, K. H. Vöge, J. Kanzow, W. Dihlmann, H. M. Mayer, U. Weber, R. Loddenkemper, E. Fleck, R. Felix:* Technik und Ökonomie der weltweit ersten Röntgen-besprechung über das öffentliche Fernsprechnetz mittels Medizinischer Desktop-Konferenz und ISDN. Akt. Radiol. 5 (1995) 346-50

17. Ricke, J., L. Kleinholz, N. Hosten, M. Richter, E. Fleck, R. Felix: Computer Conferencing Support in Radiology–how economic viability will make it the Radiologist´s workspace of the next decade. Proc. IMAC. Oahu 1995

A World Wide Web Based Access to Clinical Patient Data

Jan Thomsen, Christoph Zielinski, Dirk Emmel, Bjöm Bergh, Lutz Kleinholz and Roland Felix
Strahlenklinik und Poliklinik, Virchow-Klinikum, Humdoldt University of Berlin, Berlin, Germany

I. INTRODUCTION

The Virchow-Klinikum is one of two large university hospitals belonging to the Humboldt University Berlin, rooting back to the late 18th century. It has about 1500 beds. Like in other hospitals growing over the decades, each department has ist own proprietary information system, mostly legacy systems without compliance to any standard. Since 1988 a lot of R&D projects have been undertaken to integrate all these different department information systems and to install an overall high quality digital information infrastructure at all levels. The main goal is to enable the communication of patient related clinical and administrative data and documents over the whole campus wherever they are needed. At the network level an ATM backbone has been established which is especially useful for the transfer of radiological images and for video conferencing. To communicate data between different systems an HL7 communication server has been set up, where departmental systems are currently going to be connected to. As the general platform for deployment of and access to the documents themselves the World Wide Web technology has been chosen. The advantages of this approach are currently leading to the development of distributed information systems based on WWW through all kind of organizations all over the world, as so called *intranets*. The following paper describes how this approach has been realized at the Virchow-Klinikum Berlin with a special focus on radiology data.

II. PRELIMINARY WORK

Since 1988 a number of R&D projects in cooperation with German Telekom subsidiary DeTeBerkom has been pursued. At the starting point, the Department of Radiology, and the German Heart Institute, located on the same campus, began to install a digital infrastructure enabling a mutual exchange of all kind of clinical documents, such as EKG, radiological images, angiogramms, and related patient data, such as reports, case histories, and findings. The ARUBA project [4] aimed at providing an ATM testbed for highspeed broadband communication specifically for radiological data, but as well for exchange of documents with the German Heart Center. As a result, the Virchow-Klinikum now has a 144MB/s backbone connecting the main departments and information sources. This holds in particular for the connection of the imaging modalities and the image archive with the campus network. Most front-end PCs at the different wards, however, are still connected only via ordinary Ethernet.

Based on that network structure, the BERMED project [2] developed and realized the concept of the *Meta Patient Record*, which is basically a multimedia document management system for a heterogenouos and distributed environment. The Meta Patient Record integrates all kind of patient related documents, from textual data to images, by keeping track of the location of the original documents. At the client side, a so called Integrated Medical Application (IMA) [7] has been developed, providing a simple, intuitive access to the documents through a unified interface, relating all existing documents belonging to a particular patient together on one screen, regardless where the sources really come from. The BERMED MPR concept is a client-server hypermedia application in the true sense, aimed at providing a complete virtual electronic patient record. The client application, however, was restricted to UNIX workstations only, which makes a deployment through the whole campus nearly impossible, a fact leading naturally to the approach of the KOMET project, described later.

To make the digital infrastructure complete, in cooperation with Hewlett-Packard some other projects have been set up, among which the following two are the most important:

- A Digital Image Archive [6] is currently going to be realized, aimed at replacing the paper-film archives by the end of 1997, equipped with DICOM interfaces to the modalities.
- An HL7 communication server is installed to allow for the communication of data between all the different departmental subsystems, which are now subsequently being connected to the HL7 server. The system is based on CAInet.

Besides this, the integration of imaging modalities and other document producing systems is driven forward. Images from conventional X-Ray devices are now being digitized automatically and easily available at arbitrary places through the KOMET system.

III. THE INFORMATION INFRASTRUCTURE IN THE RADIOLOGY DEPARTMENT

At the beginning of the BERMED project the situation in the radiology department was as follows:

- Images produced by the modalities have been stored only off-line on MODs
- Data belonging to the radiological examinations, such as administrative patient data, findings, reports etc. are stored in the local RIS (called RADOS). This data contains now references to the location of the according image sequences
- The RIS also contains no references to examinations which exist for the same patient at any other departments

During 1993 to 1994 within the BERMED project a lot of hard integration work has been performed resulting in a couple of components connecting the different isolated parts. Those new components and their role within the departmental information flow have been the following:

- An ACR/NEMA spooler which transfers the images from the sources to the network file system where they are stored within a RAID system
- Triggered by this event, a spooler agent fetches the according patient examination data from the RIS and passes it to the Meta Patient Record together with the on-line location of the images. The passed data contains only a minimal amount of information necessary to match image sequences and related examination data.
- The Meta Patient Record stores this data in a dedicated small database.

The outline of the resulting basic architecture and information flow is depicted in Fig. 1. The Spooler Agent and the Meta Patient Record are the two components developed originally by teh BERMED project. The communication is realized by means of named pipes, sockets, as well as simple file interfaces. The Meta Patient Record itself was a simple prototype database developed solely for this purpose. With this general architecture, all data and documents which make up the complete radiological electronic patient record are already available online. As a user interface to this data, a UNIX based Motif client has been developed, the so called Integrated Medical Application, working in the same way on the complete different set of medical multimedia documents within the Heart Institute.

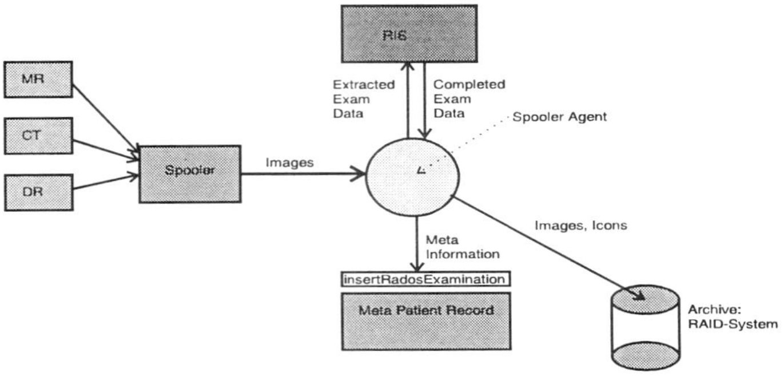

Fig.1 Information Architecture in the Radiological Department

IV. PUTTING IT ON THE WEB: THE KOMET PROJECT

The next steps of the integration process had to be taken in two directions: i) towards the integration of further subsystems, as the lab system, the pathology system, etc. at the server side, and ii) the deployment of clients throughout the whole campus, in order to make all patient documents accessible from every ward and every department. To achieve the latter, it was inevitabely to switch from the UNIX platform to the PC platform, since there are already a thousands of Pcs and dozens of Macs distributed over the whole campus. The KOMET project was established to provide a PC based client access. The primary decision was to choose the World Wide Web technology as the platform. The advantages of a WWW access are numerous, to name just four of them we consider as the most relevant to us: First, no extra client development is necessary since as clients can serve any available WWW browser, as long as it supports the HTML features utilized to structure the delivered pages. Second, it is platform independent, which is particular useful within a hospital environment as the Virchow-Kinik, where a thousands of Pcs and dozens of Macs are standing everywhere, but only very few workstations. Third, the development process is very short since the whole work is to convert the document contents into HTML format. Fourth, due to the extremely dynamic process within web technology one can always make use of the most advanced features without having to develop them by one self. In particular, this includes security features which are of course of principal importance within the hospital environment.

We started with realizing the access to the radiological image and exam data. Basically this was to provide a simple WWW database gateway to the Meta Patient Record database, since this is the central entry point to the patient information sources. The main tasks that had to be performed have been the following:

1. Installing, configuring, and administering a web server. In the beginning of the project we employed the CERN 3.0 server which had better security features compared to the NCSA server. Today, however, there are a lot of other servers commercially available which support advanced security features such as the Netscape CommerceServer or the Oracle Web Server. With both of them we are working now.
2. Designing the layout of the HTML documents, the overall document space, and the navigation possibilities between the different pages.
3. Developing the gateway to the Meta Patient Record. This has been done via relatively simple and small Perl-Scripts which connect to the MPR, build the HTML pages, read the user input from the forms, and build the next pages according to the user's selections.
4. Developing a Windows compliant helper application for the display of the ACR/NEMA images that are part of the examinations, i.e. a dedicated ACR/NEMA/DICOM viewer. This was necessary, since there was no viewer available which met the radiologists' requirements.

All HTML pages are dynamic ones, i.e. they do not exist as preformatted, static pages, but are rather built on request only based on the current user choices out of the actual data from the database. References to other documents from the pages, e.g. to the radiological images is simply done by hyperlinks. Image links are small GIF icons which show minimized view of the original ACR/NEMA images. By clicking on them the original images are transferred via HTTP and the viewer application is launched.

The access to the documents, of course, is restricted. Each user has to be registered and perform a login with password control. Additionally, to each physician a specific role is attached, which entitles him or her to have access only to his or her own patients. On the other hand, access is not restricted to users residing on the campus itself. Internal access from the campus intranet is possible as well as from anywhere else. From outside, the communication goes via ISDN lines which are connected to the hospital LAN via an ISDN router. A number of GPs in the Berlin area do have part of their patient charts administered by the Virchow-Klinikum, especially by the radiological department. They can make use of the archiving possibilities that the Virchow-Klinikum provides, for accessing the exams they let perform. Additionally, they can transmit own documents, e.g. scanned X-Ray images, and insert them into the patient chart at the Virchow-Klinikum. This is done via interactive HTML pages and HTTP transfer.

Additionally, KOMET integrates commercial PC video conferencing systems by supporting their standard interfaces. The current tendencies for DTC systems clearly point into the direction of utilizing the H.320 standard for PCs and videophones. For the sharing of applications and whiteboards the new standard T.120 will be employed. Physicians can communicate with each other by sharing e.g. the viewing application, or else by talking about a notebook which collects the relevant documents prepared by one of the partners. However, upto now it is not possible to use WWW access and videoconferencing in parallel, due to the fact that the videoconferencing system uses both available ISDN channnels. The most experience we do have is with the Intel ProShare system, which is comfortable but not sufficiently stable.

With both applications, i.e. the videoconferencing tools as well as the on-line WWW access to the patient documents together with the medical image viewer, the KOMET equipped PC is a low-cost, but sufficient to high quality solution which can be ubiquitously employed.

V. EXPERIENCES AND ONGOING ACTIVITIES

The solution as described above is now in operation within different wards. In particular, the anaesthesiologists profit a lot from this possibility. A few minutes after the X-Ray images being necessary to judge further treatment of patients under time pressure conditions have been shot and digitized they can be viewed at the local PC. For this, imaging quality is sufficient. If they want, they have all kind of other relevant information available with a few mouse clicks. Most of the physicians, internally as well as externally, are highly content with this solution. Since most of them are already familiar with World Wide Web, Netscape browser and the like, they can use the system immediately, without having to learn something new.

Performance is a critical issue, in particular with the transmission of digitized conventional X-Ray images which can have upto 8 MB, but most physicians accept this. Another critical point are the physicians' expectations concerning the layout of the document pages. If they have specific needs or wishes, we sometimes cannot fulfill them due the current limitations of HTML; however, with future HTML versions, Java and the like things will improve.

As a result from the developer's point of view, the WWW intranet/internet solution based on the digital hospital infrastructure offers a simple way for providing online access to all kinds of patient data, being truly multimedial in nature, and from almost every PC, Mac, or workstation having network access within the hospital or ISDN connection. Solutions can be developed very rapidly in close cooperation with the users, which goes both for page layout as well as the functionality with forms, buttons, icons, etc.

Our current activities concentrate on a redesign of the Meta Patient Record, on base of an Oracle RDBMS, especially for Windows NT and Sun Solaris 2.x. For the Web-DB gateway we are now switching from writing our own Perl CGI programs to employing the Oracle WebServer option which provides a very easy and secure interaction between WWW client, Web server and the database, as well as a rapid application prototyping. As a result, we will get a scalable and commercially available product, called HyperMed, which will not only have a WWW interface, but as well ODBC, SQL, DICOM, and HL7 interfaces.

REFERENCES

1. Felix R, Kleinholz L, Ohly M et al. State of the Art in Telemedicine - The Berlin Experience. *J. Europ. Radiol.* (1993); **3**: 295-303
2. Fleck E (ed.), *Open Systems in Medicine*, IOS Press Amsterdam, (1994)
3. Kleinholz L, Ohly M, Ricke J et al. Multimedia Medical Conferencing: Standards, Products, ATM, ISDN, and other Technical Perspectives. Berlin: *Proc. CAR*, (1995)
4. Kleinholz L, Ohly M, Steffens J, Fleck E, Mahr B, Felix R Broadband Telemedicine Applications: Experiences and Results of the ARUBA Project. *Proc. EUROOPT - European Symposium on Advanced Networks and Services*, Amsterdam March (1995)
5. Ohly M, Kleinholz L, Oswald H, Buggermann B, Felix R, Fleck E Open Digital Image Archives: Traffic for the Hospital ATM Infobahn. *Proc. CAR*, (1995)
6. Kleinholz L, Integrated Medical Application. In: Fleck E, ed. *Open Systems in Medicine*. Amsterdam: IOS Press (1994)

Telemedicine at the Special Olympic World Games

Henry A. Swett, M.D., Gary D. Leavitt, M.D., Vladimir Neklesa, M.D., Gregory Weltin, M.D., Morton Glickman, M.D., Lindsey Holaday, Peter Joki, M.D. and Philip Brewer, M.D.
Yale University School of Medicine, Department of Diagnostic Radiology, New Haven, Connecticut

Objective: The purpose of this study was to assess the effect of the use of telemedicine (both teleradiology and teleconferencing) to provide radiological support for a major international sporting event.

Materials and Methods: 145 radiological studies were digitized and transmitted to Yale-New Haven Hospital (YNHH). Video conferencing was implemented using 44 Mhz uncompressed video. Two radiologists interpreted all the digitized studies (1048 * 1048 * 12 bit images) and 126 of the original studies. Each reader was asked to evaluate for fracture, soft tissue swelling, old injury or other pathology. The concordance between the interpretation of the original and digitized images was evaluated. In addition, video teleconferencing between the central medical facility at the Special Olympics and the Emergency Radiology department at YNHH was available.

Results: In 126 studies, both the original films and digitized images were available for interpretation. Of these, 120 were musculoskeletal studies. For Reader 1 there was disagreement between the interpretation of the plain radiographs and digitized images in 0.8% of cases concerning the diagnosis of fracture and disagreement in 5.8% of cases concerning the diagnosis of soft tissue. For Reader 2 there was disagreement in 2.5% and 5.0% of cases concerning fracture and soft tissue swelling respectively.

Conclusion: Video teleconferencing was effectively used to facilitate communication between on-site clinicians and consultant radiologists. There was greater disagreement in the diagnosis of soft tissue swelling than fracture. This suggests that issues involving contrast may be more problematic than that of resolution. Further analysis of the data is required to determine if the discrepancies are due to reader performance or to inherent problems in digitization.

Introduction

Telemedicine encompasses a wide variety of technologies ranging from telephone consultation to teleradiology and video teleconferencing. Both teleradiology and video teleconferencing were used to provide radiological support for medical care provided for the Special Olympic World Games held in New Haven, Connecticut July 1- 9, 1995.

The Special Olympic World Games were a major international sporting event with 7200 athletes and 3000 coaches and trainers. Visiting dignitaries included President Clinton and Vice President Gore. An estimated 500,000 visitors watched events which were held at various sites in the New Haven area.

Providing medical care to the athletes, coaches and visitors was a formidable task. Residential medical stations were set up at the seven sites where athletes were housed. There were medical field stations present at all competitions. Injuries that could not be treated on site, but were not felt to require transfer to the YNHH Emergency Department were transferred to a central medical facility.

The central medical facility was comprised of an eight bed treatment area staffed with 2 physicians and 4 registered nurses. Telemedicine (teleradiology and teleconferencing) was used to provide radiological consultative services to physicians on site at the central treatment facility.

A variety of methods for transmitting digitized images have been reported. Blaine et al. used narrow-band integrated digital network and data compression [1]. Goldberg et al. used voice grade telephone lines and compressed images [2]. We used a dedicated T1 line to transmit images, similar to that described by DeCorato et al.[3].

Various degrees of resolution and contrast were provided at digital workstations for digital image interpretation. Goldberg et. al. used a 2560 * 2048 pixel display [4]. Nani used 1024 * 1024 resolution with 256 gray scale [5]. Stewart et al. used up to 4000 * 4000 pixel system [6].

Videoconferencing has been implemented with various technologies for a multitude of applications. Applications included consultation of specialists by general practitioners and in conjunction with telepathology and teleradiology [2,7,8,9].

The present study was performed to demonstrate the effectiveness of telemedicine in providing radiological consultation during a major public sporting event.

Materials and Methods

The telemedicine support of the Special Olympics consisted of three major components: on site x-ray equipment, teleradiology and videoconferencing.

On site x-ray equipment

On site radiological equipment included a portable x-ray machine (Phillips Medical System, Shelton CT.), an automatic film processor and a portable fluoroscope.

Teleradiology

The teleradiology system was comprised of a film digitizer, dedicated telephone lines and diagnostic workstations. A Lumisys 50 digitizer (Lumisys, Sunnyvale, CA) was coupled with a Siteview workstation (Phillips Medical Systems, Shelton, CT) to provide 1024 x 1024 X 12 bit resolution.

A dedicated T1 line was used to transmit the images to the radiology department. Transmission times averaged 20 - 30 seconds.

Videoconferencing

Two way video equipment was provided . No video codec was used. The system provided full motion 44 MHz uncompressed video. A video console was present at the central medical facility and at the Emergency Radiology reading room at YNHH.

Interpretation

Two radiologists interpreted both the original and digitized images. Both readers interpreted all films. Reader one was a third year radiology resident and Reader two was an attending radiologist. The digitized images were read first by both readers. The readers had manual control of window and level settings. The original films were then read at a later date and in a different order from the digitized images. No clinical history was provided. A simple questionnaire was completed for each case at both readings. The questionnaire provided for assessment of image quality and a number of possible findings, including fracture and soft tissue swelling. Unlimited time was allowed for image interpretation. At least two projections were provided and the same projections were provided for both digitized and original images.

Results

Teleconferencing

The telemedicine system was well received by the physicians stationed at the central medical facility at the Special Olympics and the consultant radiologists. No statistics were kept on the number of consultations via the video link, but positive findings were typically discussed. The video link was also used to discuss cases that did not involve transmitted images from the central facility. One example involved a patient who was transferred to the central medical facility with complaints of dizziness. The on site physician discussed the case with the Emergency physician and the Radiologist at YNHH via the video link to expedite proper imaging and treatment. The patient was then transferred to the YNHH Emergency Department for CT of the head and further management.

Teleradiology

The original radiographs and the transmitted digital images were evaluated for 126 studies. Each study was comprised of at least one image. Of the 126 studies, 120 were musculoskeletal studies with the following distribution: knee (n=22), hand, wrist or digit (n=27), ankle (n=26), tibia and fibula (n=7), nasal bones (n=2), pelvis (n=6), shoulder (n=6), elbow (n=4), forearm (n=4), acromioclavicular joints (n=2), ribs (n=2), humerus (n=1), femur (n=1) and lumbosacral spine (n=1). Five studies were chest x-rays and one was an abdominal film.

The musculoskeletal studies were analyzed to determine intra-observer disagreement between the digitized images and the original radiographs for the diagnoses of fracture and soft tissue swelling. Tables one and two show the results for diagnoses of fracture and soft tissue swelling. Positive findings were categorized as having been diagnosed in both the original and digitized studies, the digitized study only or the original study only. If a finding was found in either the digitized study or the original study, but not both, then there was disagreement between the two studies. The total number of disagreements divided by the number of studies (n=120) is the disagreement rate. The disagreement rate for fractures is 0.83% for Reader 1 and 2.5% for Reader 2. For soft tissue swelling the disagreement rate is 5.8% for reader 1 and 5.% for Reader 2.

	Reader 1	Reader 2
Both Digital and Original Images	4	4
Digital Images Only	0	2
Original Images Only	1	1

Table 1. Diagnosis of fracture using original and digitized studies.

	Reader 1	Reader 2
Both Digital and Original Images	6	4
Digital Images Only	0	6
Original Images Only	7	0

Table 2 Diagnosis of soft tissue swelling using original and digitized images.

Discussion

Telemedicine comprising video teleconferencing and teleradiology was used to provide radiological support during the 1995 Special Olympic World Games. The teleconferencing provided a convenient mode of communication between on site clinicians and referring physicians.

In assessing the utility of the teleradiology, the accuracy of the digitized images must be considered. Different groups have reported varying results concerning the accuracy of digitized images for diagnoses. Scott et al. found a system with 1,280 * 1,024 resolution inadequate for diagnosing subtle fractures [10]. Yoshino et al. also found a significant discrepancy using a high resolution system for fracture detection but attributed the discrepancies to issues involving contrast [11]. Wilson et al. found that the resolution of digitized images viewed on a 1,200 line monitor was not sufficient for diagnosing fractures [12]. Conversely DeCorato et al. found digitized images were used both reliably and efficiently for off-hours interpretation in the emergency department. The majority of disagreements between plain radiographs and digitized images were due to film reader error and only 0.4% due to an inadequate digital image. This is a similar finding to that of Goldberg et al. who also found that discrepancies between plain radiographs and digitized images were more associated with observer performance [4].

In a preliminary analysis of our data we found intra-observer disagreement for fractures of 0.83% and 2.5% for Reader 1 and Reader 2 respectively. Diagnoses of soft tissue swelling had an intra-observer disagreement of 5.8% and 5.0% for Reader 1 and Reader 2 respectively. The rate of disagreement concerning soft tissue swelling may suggest that issues of contrast are actually more problematic than issues concerning resolution. Further analysis is necessary to determine whether the discrepancies were due to observer performance and proper use of the digital workstations or inherent problems in digitization.

1. Blaine, G.J., *et al.*, *Teleradiology via narrow-band integrated services digital network (N-ISDN) and Joint Photographic Experts Group (JPEG) image compression.* J Digit Imaging, 1992. **5**(3): p. 156-60.

2. Goldberg, M.A., *et al.*, *Making global telemedicine practical and affordable: demonstrations from the Middle East.* Ajr Am J Roentgenol, 1994. **163**(6): p. 1495-500.

3. DeCorato, D.R., N.J. Kagetsu, and R.C. Ablow, *Off-hours interpretation of radiologic images of patients admitted to the emergency department: efficacy of teleradiology.* Ajr Am J Roentgenol, 1995. **165**(5): p. 1293-6.

4. Goldberg, M.A., *et al.*, *New high-resolution teleradiology system: prospective study of diagnostic accuracy in 685 transmitted clinical cases.* Radiology, 1993. **186**(2): p. 429-34.

5. Nani, M.T., *et al.*, *[Teleradiography for diagnosis in emergency care. A clinical experience]. [Italian].* Radiol Med (Torino), 1992. **84**(4): p. 451-4.

6. Stewart, B.K., S.3. Dwyer, and H. Kangarloo, *Design of a high-speed, high-resolution teleradiology network.* J Digit Imaging, 1992. **5**(3): p. 144-55.

7. Brismar, B., *[Hospital without borders--visions of telemedicine]. [Swedish].* Nord Med, 1995. **110**(8-9): p. 209-10.

8. Mun, S.K., *et al.*, *Teleradiology/telepathology requirements and implementation. [Review].* J Med Syst, 1995. **19**(2): p. 153-64.

9. Swett, H.A., *et al.*, *Telemedicine: delivering medical expertise across the state and around the world.* Conn Med, 1995. **59**(10): p. 593-602.

10. Scott, W.J., *et al.*, *Subtle orthopedic fractures: teleradiology workstation versus film interpretation.* Radiology, 1993. **187**(3): p. 811-5.

11. Yoshino, M.T., *et al.*, *Diagnostic performance of teleradiology in cervical spine fracture detection.* Invest Radiol, 1992. **27**(1): p. 55-9.

12. Wilson, A.J. and J.C. Hodge, *Digitized radiographs in skeletal trauma: a performance comparison between a digital workstation and the original film images.* Radiology, 1995. **196**(2): p. 565-8.

International Telemedicine: 18 Months Experience

Mark A. Goldberg, M.D., Hassan S. Sharif, M.D. and
Ricky J. Richardson, M.D.
American Telemedicine International, Cambridge, Massachusetts and
WellCare Holdings, N.V., Netherlands
Daniel I. Rosenthal, M.D., Giles W. Boland, M.D.,
Maria Lopez-Bresnahan, M.D. and Joseph C. Kvedar, M.D.
Massachusetts General Hospital, Boston, Massachusetts
Michael T. Modic, M.D.
Cleveland Clinic Foundation, Cleveland, Ohio

Introduction

The purpose of this abstract is to review 18 months of operational experience with an international telemedicine network connecting U.S. medical centers to sites in the Middle East including Saudi Arabia, Jordan, and Lebanon. The network currently includes Massachusetts General Hospital (MGH) and the Cleveland Clinic Foundation (CCF) as providers. There are currently five transmission sites operational in the Middle East. Clients include patients, physicians, hospitals, and insurance companies in the various countries.

Our initial endeavor focused on the delivery of teleradiology services to the Middle East. However, early feedback from patients and physicians indicated that while access to high quality, subspecialized radiologic expertise was appealing, it was insufficient. In addition, patients and physicians wanted access to medical and surgical subspecialists who could provide input into the further diagnosis and management of disease processes. In many instances, patients and physicians were interested in learning whether there were new treatment options available in the United States for a known condition. In other cases, the diagnosis or treatment plan was uncertain and a second opinion was desired. In order to address this need we developed a service referred to as patient management consultations (PMC's).

One of the principal implementation challenges for this service related to limitations in the readily accessible telecommunications infrastructure which consisted of voice grade phone lines. The available infrastructure made real-time interactive video conferencing impractical. For high-resolution image transmission, a combination of inverse multiplexing and wavelet-based image compression has been used. Other challenges have included time differences (8 hour difference from EST), staggered work weeks (different weekends and holidays observed), and obtaining support from local physicians and decision makers.

Materials and Methods

Services included teleradiology (for primary interpretations or second opinions) and patient management consultations. For teleradiology, images are acquired using a film digitizer station (American Telemedicine International; Cambridge, MA) at a resolution of 1664 x 2020. The digitizer station integrates a Lumisys 150

(Sunnyvale, CA) laser scanner with a Macintosh PowerPC 610 (Apple Computer, Cupertino, CA) to capture history and demographic information. Following acquisition, the demographic information is stored in an associated database (Sybase, Emeryville, CA) on a Sun SparcStation 10 (Sun Microsystems, Mountain View, CA). Prior to transmission, images are compressed using a wavelet-based algorithm with target compression ratios of 20 : 1 for digitized radiographs and 10 : 1 for CT/MR. Inverse multiplexing is used to combine phone lines for increased throughput at high volume sites. Because of the frequency of dropped lines and the size of the data files being sent, the telecommunications equipment is configured with error detection and correction technology that allows an interrupted transmission to pick up at the point of failure rather than restarting from the beginning of the file.

Medical histories, laboratory results, and other components of the medical record (e.g., EKG, EEG, etc.) are transmitted by fax to support patient management consultations. Pathology material is sent by courier pending implementation of telepathology. All case material, including medical information and images, is routed via American Telemedicine International (ATI) in Cambridge, MA. ATI takes responsibility for managing the flow of information over the network and distributing case material to the participating institutions. ATI has remote dial-up support capabilities to assist users, provide software upgrades, and diagnose problems if technical difficulties arise. Twenty-four hour support is provided 365 days per year.

At the provider sites, radiologic images are displayed on high-resolution 1792 x 2252 diagnostic workstations (American Telemedicine International, Cambridge, MA). Case material is triaged to an appropriate specialist at one of the provider institutions. For PMC's, the consultant is informed of any associated teleradiology or pathology material that has been sent. After review of the available information, the consultant provides a formal note that recapitulates the available information, makes recommendations for further treatment or management, and, when necessary, requests that additional information be obtained. Reports from radiologists, pathologists, and consultants are transmitted back to ATI by fax or E-mail, and then forwarded to the requesting site in the Middle East.

Results

Over 1,350 teleradiology and 350 patient management consultations have been performed. For image transmission, the mean compression ratio was 22.1 and transmission times averaged 3.1 min using two phone lines at a cost of approximately $7.00 per image. The average radiologic study consisted of 4.6 images (including digitized, laser-printed CT and MR films). For teleradiology, the average turn-around time was 28 hours. The image transmission system has been extremely robust with an up-time of > 98% including all sites in the U.S. and the Middle East.

For PMC's, the mean turn-around time was four days (median 3 days). Orthopedics, neurology, and neurosurgery account for nearly 50% of all PMC's, with a wide variety of other specialties represented in smaller numbers (Figure 1). Approximately, one-fifth of patients expressed an expectation that they would travel abroad for additional medical care prior to PMC's, but only 4% actually traveled overseas after receiving a telemedicine consultation. In 10-15% of cases, the consultant required additional information before a final consultation report could be rendered. The nature of the additional information requested ranged from more detail concerning medical history or physical findings to additional laboratory testing, imaging studies, or biopsies. Patient management consultations were accompanied by radiology in 80% of cases and by pathology material in 5-10% of cases.

At the outset, participating physicians expressed concern that the disease processes may be obscure or unfamiliar to U.S. physicians. This has not proven to be the case, with the vast majority of disease processes being common to Western medical practice.

International Patient Management: Distribution by Specialty

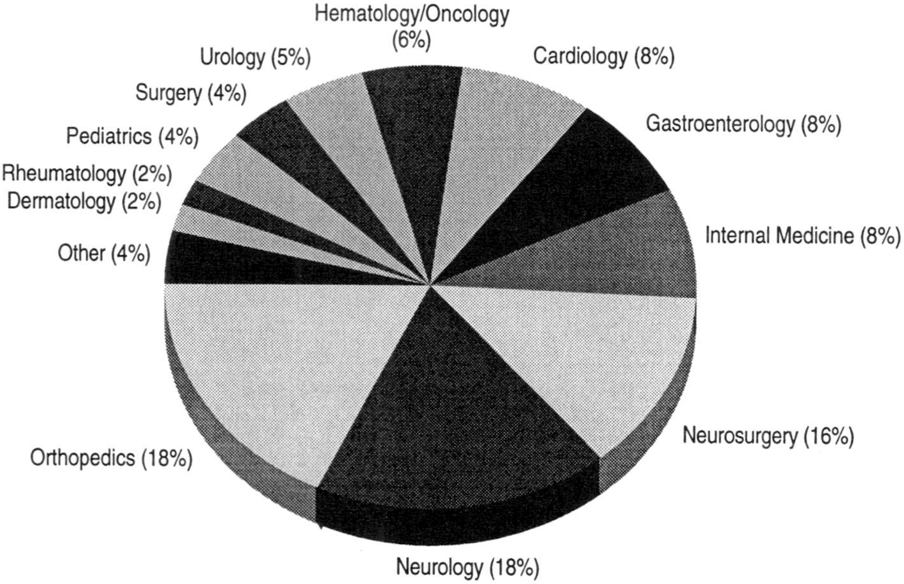

Figure 1. Pie chart shows distribution of patient management consultations by specialty. Neurology, neurosurgery, and orthopedics account for approximately 50% of cases.

Discussion

Without the use of image data compression, transmission of a single digitized radiograph would take in excess of one hour using a voice grade phone line. Lossless compression can be used, but this technology is limited to achieving compression ratios in the range of 1.5 : 1 to 3 : 1 [1]. Compression ratios in the range of 10 : 1 are required to have a substantial practical and economic impact on teleradiology systems. Combining wavelet-based compression at ratios up to 20 : 1 and inverse multiplexing (to combine two phone lines) we have achieved transmission times of approximately 3 minutes per image. While the concept of lossy compression may not be immediately embraced, there is substantial evidence that lossy compression algorithms can be implemented without sacrificing diagnostic image content [2-6]. Our experience to date includes the successful transmission of over 5000 compressed images from the Middle East.

Teleradiology is, by far, the most mature of telemedicine subspecialties, whereas telepathology is in a relatively earlier stage of development. Considerable debate continues over the optimal approach to delivering telepathology services with the two main alternatives being store and forward of selected static images versus real-time video microscopy. With video microscopy, the consultant is able to manipulate a remotely located microscope via robotics [7, 8]. Whatever the ultimate solution, it seems likely that some percentage of material will still need to be sent physically to allow special stains or other types of specialized analysis. Pathology services are an indispensable component of comprehensive patient management consultations.

The telemedicine project discussed in this abstract differs considerably from most of the pilot and demonstration projects in the United States [9]. Many projects in the U.S. have relied heavily on subsidies from federal, state, and local agencies as well as from industry (particularly the telecommunications industry). Several of the these projects have implemented high-end, bandwidth-intensive applications, only later attempting to determine if these systems deliver cost-effective health care. Many projects have been technology driven, rather than customized to user needs. As a self-sustaining undertaking, our enterprise has required the use of practical and cost-effective technologies. While we recognize the value of interactive video conferencing in some forms of telemedicine, we have found that store and forward technologies can be used to satisfactorily address a broad array of medical problems. We have been surprised that only a small number of consultations result in follow-up telephone conversations between the referring physician and the consultant (< 5%). It is anticipated, however, that the role of video conferencing in our system will expand with further decreases in the cost of the technology and of bandwidth.

While the cost-benefits of this program are not yet quantified, it is clear that the ability to minimize costly transfer of patients to overseas medical institutions is a substantial economic benefit.

Conclusion

Telemedicine services can be delivered affordably over existing telecommunications infrastructures using a store and forward approach. Significant added value has been delivered by the patient management consultation service. We are in the process of aggressively expanding the geographic scope of the network and the variety of media that can be transmitted.

References

1. Gillespy TI, Rowberg AG. Displaying radiologic images on personal computers: Images storage and compression — part 1. J Digit Imaging 1993; 6:197-204.

2. MacMahon H, Doi K, Sanada S, et al. Data compression: effect on diagnostic accuracy in digital chest radiography. Radiology 1991; 178:175-179.

3. Sayre JW, Ho BKT, Boechat MI, Hall TR, Huang HK. Subperiosteal resorption: effect of full-frame image compression of hand radiographs on diagnostic accuracy. Radiology 1992; 185:599-603.

4. Aberle DR, Gleeson F, Sayre JW, et al. The effect of irreversible image compression on diagnostic accuracy in thoracic imaging. Invest Radiol 1993; 28:398-403.

5. Goldberg MA, Pivovarov M, Mayo-Smith WW, et al. Application of wavelet compression to digitized radiographs. AJR 1994; 163:463-468.

6. Cosman PC, Davidson HC, Bergin CJ, et al. Thoracic CT images: effect of lossy image compression on diagnostic accuracy. Radiology 1994; 190:517-524.

7. Black-Schaffer S, Flotte TJ. Current issues in telepathology. Telemedicine Journal 1995; 1:95-106.

8. Weinstein RS. Static image telepathology in perspective. Hum Pathol 1996; 27:99-101.

9. Perednia DA, Allen A. Telemedicine technology and clinical applications. JAMA 1995; 273:483-488.

SESSION 9

PACS Integration

Co-Chairs:

Atsuko Heshiki
John B. Strauss

Performance Improvements in PACS

Janice C. Honeyman, Meryll M. Frost, Walter Huda and Edward V. Staab
Department of Radiology, University of Florida, Gainesville, Florida

1. Introduction

Early Picture Archiving and Communication Systems (PACS) achieved their goals of storing digital images and making them available to requesting sites, however, the performance and functionality of many systems have not met the expectations of the users. Most Radiologists do not have time to move new and comparison studies to the workstation for review or diagnosis and would prefer automatically study routing. When a Radiologist does need to move a study to a workstation from an archive, the study should be easy to find with rapid transfer. Both automatic routing and archive queries require that accurate and complete representation of patient and study information be present in the database, which is difficult to implement with manual data entry. The performance of an archive retrieve command can be compromised by inefficient software, inadequate numbers of read devices, and the use of off-line storage methods. In order to enhance the current systems to meet the minimum levels of acceptability, rapid retrievals from archives must be achieved, a Radiology Information System (RIS) interface must be added, automatic routing of studies must be implemented, and a staged, distributed archive architecture must be developed. [1,2]

The expanding PACS installations at the University of Florida are being enhanced to support the functionality described above. A large distributed archive is in the final stages of development which will optimize the performance of retrievals. The combination of magnetic intermediate storage logically networked to the workstations most likely to request studies and long term tape storage is designed to allow fast access to approximately 85% of the studies with virtually unlimited long term storage.

An investigational RIS interface allows direct, automatic download of patient demographics and study information into the database on a Kodak Computed Radiography Unit at the time a study is ordered. The same interface is used to verify the patient information as studies are moved from Dicomit Ultrasound PACS units to the archives, workstations, and printers. Information provided in the interface directs the routing of images to the correct workstation and archives and provides complete and correct patient and study information.

This paper describes the new archive architecture and information infrastructure designed to improve PACS performance at the University of Florida.

2. Archive

Utilizing the acquisition and retrieval data accumulated over several years, a new strategy for archiving has been developed. Our studies indicate that approximately 85% of all retrievals occur within the first 4 to 6 months from the date of the previous study. Three medium term magnetic disk archives are being added to store studies for up to six months in an effort to improve performance for up to 85% of retrievals. The medium term archives are logically linked to specific reading areas, initially abdominal (with ultrasound), chest (with pediatric), and neuroradiology (with musculoskeletal radiology). Additional medium term archives will be added as needed. The parallel nature of this design allows rapid study access for each of the organ based areas in our department.

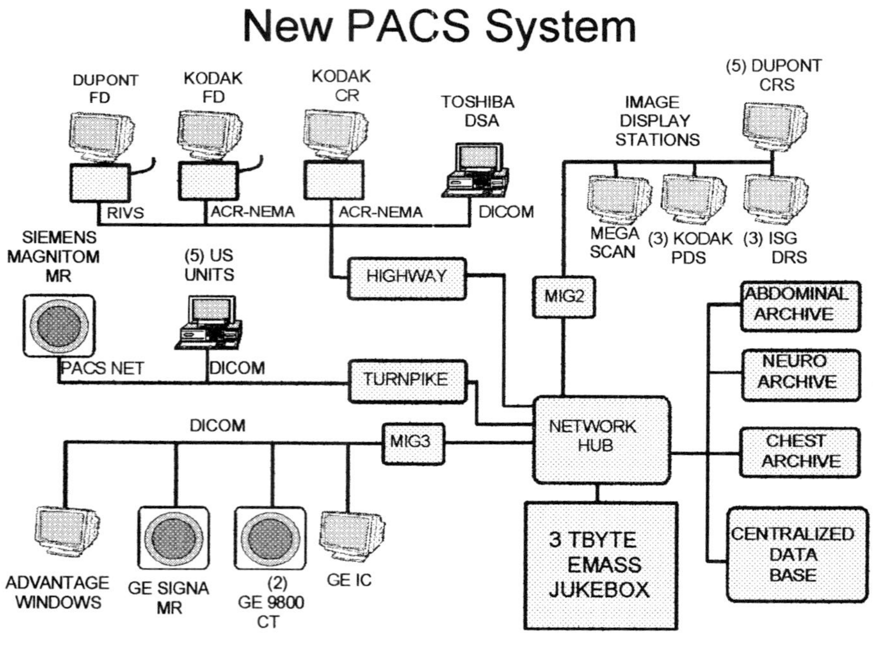

Figure 1: New Archive Architecture at the University of Florida

The capacity of each medium term archive is 81 Gbytes for medium term storage and 9 Gbytes for short term storage. The short term storage is mirrored to guarantee secure storage until studies are moved to both the medium term and long term archives. Mirrored storage is a less expensive alternative to a Redundant Array of Inexpensive Drives (RAID). Studies are stored with a 2:1 non-destructive compression algorithm. The single long term tape archive from EMASS has an initial capacity of 3 TeraBytes uncompressed (6 TeraBytes compressed with non-destructive compression) The jukebox has to total capacity of uncompressed 14 TeraBytes for future expansion. The hardware consists of an ABBA/E jukebox with two hexatower storage compartments, 6 Digital Linear Tape (DLT) tape drives, a 10 Gigabyte RAID drive for rapid acquisition and retrieval staging, and a Silicon Graphics CHALLENGE DM processor with 2 CPUs. This system was selected because the robotics can handle almost any storage media available now or in the future. The initial selection of DLT can easily be upgraded to include VHS, D2, or optical media. [3,4]

The central database is implemented on an Oracle Relation Database Management System (RDBMS). A query to the database directs a retrieval from one of the distributed archives automatically and invisibly to the user.

3. RIS

Routing and prefetching algorithms require accurate and complete study information which is frequently not available when manual data entry is employed. An RIS interface is crucial to improving the operation of a PACS. [5,6]

The RIS used by Shands Hospital and the University of Florida was developed by Community Health Computing and has been in place for more than six years. Although a Health Layer Seven (HL7) interface was implemented to allow communication between the RIS and the Hospital Information System, there was no provision for communications with PACS. The RIS system was extensively customized by Shands Information Services personnel and was serviced almost solely on-site. The system had to be further customized to meet the needs of this project by on-site programmers.

In order to meet our requirements, an event driven system was needed that transmitted information to PACS when studies were ordered. On analysis of the RIS, it was found that placing an order triggered the printing of a request form in the Radiology Department. An additional action was implemented that sent a packet of information to a PACS RIS-server when an order was placed.

The PACS RIS-server running on a Sun Sparcstation, has both a single threaded RS-232 connection to the RIS and a socket based ethernet interface to PACS clients. There are two modes of operation of the system, the automatic application described above and a real-time application. In the real-time application, client computers with bar code readers submit a query to the RIS-server based on the accession number. The parent process mallocs shared memory space for the response and forks a child process to handle the RS-232 request. When a response is returned, the child stores the data in the shared memory space and informs the parent that it is complete. Both the real time and the automatic operation store the packets for use of PACS processes in a relational database. [7,8]

All RIS packets are stored in MiniSQL (mSQL, copyright, 1993 - 1995 David J. Hughes, developed as part of the Minerva Network Management Environment), a lightweight database engine suitable for applications requiring short term database storage with non-complex query requirements. Data remain in the database for approximately one week after which they are automatically purged as space is needed. The data structure allows each patient to have multiple orders with the medical record number acting as the key between the two and used as the join field. The accession number is a unique number that identifies the study and patient in the RIS and which is frequently referred to as the accession number. A Unix time stamp is attached to each record in the database to allow oldest record first deletions. As orders are inserted into the database, if the medical record number matches an existing patient, the time stamp attached to the patient information is updated to match the new order. Otherwise, the new patient record is inserted.

The first clinical application for the RIS / PACS interface is in the Ultrasound division. Ultrasound PACS has been implemented using the Dicomit PACS system. Dicomit uses a frame grabber on each Ultrasound unit with optical character recognition to identify the patient name and medical record number. Images are transferred to the PACS autorouter using DICOM 3.0 protocols where they are sent to an archive, a Kodak PDS workstation, a Kodak XLP laser camera, and/or a Werkswriter paper printer (Softwerks, Inc., Gainesville, Fl). Ultrasound studies are either interpreted in the adult or pediatric ultrasound areas. Pediatric radiologists prefer to have either paper or film hard copy printed because of the distance between the ultrasound area and the pediatric reading room. When the radiologist is in the ultrasound area, he or she would have to walk to the other end of the department to view the study on the workstation so hard copy is frequently used during the performance of the study with soft copy used for diagnostic interpretation.

In the original implementation, studies sent to the autorouter were matched by medical record number and name to entries in the mSQL database. Errors introduced by optical character recognition and human data entry caused errors in routing. To improve matching the study to the database, a barcode reader has been attached to the Dicomit units. The accession number from the request form is barcoded into the system and added to the DICOM header in group x10, element x1000 - Other Patient Ids, in index 2 (out of the possible 1 - 10). The addition of this field to the study allows 100% match of image data and RIS information for Ultrasound.

Although the addition of the barcode reader to the ultrasound PACS and the RIS / PACS interface assures accurate information for storage and routing of studies it does not solve the efficiency problems associated with requiring technologists to manually enter data. In a parallel effort, the RIS packets were sent to an experimental interface developed by Kodak Health Imaging Systems as a potential information server to the Kodak CR Quality Control Workstation (QCW) where CR images can be displayed and routed after the plate has been read.

In addition to the RIS interface storing information in the mSQL database, packets for studies that could be performed using CR were identified by the procedure description code and were routed to the Kodak's information interface to the QCW running on a PACS routing workstation. The RIS-server moved the appropriate study information to a process which converted the packets to match the requirements of the Kodak interface and Kodak processes moved the information to the QCW.

When a technologist finished a CR study, he or she barcoded the patient's medical record number and the full patient demographics were selected to be attached to the image associated with a CR plate. This eliminated a tedious data entry task for the technologist and increased technologist's efficiency.

Results - RIS / US PACS interface

In the first five months of operation, the Ultrasound PACS acquired and stored over 3100 studies. When a study could not be matched to an mSQL entry, a message was sent to an E-mail address with the details of the problem. Greater than 95% of all studies were matched to an entry in the mSQL database.

Results - RIS / CR interface

Randomly selected radiology study request forms were collected over a four day period. The following information fields were checked against the information loaded on the QCW by the RIS-server: patient medical record number, patient name, date of birth, requesting physician name, and patient bed number. A total of 67 exams were inspected. Of these 59 were found correct in all fields checked. The other eight patients had had subsequent examinations ordered and the QCW had been updated. The flat file format of the database in the QCW allowed information from only one request form to be stored at any time and although the patient's name was correct, the location, study description, study accession number, and requesting physician could be incorrect if additional studies were requested before an earlier one was completed. In all cases the patient information (name, medical record number, date of birth) were correct. [9]

4. Summary and Conclusions

For the organ based paradigm used at the University of Florida, the distributed data model utilizing fast medium term archives and a single large long term archive provides efficient and rapid storage and retrieval of diagnostic medical images.

An RIS / PACS interface has been successfully integrated into two PACS applications at the University of Florida and will be expanded to work with other modalities and with greater functionality. The interface developed at the University of Florida was based on a custom design using a legacy RIS. The software was designed in modules so only the connection to the RIS will have to be changed when the new system is installed and an HL7 interface is available. The communication within the PACS networks and data storage in the mSQL database will not change, making the transition possible with a minimum of effort.

The RIS interface to the Kodak Health Imaging system's CR unit was experimental and is not a current product. The connection, however, as a proof - of - concept was successful and all manufacturers of image producing equipment should be encouraged to provide standard methods to interface with information systems to improve efficiency of use and data accuracy.

5. References

1. Wilson DL, Smith DV, Rice B. "Intelligent prefetch strategies for historical images in a large PACS",SPIE, Vol 2165, 1994.

2. Honeyman JC,Frost MM,Staab EV, Bidgood D. " Clinical and Research PACS Implementation and Evaluation",IMAC91, 1991.

3. Frost MM, Honeyman JC, Staab EV. " Image Archive Evolution at the University of Florida", IMAC95, (in press).

4. Frost MM, Honeyman JC, Staab EV. "PACS archive strategy utilizing a three-terabyte jukebox",*SPIE Medical Imaging,* 1996, (in press).

5. Reynolds RA, Strickland NH, Bruckner PM, Mayer R, Niggemann M. "Matching images from digital modalities to exams scheduled via RIS or PACS", *SPIE Medical Imaging*, 2435, 340 - 346, 1995.

6. He Y, Huang LJ, Valentino DJ, Wingate WK, Avizienis A. "Fault tolerance techniques to assure data integrity in high-volume PACS image archives", *SPIE Medical Imaging*, 2435, 378 - 386, 1995.

7. Honeyman JC, Frost MM, Staab EV. "On-Line Medical Record / RIS / PACS interface", *SPIE Medical Imaging*, 2165, 179 - 184, 1994

8. Honeyman JC, Frost MM, Moser R, Huda W, StaabEV. "RIS Requirements to Support a PACS Infrastructure", *SPIE Medical Imaging*, 1996 (in press).

9. Huda W, Honeyman JC, Rill L., "Technical Evaluation of the Kodak 400 CR system", *A Report to Kodak Health Imaging Systems*, pp. 1 - 33, July, 1995.

Cost Effectiveness of a Phased Approach to Implementation of a PACS Network in a Level One Trauma Center

Quentin Anderson, M.D. and Mary Shaw, B.S.
Medical Imaging Department, Hennepin County Medical Center,
Minneapolis, Minnesota

In a traditional film based system, the management and distribution of X-rays and reports is labor intensive and has varying degrees of effectiveness. In fact, we consistently failed in the areas that needed the information the most: the Emergency Department, the Intensive Care Units, and the Operating Rooms. Over the past ten years the support staff in the Department of Medical Imaging quadrupled (Figure 1). Despite these efforts 8% of our films were unavailable for review.

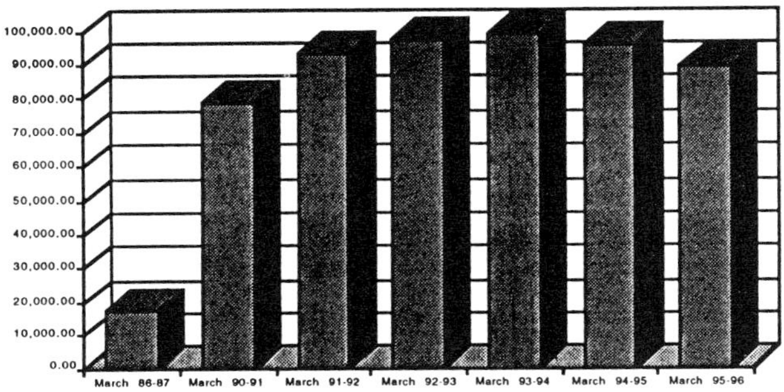

Paid Hours for Support Staff

Fig 1.

Converting to a digitally based system where images and information are available at any time, in any place for our clinicians was clearly the solution. However, to convert the entire department to a digital format would require a significant up front capital outlay. A modular approach, (budgeted expenses) would spread cost over time.

To decide the order of implementation, a financial analysis was performed to determine the cost of providing services in the areas that had the highest problems i.e. the Emergency Department, Intensive Care Units and the Operating Room. Our cost analysis included the current cost of film production (direct film, processing and archival costs), lost films, film retakes, unbilled studies and associated personnel costs to maintain the film based system.

Our digital PAC's system has been operational in the ICU's for the past 12 months and the results of our initial efforts have been rewarding. Exam retakes in the ICU's have been significantly reduced from 12% to 1.2%. The concurrent image capture distributions for the ICU studies has reduced the technologist travel time by 158 minutes a day (0.46 FTE). This has resulted in less staffing in the Emergency Department. This factor is reflected in (Figure 2).

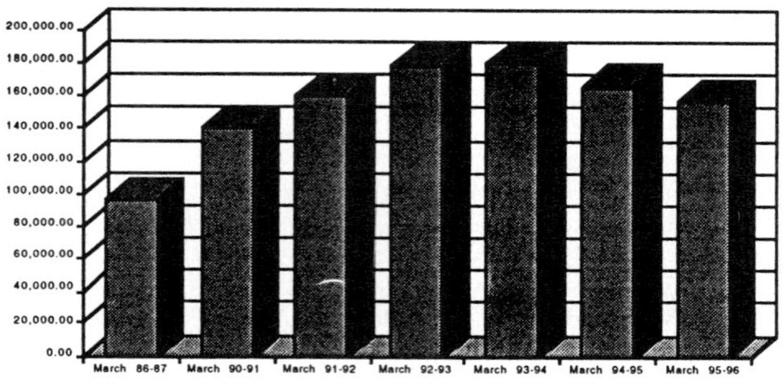

Paid Hours for Technical Staff

Fig 2

While our workload has remained the same, the number of paid hours has been steadily decreasing. Similar analysis of our daily log of incomplete exams, (films completed but not reported) shows the same trend. Figure 3 shows our incomplete exam studies did not change from 1992 until 1996 when we completed the digital conversion of the Intensive Care Units.

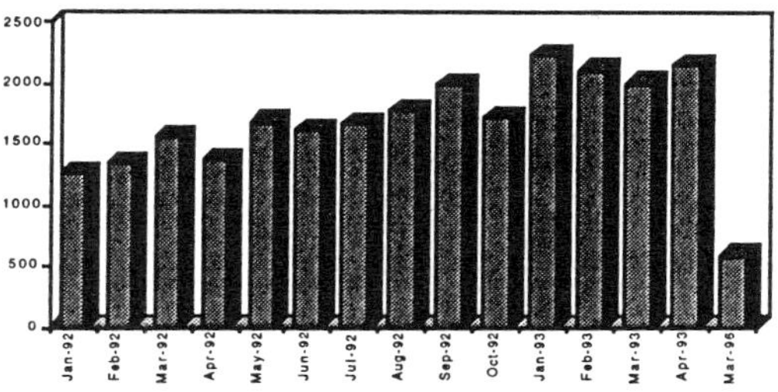

Incomplete Exams

Fig. 3

An analysis of the time spent traveling to and from the Medical Imaging Department by non-radiology physicians demonstrated a time savings. Prior to installation of the ICU digital PAC's system, the estimated daily travel time was approximately 90 minutes. This has essentially been eliminated which results in a 6-12 hour per FTE per week time saving. This time has been redirected to patient care rather than non-productive data gathering.

Film costs are steadily decreasing as film is eliminated. A significant decrease in this expense will occur with the conversion of the Emergency and Orthopedic Departments.

Our modular PAC's system was initially designed for high quality review monitors. In the next 30 days we will be adding low cost reference monitors for wider application and distribution. The high quality monitors can be used for diagnostic purposes and the low cost monitors which have excellent resolution meets the clinical need of a viewbox in the hallway.

We are also integrating our RIS report system into the PAC's Image Management System. This will allow us to place a short, typed text report with the soft copy image (object management). These two additions will allow us to distribute image and text at one work station, with low cost and improved data distribution.

The remaining key issue for a filmless department focuses on the film archive. This must be digitized. We are currently formulating our policies for digitizing the film archive such that the film base archive will be available on the digital PAC's network.

With these two applications, reconfiguration of high quality and low cost monitors plus film archiving we can rapidly progress with our modular conversion. We are planning for conversion to digital radiography in the Emergency Department, Operating Rooms and the Orthopedic Clinic within the next 120 days.

Converting film library systems to digital PAC's systems requires a unified modular approach. We have now designed our floor plan and procedures to implement digital imaging throughout the Department and satellite locations.

In closing, our business decision and proforma were based on resolving problems and cost analysis. We have resolved one of our three critical care network problems, the Intensive Care Unit. This initial conversion process gave us insight to identify and resolve issues and processes. We have documented favorable cost recovery with paid technical and support hours plus additional benefits of improved turnaround time of incomplete exams and reduction in non-radiology physician travel time.

We believe we made the correct decision.

ICU Display Station Impact and Utilization Studies

Katherine P. Andriole, M. Luigia Storto, Gordon Gamsu and Ronald L. Arenson

Laboratory for Radiological Informatics, Department of Radiology
University of California at San Francisco, San Francisco, California

ABSTRACT

Changes in health-care professional behaviors as a result of the introduction of a picture archiving and communication system (PACS) display station to an adult medical-surgical intensive care unit (ICU) are investigated via pre- and post-PACS workstation placement evaluations. ICU display station utilization and the impact on clinical operations are also examined. Parameters measured both pre- and post-PACS ICU display station placement include the number of films per patient day, the number of clinician reviews of a patient's images per day and the percentage of images on which the unit interacts with a radiologist. The elapsed times from the time of exposure to the time of: image review by the referring physician, radiologist-unit interaction and clinical action based on image information are also measured. Results of the pre-PACS display station placement found: the average number of films per patient day to be 1.30 ± 0.60, the average number of clinician reviews of a patient's images per day to be 2.18 ± 1.35 and the percentage of time which the ICU clinicians interact with a radiologist to be 27.4 %. Post-PACS measurements of the same parameters include: 1.09 ± 0.69 films per patient day, 2.00 ± 4.80 clinician reviews of images per day and 28.9% interaction with radiology. The average elapsed times from the time of exposure to the time of image review by the non-radiologist clinician measured 2 hours 32 minutes ± 1 hour 50 minutes pre-PACS and 1 hour 35 minutes ± 56 minutes post-PACS; the time to radiologist-unit interaction averaged 1 hour 42 minutes ± 2 hours 3 minutes pre-PACS and 1 hour 56 minutes ± 1 hour 23 minutes post-PACS; the average time to clinical action measured 3 hours 21 minutes ± 3 hours 24 minutes pre-PACS and 2 hours 6 minutes ± 1 hour 46 minutes. The results of this investigation suggest that the introduction of a PACS display station in the ICU may reduce the number of exams per patient day, decrease the elapsed time from the time of exposure to the time of image review by the unit clinician, and improve the time to clinical action. Note, however, that it does not appear to change the percentage of total images on which the unit interacts with a radiologist.

1. INTRODUCTION

Several groups, most notably the University of Pennsylvania and Duke University, have examined the effect of a digital imaging network on physician behavior in an intensive care unit (ICU), time comparison of ICUs with and without digital viewing systems and strategies for experimental design of ICU picture archiving and communication system (PACS) station technology evaluation studies.[1-9]

The purpose of this investigation is to measure, analyze and present objective data obtained during continuous clinical operation, documenting the direct results of placing a PACS display station in an adult Medical-Surgical ICU on: physician and radiologist behavior, the time to clinical action and the number of exams performed per patient day. These measures, along with display station utilization studies, may give further insight into ICU workstation design and potentially elucidate cost-effectiveness issues.

2. MATERIALS AND METHODS

All unit portable examinations at our institution are performed with computed radiography (CR). Primary diagnosis is done by reading CR hardcopy. Prior to placement of a PACS display station in the ICUs (pre-PACS), films are often duplicated for the purposes of unit review. The pre-PACS period spanned a two-week period prior to placement of the display station in the adult medical-surgical ICU. The post-PACS phase included two weeks after placement of a work station up in the intensive care unit, to which images of patients admitted to the ICU are sent. The post-PACS period was preceded by three months of extensive monitoring and testing of image delivery to the display station and work station reliability, as well as end-user display station training.

Parameters measured both prior to placement of a PACS display workstation in the ICU and after placement of the display station in the unit (post-PACS) are summarized in Table 1. They include the number of films per patient day, the number of clinician reviews of a patient's images per day and the percentage of images on which the unit interacts with a radiologist. The elapsed times from the time of exposure to the time of: image review by the referring physician, radiologist-unit interaction and clinical action based on image information are also measured.

The number of clinician reviews of a patient's images and the time of image review, as well as the number and time of Radiology-ICU interaction were obtained utilizing a motion activated video camera placed in the chest reading room, aimed at the alternator dedicated

MEASURED PARAMETERS
Films per Patient Day
Clinician Reviews of a Patient's Images per Day
% Images on which the ICU Interacts with Radiology

ELAPSED TIME FROM TIME OF EXPOSURE TO TIME OF
Image Review by Non-Radiologist Physician
Radiologist-ICU Interaction
Clinical Action based on image information

Table 1. Parameters and elapsed times measured both pre- and post-PACS ICU display station placement.

entirely to the medical-surgical ICU under study. Clinical action data was obtained from review of patients' charts and day sheets in the unit, and unit clinician/nurse daily survey forms. Additionally, in the post-PACS phase, the number and times of ICU reviews of a patient's images were obtained via a computer workstation function utilization tracking program.

The medical-surgical ICU display station utilized in the post-PACS phase is an ISG workstation (ISG Technologies, Inc. Ontario, Canada) developed jointly by ISG and the University of California at San Francisco (UCSF) Laboratory for Radiological Informatics (LRI). It consists of two medium resolution (1280 by 1600 line) monitors. Patient demographics and radiology reports (both preliminary and final) appear on the left monitor, as does the most recent image of a selected patient, resident in the unit. Previous or historical images are displayed on the right monitor and can be paged through in full screen resolution or viewed in half-, quarter-, eighth-, etc. minified versions. Display functionality includes interactive window and level (or contrast and brightness) modification, zoom (magnification), pan or scroll, image rotation, and gray scale reversal.

3. RESULTS and DISCUSSION

An analysis of ICU display station utilization or viewing activity in the adult medical-surgical unit over a typical 24 hour period documents that the workstation was accessed at every hour of the day except at 4 AM, with the heaviest usage during pre-morning (AM) rounds, during morning/work rounds and during afternoon (PM) sign-out rounds.

The most frequently used workstation tools were the interactive window (contrast) and level (brightness) functions for modification of the gray-scale look-up table in real time. Adjustment of window and level were utilized during viewing of 75.2 % and 57.8 % of images respectively.

Review of a patient's previous images was used 56.2% of the time. The zoom, inverse grayscale (i.e., "black bone" image view) and viewing of the radiology report were accessed less frequently (on 20.7 %, 11.7 % and 10.4 % of images viewed, respectively).

The average results for the parameter measurements of the number of films per patient day, the number of clinician reviews of a patient's images per day and the percentage of time the unit interacts with a radiologist are shown in Table 2, for both the pre-PACS phase (prior to the placement of the PACS display station in the ICU) and the post-PACS phase (after placement of the PACS workstation in the ICU).

Note that the number of films per patient day prior to placement of the PACS display station up in the ICU averaged one to two images per day (1.30 ± 0.60), while after placement of the PACS workstation up in the ICU the average number of films per patient was slightly less (1.09 ± 0.69). Also, pre-PACS measurements of the number of clinician reviews of a patient's images per day averaged one to three viewings per day (2.18 ± 1.35), with the post-PACS measurement averaging roughly the same number of viewings of a patient's images per day or slightly increased viewing (2.00 ± 4.80). Note, however, that the percentage of images on which the unit consulted with a radiologist was roughly the same for the pre- and post-PACS phases (27.4 % and 28.9 % respectively).

AVERAGE	PRE-PACS RESULTS	POST-PACS RESULTS
# Films / Patient Day	1.30 ± 0.60	1.09 ± 0.69
# Clinician Reviews of Images / Day	2.18 ± 1.35	2.00 ± 4.80
% Time Unit Interacts with Radiologist	27.4 %	28.9 %

Table 2. Average results for parameter measurements pre- and post-PACS, including the number of films per patient day, the number of clinician reviews of a patient's images per day and the percentage of images on which the unit interacts with a radiologist.

The average results for the elapsed times from the time of exposure: to the time of image review by the non-radiologist clinician, to the time of unit-radiology interaction and to the time of clinical action based on nformation ascertained from a patient's images are shown in Table 3, for both the pre-PACS phase and the post-PACS phase.

Note that the average elapsed time from the time of exposure to the time of image review by the non-radiologist clinician was significantly less after placement of the PACS display station up in the unit (2 hours 32 minutes ± 1 hour 50 minutes pre-PACS and 1 hour 35 minutes ± 56 minutes post-PACS), as was the time to clinical action based on the image information (3 hour 21 minutes ± 3 hours 24 minutes pre-PACS and 2 hour 6 minutes ± 1 hour 46 minutes post-PACS). The time of the radiologist-unit interaction remained roughly the same (1 hour 42 minutes ± 2 hours 3 minutes and 1 hour 56 minutes ± 1 hour 23 minutes pre- and post-PACS respectively).

AVERAGE ELAPSED TIME

	PRE-PACS RESULTS	POST-PACS RESULTS
Image Review by Non-Radiologist		
	2 h 32 min ± 1 h 50 min	1 h 35 min ± 56 min
Radiologist-Unit Interaction		
	1 h 42 min ± 2 h 3 min	1 h 56 min ± 1 h 23 min
Clinical Action		
	3 h 21 min ± 3 h 24 min	2 h 6 min ± 1 h 46 min

Table 3. Average elapsed times measured pre- and post-PACS, including the elapsed time from the time of exposure to: the time of image review by the non-radiologist clinician, the time of unit-radiology interaction and the time of clinical action based on the image information.

Statistical analysis tests (*p* values) of the significance of the difference of the mean values of the parameters measured prior to placement of the PACS display station in the ICU and the mean values measured after placement are shown in Table 4. The difference in means is statistically significant for a reduction in the number of films per patient day post-PACS and for a reduction in the elapsed time from the time of exposure to the time of image review by the non-radiologist ICU clinician post-PACS. Although a reduction in the time to clinical action was clearly seen after placement of the PACS display station in the ICU, the result was not statistically significant, due to the small sample size for this parameter.

4. SUMMARY

In this study to assess the changes in health-care-professional behavior as a result of placement of a PACS display station in the medical-surgical intensive care unit, and to assess ICU workstation utilization and the impact on clinical operations, via pre-and post-PACS evaluations, the following may be concluded. Introduction of a PACS display station in the ICU may reduce the number of exams per patient day, decrease the elapsed time from the time of exposure to the time of

Test of Significance of Differences of Means (*p* vales)	
# Films / Patient Day	$p = 0.0005$*
# Reviews of Patient's Images / Day	$p = 0.30$
% ICU Interacts with Radiology	$p = 0.75$
Time to Image Review	$p < 0.00001$*
Time to Radiology-ICU Interaction	$p = 0.56$
Time to Clinical Action	$p = 0.11$
	* Statistically Significant

Table 4. Resulting p values for the test of significance of the difference of means for parameters measured pre- and post-PACS.

review by the unit clinician, and improve the time to clinical action. Note, however, that it does not change the percentage of total images on which the unit interacts with a radiologist.

5. ACKNOWLEDGMENTS

The authors would like to thank Jonathan Go of ISG Technologies, Inc., Ontario, Canada, for his contributions to this study and acknowledge the support from Fuji Medical Systems U.S.A., Inc.

6. REFERENCES

1. Arenson RL, Seshadri SS, Kundel HL, *et al.* "Clinical evaluation of a medical image management system for chest images." *AJR* 150:55-59, Jan. 1988.
2. DeSimone DN, Kundel HL, Arenson RL, *et al.* "Effect of a digital imaging network on physician behavior in an intensive care unit." *Radiology* 169:41-44.
3. Humphrey LM, Fitzpatrick K, Atallah N, and Ravin CE. "Time comparison of ICUs with and without digital viewing systems." *SPIE, Medical Imaging 1992.* Vol. 1654:402-407.
4. Kundel HL, Seshadri SS, Carey B, Kishore S, *et al.* "Display station utilization in a PACS serving the medical intensive care unit of the Hospital of the University of Pennsylvania." *SPIE, Medical Imaging 1992.* Vol. 1654:424-427.
5. Kundel HL, Seshadri SS, Langlotz C, Kishore S, *et al.* "Strategies for the clinical evaluation of PACS: experience with experimental design in a medical intensive care unit." *SCAR94.* pp. 614-619.
6. Kundel HL, Seshadri SS, Shile PE, Polansky M, *et al.* "Evaluation of PACS in a medical intensive care unit: the effect of computed radiography." *SPIE, Medical Imaging 1994:* Vol. 2165:481-487.
7. Horii S, Kishore S, Feingold E. Stevens JF, *et al.* "Intensive care unit workstation usage: digitized film versus phosphor plate imaging." *SPIE, Medical Imaging 1995.* Vol. 2435:286-293.
8. Langlotz CP, Cleff B, Even-Shoshan O, Bozzo M, *et al.* "The incremental cost of PACS in a medical ICU." *SPIE, Medical Imaging 1995.* Vol. 2435:294-301.
9. Kundel HL, Seshadri SS, Langlotz CP, Horii S, *et al.* "Prospective comparison of the usage of conventional film and PACS based computed radiography for portable chest x-ray imaging in a medical intensive care unit." *SPIE, Medical Imaging 1995.* Vol. 2435:302-309.

Utilization of PACS in the Practice of Vascular Surgery

Bruce Reiner, M.D., Eliot Siegel, M.D., Frank Hooper, Sc.D., Zenon Protopapas, M.D., Stephen Pomerantz, M.D., Lois Killewich, M.D. and Michael J. Maroney, M.D.

Department of Radiology and Vascular Surgery, Baltimore Veterans Affairs and University of Maryland Medical Centers, Baltimore, Maryland

Objective: To determine the acceptance and clinical applicability of imaging studies displayed on a Picture Archiving and Communications System (PACS) in the practice of Vascular Surgery.

Materials and Methods: Comprehensive questionnaires and interviews were conducted with physicians and nurses engaged in the practice of Vascular Surgery at the Baltimore VA Medical Center, where PACS has been in routine, hospital wide operation for over two years. The perceptions of clinical staff were assessed as to the efficacy of PACS in comparison to conventional film-based images.

Results: There was overwhelming consensus amoung the Vascular Surgery staff that PACS strongly enhanced their clinical practice, both in and out of the operating room (OR). Vascular Surgeons rely heavily on image display in the OR to direct the approach and course of surgery. PACS offers unique intraoperative imaging capabilities including rapid image retrieval with enhanced archiving, cine review, high resolution images, and the ability to obtain direct quantitative measurements of vessel caliber and degree of stenosis. The increased accessibility and availability of images throughout the hospital allows for dramatic improvements in time management with overall improvement in patient care.

Conclusion: PACS has positively impacted on imaging capabilities in the practice of Vascular Surgery both in and outside of the operating room, and is strongly preferred by clinicians over conventional film-based alternatives.

Introduction: The Baltimore Veterans Affairs Medical Center (BVAMC) is a 300 bed teaching hospital which operates a large-scale, hospital wide PACS (Loral Medical Imaging Systems, Chicago, IL.), with filmless operation for the past two years. Fourty-three Macintosh (Apple Computer, Cupertino, CA) workstations are located throughout the hospital interfaced with Angiography, CT, MRI, Ultrasound, Nuclear Medicine, fluoroscopy, and general radiography.[1,2]

To date, little has been written regarding PACS utilization in the operating room, specifically as it pertains to the practice of Vascular Surgery. This study was undertaken to determine the clinical efficacy of PACS and to determine what unique requirements and modifications could be implemented to better assist the vascular surgeon in their everyday practice.

Materials and Methods: Comprehensive questionnaires and interviews were conducted to evaluate the utilization, acceptance, and expectations of PACS compared with conventional film based systems in the practice of Vascular Surgery at the Baltimore VA Medical Center. Fifteen vascular surgery personnel were randomly chosen, consisting of seven physicians and eight nurses, with a wide range of medical and PACS experience.

Results are summarized in tables 1 and 2. Quantitative responses in evaluating the impact of PACS included positive, negative, or no effect when compared with conventional film based images. A subjective score for positive or negative responses was assigned in a range of 1 to 5 with 1 being low, 3 moderate, 5 high. Data from additional open-ended questions was reviewed and incorporated into the discussion section of the text.

Results: There was consensus amoung the entire Vascular Surgery staff that PACS strongly enhanced their clinical practice, both in and out of the operating room. When comparing the experience of PACS with conventional film based imaging, all survey parameters evaluated were felt to be positively affected after the introduction of PACS.

While Angiography was the primary imaging modality utilized in the study group, plain radiography was also reported to be enhanced by PACS capabilities. Reported increases in image accessbility, report turnaround time, and improved archiving resulted in overall reduction in frequency of radiologist consultations for plain films. No corresponding reduction in consultations with Angiography were reported comparing PACS with film based images.

A commonly reported strength of PACS by physicians was the ability to perform instantaneous image review at various locations throughout the hospital, significantly enhancing work efficiency and time management. Utilization of tools on the PACS workstations was one of the many factors accounting for improvement in image quality, amount of useful information, and confidence in making diagnoses.

One common complaint unique to nursing personnel was the reported difficulty in learning to use PACS as well as maintaining computer skills. Limited and infrequent use of PACS by nursing staff was cited as the principle problem and the request for regular inservices was made.

Response According to Occupation: Physicians vs. Nurses

Survey Parameter	Percent with Positive Response	Median Subjective Score
Image Quality	71%	4
Availability of Images	86%	5
Amount of Useful Information	100%	4
Time Spent Retrieving Images	86%	3.5
Time Required to Interpret	71%	3
Confidence in Making Diagnosis	57%	4.5
Quality of Patient Care	71%	4
Overall Impression of Image Review in OR	71%	4
Duration of OR Cases	33%	4

Table 1: Physician Responses

Survey Parameter	Percent with Positive Response	Median Subjective Score
Image Quality	100%	4.5
Availability of Images	88%	4
Time Spent Retrieving Images	100%	4.5
Overall Impression of Image Review in OR	100%	5
Duration of OR Cases	100%	4

Table 2: Nurses Response

Discussion: Previous studies[2,3] have described the multitude of potential benefits offered by PACS including better image management with fewer lost and unread studies, use of computer enhancement to produce consistently higher quality images, ability to provide real-time image interpretation, easier access to images for clinicians, reduced radiation doses, and teleradiology.

Initial reports of PACS cost-effectiveness were somewhat controversial[4,5] and ignored the "hidden" costs to the healthcare system resulting from inefficiencies inherent to traditional film archival systems.[5-7] Additional non-monetary effects also to be considered include improved diagnostic accuracy, more timely diagnosis, and improved image in the marketplace[8].

Additional advantages of PACS were identified in this study unique to the intraoperative setting including a decrease in film retake rates and increased image turnaround time for intraoperative angiograms. Several members of the Vascular Surgery team also reported overall reduction in stress levels during surgery related to improved accessibility and quality of images, along with overall reduction in duration of surgery.

As one would expect, perceptions of the respondents differed depending upon occupation and level of training. Nursing personnel tend to focus on advantages in archiving, image retrieval, and overall time savings leading to enhanced patient care. Physicians tended to focus on the unique image manipulation capabilities of PACS including depiction of distal branch vessels with zoom and magnification, window/level adjustment, and black/white reversal. The ability to utilize cine function as well as obtain direct linear and area measurements were also functional improvements cited by surgeons.

Recommended future modifications to enhance PACS in the practice of Vascular Surgery include implementation of color flow and doppler ultrasound images, 3-D reconstruction for CT and MRI vascular studies, and addition of surgical atlases for anatomic review.

References

1 Pomerantz SM, Siegel EL, Pickar E, et al: PACS in the Operating Room: Experience at the Baltimore VA Medical Center. Proceedings of IMACS Conference August 1995 (In Publication)

2 Siegel EL, Diaconis JN, Pomerantz S, et al: Making Filmless Radiology Work. J. Digit Imag 8:151-155, 1995

3 Siegel EL: Plunging into PACS. Diagnostic Imaging 15:69-71, 1993

4 Gray JE, Karsell PR, Becker GP, et al: Total Digital Radiology: Is it Feasible? Is it Desirable? AJR 143:1345-1349, 1984

5 Saarinen AO, Haynor DR, Loop JW, et al: Modelling the Economics of PACS: What is Important Proc SPIE 1093:62-73, 1989

6 Mun SK, Horii S, Benson H, et al: Experience with Image Management Networks at Three Universities: Is the Cup Half-Empty or Half-Full? Proc SPIE 1093:194-201, 1989

7 Straub WH and Gur D. The Hidden Costs of Delayed Access to Diagnostic Imaging Information: Impact on PACS Implementation. AJR 155: 613-616, 1990

8 Hilsenrath PE, Smith WL, Berbaum KS, et al: Analysis of the Cost-Effectiveness of PACS. AJR 156:177-180, 1991

Effective Productivity of Picture Archiving and Communication System in the Interpretation of Computed Tomography Exams

Bruce Reiner, M.D., Eliot Siegel, M.D., Frank Hooper, Sc.D., Zenon Protopapas, M.D., Stephen Pomerantz, M.D., Andrew Dahlke, M.D. and Davis Rallis, M.D.

Department of Radiology, Baltimore Veterans Affairs and University of Maryland Medical Centers, Baltimore, Maryland

Objective: To compare radiologist productivity in the interpretation of CT images using hard copy film vs. soft copy using a PACS computer workstation.

Materials & Methods: One hundred CT exams were randomly collected over a three week period and independently reviewed by four board certified radiologists experienced in PACS. Determinations were made as to the amount of time required to retrieve, evaluate, and dictate the individual CT examinations. Time-comparison was made between soft copy interpretation (using a 2,048 x 1,536 pixel monitor) vs. conventional hard copy interpretation viewed on a viewbox with images obtained at multiple window and level settings.

Results: There was a reduction in the overall time of interpretation using PACS computer workstation when compared with conventional hard copy images. Factors accounting for the improvement in radiologist productivity using PACS included rapid availability of a wide range of window/level settings, ability to perform direct measurements of size and attenuation values, and rapid retrieval of prior studies for direct comparison. These improvements in productivity were best exemplified in complicated cases requiring comparison with multiple prior exams.

Conclusions: The productivity in CT interpretation is improved using PACS when compared with conventional hard copy images. This translates into greater patient throughput, enhanced time efficiency, and greater radiologist availability for patient and physician consultations.

Introduction: Prior studies[1,2] have reported the multitude of advantages associated with PACS when compared with conventional film-based operation. These advantages include improved archiving, easier accessibility of images for both clinicians and radiologists, reduced average radiation doses, teleradiology capabilities, and the ability to perform image enhancement to produce higher quality images.

Little to date [3-5] has been written regarding issues of radiologist productivity, specifically as it pertains to the interpretation of CT exams. These productivity issues are of particular importance in today's economic climate where the cost-effectiveness of PACS remains in doubt [6,7].

This study was undertaken to determine if radiologist efficiency gains could be achieved in the routine interpretation of CT exams. At the same time, we wanted to determine if interpretation accuracy would be significantly altered with the use of PACS.

Materials and Methods: During a three week period, 100 CT exams were randomly collected for inclusion in the study. CT exams were obtained with either a Picker PQ-2000 spiral scanner (Picker International, Cleveland, OH) or a GE High Lite Advantage Scanner (General Electric Medical Systems, Milwaukee, WI). The CT scanners have DICOM digital image communication interfacing with a hospital wide PACS system.

All exams were reviewed by four board certified radiologists experienced with PACS. The exams evaluated multiple organ systems including head, sinus, orbit, chest, abdomen and pelvis. Interpretations were made using both conventional film-based (hard copy) images and images displayed on PACS (soft copy), consisting of a four-monitor 2.048 x 1,536 pixel Macintosh II (Apple Computers, Cupertino, CA) workstation.

Time-motion analysis was performed recording each step in the process of image review and interpretation. An independent observer recorded time measurements for image retrieval, display, evaluation, and report dictation. The number of window/level adjustments and tools used during soft-copy interpretation were also recorded. Following completion of image interpretation and dictation, the interpreting radiologist was asked to fill out data sheets for each exam, which was subsequently used to access interpretation accuracy.

All reading was done in a customary fashion with prior comparison studies and reports made available at the time of interpretation. Any interruptions occurring during the timing study were recorded and factored into final data analysis.

Results and Discussion: Time analysis demonstrated a reduction in the overall time of CT interpretation when using PACS computer workstation compared with conventional hard copy images. As one would expect, there was some variation in time savings depending upon the type and complexity of the exams being reviewed. While the actual time measurements varied between radiologists, the degree of time savings remained fairly consistent.

No significant differences in overall interpretation accuracy was demonstrated comparing PACS to film interpretation. Radiologists tend to review images at a greater number of window/level settings when using the PACS workstations, but this had no significant effect on overall accuracy. Soft-copy interpretation allowed for direct measurements to be obtained (size and attenuation values), which led to enhanced radiologist productivity, particularly in complicated cases requiring multiple measurements.

Prior work[8] has shown the time to display images is slightly longer with PACS when compared with film, but this is offset by advantages of PACS including fewer interruptions, increased accessibility of old exams and reports, and the ability to perform rapid measurements and window/level adjustments.

Recent improvements in software design have allowed for greater efficiency of CT interpretation. One such improvement is the ability to automatically retrieve and display pertinent comparison studies and reports. This obviates the need for additional time-consuming steps previously required by the radiologist.

An additional item leading to enhanced radiologist productivity is the addition of a second workstation in the CT reading room. Previously when clinicians consulted for image review, the radiologist had to abort the exam being reviewed in order to review the study in question. The addition of a second monitor allowed the radiologist to assist the clinician with another study without closing the exam being interpreted.

Conclusion: The productivity in CT interpretation is improved using PACS when compared with conventional hard copy images. This translates into greater patient throughput, increased radiologist availability, and enhanced time efficiency.

References

1 Siegel EL: Plunging into PACS. Diagnostic Imaging 15:69-71, 1993

2 Siegel EL, Diaconis JN, Pomerantz S, et al: Making Filmless Radiology Work. J. Digit Imag 8: 151-155, 1995

3 Beard DV, Hemminger BM, Denelsbeck KM, et al: How Many Screens Does a CT Workstation Need? J. Digit Imag 7: 69-76, 1994

4 Hirota H, Shimamoto K, Yamakawa K, et al: Clinical Evaluation of Newly Developed CRT Viewing Station: CT Reading and Observer's Performance. Computerized Medical Imaging and Graphics 19: 281-285, 1995

5 Kato H, Kubota G, Kojima K, et al: Preliminary Time-Flow Study: Comparison of Interpretation Times Between PACS Workstations and Films. Computerized Medical Imaging and Graphics 19: 261-265, 1995

6 Hilsenrath PE, Smith WL, Berbaum KS, et al: Analysis of the Cost-Effectiveness of PACS. AJR 156: 177-180, 1991

7 Langlotz CP, Even-Shoshan O, Seshadri S.S. et al: A Methodology for the Economic Assessment of Picture Archiving and Communication Systems. J. Digit Imag 8: 95-102, 1995

8 Siegel ES, Dransfeld J : Impact of PACS on Radiologist Productivity, Poster Session, RSNA 1994, November 28, 1994

The Experience of Interpreting Soft-copy Emergency Department Computed Tomography Studies at a Major Medical Center

H. Dao and J. Stracener
Department of Radiology, Brooke Army Medical Center, San Antonio, Texas

Brooke Army Medical Center(BAMC) is a level I trauma center in San Antonio, Texas, which has metropolitan population of 1.5 million. BAMC consists of two separate hospitals located one mile apart. In the fall of 1992, MDIS (Medical Diagnostic Imaging Support System), a hospital-wide RIS/PACS (Radiology Information System/Picture Archiving and Communication System), was installed by Loral Medical Systems (Hoffman Estates, Illinois). By July 94, all CT studies were made available on PACS immediately following completion of the exam. All imaging studies currently are transferred non-compressed with a 32-bit wide data stream using the DICOM standard. The mean transfer time for each CT image from the GE 9800 CT scanner (Milwaukee, Wisconsin) is 8 seconds. From August 94 to February 96, the Emergency Department (ED) requested an average of 212 CT studies per month (range 174-275, total 4033, median 210). The average percentage of the CT studies ordered by the ED can be categorized as follows: 68.2 % head CT, 18.3 % chest/abdominal/pelvic, 6.4 % spine, 7.1 % others (facial, orbits, or musculoskeletal).

At our institution, emergent CT scans are performed at a site adjacent to the ED. Due to the availability of the hospital-wide RIS/PACS, it is not necessary for a radiologist to be physically present to monitor the exam while it is being performed. Overall departmental efficiency has improved since the introduction of PACS. First, the radiologist can continue with his/her normal work duties and interpret the emergent CT scans as they are completed without leaving the work area. This is especially important since the ED CT scanner is located in a separate building outside one hospital and one mile away from the satellite hospital. Second, the radiology technologist can spend a greater amount of time scanning patients, instead of printing all the required images with the various window and level settings. Additionally, it is not necessary for the technologist to bring the CT exam to the radiologist for review and interpretation. The estimated time savings to the technologist is 15 minutes per each CT study. An additional savings of 10 minutes can be realized by the radiologist since each abnormal CT scan can be reviewed simultaneously by both the radiologist and the ED physician on the PACS monitors. The overall time savings for both the radiologist and the technologist for each abnormal CT exam is 25 minutes.

Another advantage is that the PACS workstation monitor is simple to use. Preset window and level settings are available on the PACS workstation allowing for expeditious review of the entire CT scan. Without the need for hard copy images, significant monetary savings to the annual radiology budget is realized. The approximate savings in film cost is $28,000 per year from ED CT scans (each sheet of film costs $1.15). The radiologist, with the use of the computer workstation, can magnify, measure the size, or determine the Houndsfield units of any structure. The convenience of the radiologist having the ability to perform these functions during image interpretation leads to increased efficiency and speed of interpretation of studies. Also, the need to retrieve and review raw data on magnetic tapes is eliminated. In instances in which prior CT exams are available for comparison, these old studies are easily retrieved from the PACS storage archive, usually within one to three minutes. Problems inherent to a traditional film storage system, such as missing films or films unavailable because they are in the possession of a consulting physician, are eliminated. Additional time savings also are realized since the technologist or file room personnel do not need to locate the older exams. In addition, the ability to review old studies and to compare images from other imaging modalities allows for more accuracy in diagnosis. For difficult cases, the interpreting radiologist can solicit a second opinion from another staff radiologist at either hospital.

The PACS system has proven to be extremely reliable. The downtime for the MDIS system has averaged only 1.2 hours per month since August 94 (for a total of 24 hrs over the nineteen month period). Most importantly, through the use of PACS monitors in the ED, discussion of pathology is facilitated since both the radiologist and the ED physician review the same images simultaneously, despite their physical separation. This improves communication between the ED physician and the radiologist. A random survey of BAMC ED physicians reveals that the majority (75%) prefer the current system of soft copy reading on MDIS because of the ability to review and discuss the study simultaneously with the radiologist.

A major disadvantage of reading studies on PACS monitors is the relatively long time, from random timing surveys, to display a study (usually 40-45 seconds for a head CT) compared with hanging films on a rotator (usually 20-25 seconds for a head CT). However, in January 96, both software and hardware upgrades were installed. The hardware upgrade consisted of changing the individual workstation driver from Apple Macintosh IIfx computer(Cupertino, California) to Apple Macintosh Quadra 950 computer and adding more memory to the main controlling computer. Subsequently, the average display time for a head CT has decreased to 15 - 20 seconds. The computer's response time to manipulation of the image, such as changing contrast level and window, has been cut in half.

Another disadvantage in using the PACS system is the relatively high cost of the workstation (approximately $20,000 for each high-resolution 2K video monitor). Each workstation has a maximum of four adjacent high-resolution 2K monitors. The four monitor configuration makes direct comparison with old studies more time consuming when compared to using a film alternator. Additionally, at present, the system cannot transfer coronal/sagittal reformatted CT images and scout scanograms directly into MDIS. A minor disadvantage of PACS is the radiologist's learning period required to be proficient in soft copy image interpretation. The average training period includes a two hour training session and several more hours of one-on-one applications on the workstation with a trained user of the PACS.

In conclusion, the ability to read emergency department CT scans on computer workstation monitors has enhanced the efficiency of our radiology department. Review of the emergent CT studies is more expeditious for both the radiologist and the ED physician. Additionally, the use of soft copy imaging has improved communication and staff interaction between the radiologist and clinician due to the ability to simultaneously review the images while telephonically discussing the results of the study.

PACS in the Operating Room and Clinic: Efficacy for Orthopedic Surgeons

Stephen M. Pomerantz, M.D., Eliot L. Siegel, M.D., Zenon Protopapas, M.D., Bruce Reiner, M.D. and Elliott Pickar, M.A.
Baltimore Veterans Affairs Medical Center, Baltimore, Maryland
University of Maryland Medical System, Baltimore, Maryland

Successful implementation of a hospital-wide Picture Archiving and Communication System (PACS) requires addressing the specific needs of the clinicians and their staffs.[1] Acceptance of a PACS requires a level of functionality equivalent to or better than the film based system it replaces. During a preliminary study of the efficacy of the PACS at the Baltimore Veterans Affairs Medical Center (BVAMC) for surgeons and staff in the OR and clinic,[2] it became evident that orthopedic surgeons in particular had very specialized imaging needs and therefore had specialized requirements for the PACS. In the current study, we specifically evaluated the ability of the BVAMC PACS to meet the needs of orthopedic surgeons and provide suggestions to improve design of future systems.

The BVAMC is a 300 bed teaching hospital which has operated a hospital-wide PACS (Loral Medical Imaging Systems, Chicago, IL) for approximately 2 ½ years.[3-5] Forty-two PACS workstations utilize a Macintosh (Apple Computer, Cupertino, CA) IIFX or Quadra 950 system. These are distributed throughout the BVAMC including the diagnostic imaging department, patient-care wards, conference rooms, surgical and medical outpatient clinics, intensive care units, emergency room, and the operating room (OR). Workstations are linked by fiberoptic cable to a central server using a proprietary network protocol which enables rapid imaging display. Images are initially stored on-line for approximately two to three weeks after acquisition on a central high performance image file server. Studies are then archived to an optical jukebox with slightly longer retrieval times.

One of the eight BVAMC operating rooms is dedicated for use by the orthopedic surgeons, although occasionally cases are performed in other rooms. All of the general purpose ORs contain a two-monitor (1150 by 880 pixel, landscape) workstation. (Diagnostic workstations in the radiology department have four 1536 by 2048 pixel, portrait monitors). The orthopedic surgery outpatient clinic consists of eight patient examination rooms served by a "team room" containing a two monitor (1024 by 1280 pixel, portrait) workstation.

Interviews were conducted with 11 orthopedic surgeons (3 attendings and 8 residents) who have had experience with the BVAMC PACS as well as with the film based environment in the adjacent University of Maryland Hospital. The surgeons were asked to describe those elements of the PACS that exceeded, were equivalent to, or were inferior to a film based system. Suggestions for improvement were solicited. Additionally, orthopedists were directly observed by radiologists in the OR and orthopedic outpatient clinic.

In the operating room, many of the orthopedic surgeons' comments and suggestions were similar to those of other surgical subspecialties.[2] Workstation placement is felt to be suboptimal. The workstation in the orthopedic OR (Figure 1) is directed away from the OR table making direct observation during a procedure impossible. Optimal positioning was not anticipated when the room was designed and the fiberoptic connections installed. The surgeons suggested placing the monitors on ceiling-attached articulated arms so that their position could be varied according to need. If necessary, they could be brought up to the OR table at eye level when desired. Only a minority of the surgeons desire more

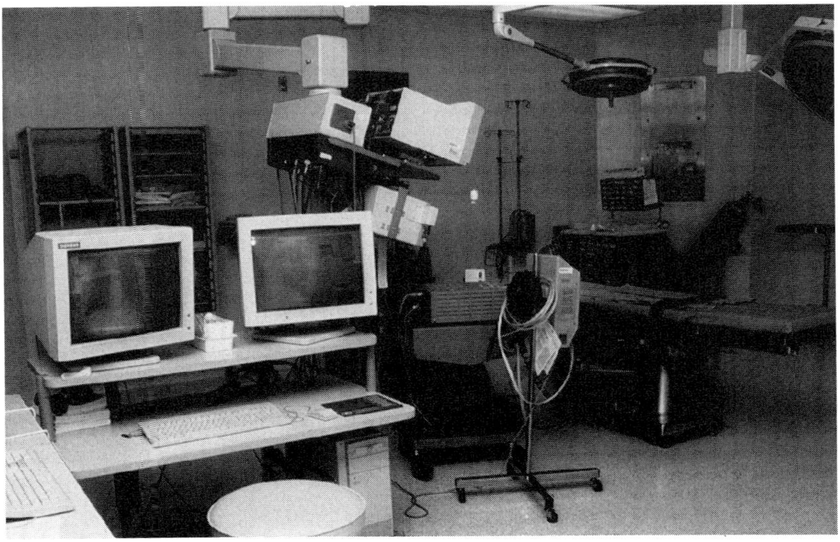

Figure 1. Two monitor (1150 by 880 pixel) PACS workstation in the orthopedic operating room. Surgeons cannot directly view the monitors from the operating table. Optimal positioning of the workstation was not anticipated in the original room design and fiberoptic connection site selection. Orthopedic surgeons have requested that monitors be suspended from ceiling-mounted articulated arms for variable positioning.

than two monitors per workstation in the OR (and clinic). Orthopedists find glare to be detrimental to image review and requested monitor design modification. A foot pedal operated dimmer switch for room and OR table lights would be of value. Workstation operation with regard to image manipulation and image navigation is believed to be unnecessarily complicated which is particularly detrimental in the pressured OR environment. Simplified, intuitive controls are desired. Workstations are operated by the surgeons before the procedure or by nurses or other OR personnel during the procedure. Alternatively, the surgeon may put on a second set of gloves to use the workstation or "break scrub" entirely. Half of those surveyed felt that sterile controls on the OR table or voice activated commands (such as "next Image" or CT bone settings") would be of value.

A major drawback of the PACS in the OR for the orthopedic surgeons is the inability to properly use prosthesis templates. In the traditional film based environment, a plastic template provided by the prosthesis manufacturer is placed over the joint on the film to estimate the correct component size. This assures that the proper hardware can be ordered prior to surgery if not already in inventory. The joint is again "templated" in the OR to assure proper sizing. All templates are designed specifically for film with a 15% magnification adjustment. Orthopedists find the templates unreliable with the PACS. Several surgeons related attempts to display a radiograph with a 1:1 aspect ratio, laying the plastic template over the screen. They have found this to be unreliable and have requested PACS generated hard copy for this purpose which has also been found to be unreliable for size estimation. Almost all prosthesis sizes are simply estimated without the use of templates. Although this has not caused any problems according to the surgeons, a solution to this problem would be welcomed. Suggestions include having templates programmed into the PACS software. However, surgeons would be most comfortable with hard copy capability with the magnification identical to traditional film.

Orthopedic surgeons are unable to view the specialized extended images used for procedures such as correction of scoliosis or leg length discrepancy. In a film based system, an image typically composed of three or more linked film sheets exposed in a single long cassette would be displayed. Surgeons have had to do without these long length images or have had to specially request traditional hard copy images. It was believed by the orthopedists that a monitor capable of displaying the entire spine to scale would be impractical. However, software capable of linking contiguous images and displaying them at reduced scale, perhaps on an extended size monitor would be a possible solution. Image measurements would necessarily be required to be accurate despite changes in scale.

The majority of orthopedic surgeons believe that interactive three dimensional (3D) image display and manipulation capabilities for preoperative planning and intraoperative roadmapping would be an significant advantage of the PACS over film. They feel that this is a capability particularly suited to their subspecialty due to the assistance provided in such procedures as complex acetabular reconstruction. Currently, the PACS workstations can provide 3D image display through the display of rapid sequential images (cine). Three dimensional reconstructed images from CT or MRI studies can be displayed any PACS workstation in the form of rotating images. To date, this ability has not been frequently utilized. Although surgeons have viewed reconstructed images in the radiology department, interviews revealed that many were not aware that when requested, the datasets could be exported to the PACS. They suggest when image reconstruction is requested, images should be automatically exported to PACS. Interactive manipulation of images at the PACS workstation is also seen as a potential benefit.

Depending on the size of the retrieval queue, obtaining images from the optical disk jukebox may be delayed to an unacceptable degree during a surgical procedure. This has been avoided by having members of the surgical team and/or members of the OR staff "fetch" images in advance. Often the images are already "on-line" because they are either current (the exam has been performed within 2-3 weeks) or have been previously retrieved for preoperative review. The orthopedists have requested more rapid retrieval through software/hardware modification and through automatic retrieval when a patient is admitted to the hospital or scheduled for surgery.

Most intraoperative images are obtained with a portable C-arm X-ray machine. They are frequently used to confirm positioning of bones, joints, and hardware. The C-arm is not linked to the PACS and the orthopedic surgeons expressed no need to archive these images. When radiographs are obtained with a conventional portable x-ray machine, surgeons describe frequent delays in viewing the images on PACS. This may be due to the relatively inconvenient location of the image readers. Placing them adjacent to the OR suite would be helpful. Additionally, automated display would obviate some of the problems the surgeons and staff have when attempting to find the images in the system.

The hectic pace of the orthopedic outpatient clinic presents a substantial challenge to a hospital-wide PACS. Issues critical in the OR such as workstation hardware and software complexity, monitor glare, and retrieval time are also important in the clinic. The major drawback to the use of PACS in the BVAMC clinic is delays caused by having eight examination rooms served by only a single PACS workstation. Whereas in a film environment, images can be reviewed quickly on lightboxes potentially present in each of the examination rooms, there is a constant wait for the workstation. This becomes a particular problem when a complicated case with multiple studies ties up the workstation for a long period of time. Frequently, a workstation in an adjacent clinic will be utilized but this is not felt to be a satisfactory solution. The surgeons would like to see *at least* two workstations in the orthopedic clinic. Another drawback of only having a workstation in the team room is that the physician often likes to show the patient his or her films to help illustrate their medical problem as well as to help in demonstrating proposed treatment. This is usually precluded by the current setup. The major advantage of the PACS to the orthopedists in their outpatient clinic is image availability. Although there were many complaints about long retrieval times for images archived to optical disk when the PACS was first implemented, this has diminished to some degree due to prefetching by the orthopedic staff. However, the orthopedists relate a relatively high rate of film loss or inability to locate films in the traditional non-PACS hospital. The ability to essentially always locate images was cited by the majority of the orthopedic surgeons as a significant advantage of PACS.

Although formal training is offered to surgeons and staff, none of the orthopedic surgeons interviewed had taken advantage of the opportunity. Reasons given included time constraints, "inertia", and not knowing about the training. Residents typically rotate through the BVAMC in three month blocks. The residents and their attendings related that the lack of training and the short periods of PACS use preclude using the system to its potential. It was evident to the radiologist observers that many "deficiencies" of the system as described by the orthopedists such as occasional poor image quality are actually a function of poor training. Although admitting to a lack of training, all of the orthopedists stress that in order for the system to be more useful, it must be more intuitive and require less training.

Miscellaneous issues pertinent to the orthopedic surgeons were raised during interviews and by observation. One such issue is the inability to superimpose images on the PACS. Frequently, in a film environment, pre and post reduction films will be superimposed to assess changes. Modifications of software to allow this would be of value. Some images such as frontal views of the pelvis must be reduced in overall size to include all portions of the image due to the geometry of the screen. Larger monitors would help with this although only one surgeon found it to be a problem. The orthopedic surgeons are generally satisfied with image quality although many felt that resolution was somewhat diminished when compared to an excellent film image. They believed that the small compromise in resolution was compensated for by the image enhancement abilities such as contrast modification and magnification. Additionally, they state that they cannot be assured of an "excellent " image in a film based environment. One of the hand surgeons was concerned that the resolution of the monitors in the OR and clinic is lower than those in the radiology department. He believes that because orthopedic surgeons often interpret their own images without reviewing the radiology report or consulting with a radiologist, they should have the best monitors possible. In a related issue, many of the orthopedists do in fact read the typed radiology interpretations that are available on-line. There is a several day delay until these are available due to the time it takes to transcribe the dictated report. Several of the orthopedic surgeons said that it would be helpful if the audio file from the dictation were available on the PACS as soon as the study is dictated. This would allow more input of radiologists than is typical in the film environment.

There was overall satisfaction with the PACS and only one of the orthopedic surgeons interviewed would go back to a film environment if given the choice. There was definitely a lower level of satisfaction however, when orthopedic surgeons were compared to the other surgical subspecialties in general. In order to fully satisfy the most particular end users of PACS technology such as the orthopedic surgeons, everyday routine experience with PACS such as at the BVAMC must be monitored in order to make modifications in imaging protocols as well as software and hardware design and implementation.

References

1. Gur D, Fuhrman CR, Thaete FL: Requirements for PACS:Users' perspective. Radiographics 13:457-460 1993

2. Pomerantz SM, Siegel EL, Protopapas Z, et al. Experience and design recommendations for picture archiving and communication systems (PACS) in the surgical setting. J Digit Imaging, In Press

3. Siegel EL: Plunging into PACS. Diagn Imaging 15:69-71 1993

4. Siegel EL: Impact of filmless radiology on the Baltimore VA Medical Center. Proceedings of the 1995 Military Telemedicine Symposium, IEEE Computer Society Press, in press.

5. Siegel EL, Diaconis JD, Pomerantz SM, et al: Making filmless radiology work. J Digit Imaging 8:151-155

PACS in the Emergency Room: Experience at the Baltimore VA Medical Center and Design Considerations for the Future

Zenon Protopapas, M.D., Eliot L. Siegel, M.D.,
Stephen M. Pomerantz, M.D., and Bruce I. Reiner, M.D.

Department of Radiology and Nuclear Medicine, Baltimore VA Medical Center,
Department of Radiology, University of Maryland Medical School, Baltimore, Maryland

Elliott Pickar, M.A.

Department of Radiololgy and Nuclear Medicine, Baltimore VA Medical Center, Baltimore, Maryland

Robert J. Doherty, M.D.

Department of Emergency Care Services, Baltimore VA Medical Center, Baltimore, Maryland

The Baltimore Veterans Affairs (VA) Medical Center is a 300 bed tertiary referral medical facility providing medical services for the veterans in Maryland. The annual outpatient visits at the medical center number approximately 260,000 with 7,500 admissions. These result in a total of 60,000 imaging studies annually. The Baltimore VA has a "full service" emergency room which orders approximately 10,000 imaging studies per year. Since the VA emergency room does not routinely make itself available to the general public, there is a disproportionately small percentage of major trauma cases such as motor vehicle accidents.

The Baltimore VA Medical Center utilizes a large scale PACS (Picture Archival and Communication System). This was installed in June of 1993 and has been in continuous operation for three years with hospital-wide "filmless operation" for more than two years. All interpretation of imaging studies is performed using the PACS workstations and all conventional radiographic examinations are performed using computed radiography. Forty-three imaging workstations (Loral Medical Imaging Systems, Chicago) are located throughout the hospital. Additionally, there is a bi-directional interface with the hospital information system.

The two imaging workstations in the emergency department utilize Macintosh (Apple Computer, Cupertino, CA) Quadra 950 systems, each with two (1024 x 1280 pixels) monitors. One of these is located in an office designated for the ER physician staff where the ER personnel have the ability to darken the room and where there is access to the hospital information system. The other workstation is located in the central emergency room working area near the entrance to the ER.

All studies are available as soon as they have been completed and processed and are easily accessible to the ER staff. Images can be viewed simultaneously by multiple radiologists or clinicians in different locations.

The immediate availability of images in the ER setting is particularly important because of the large percentage of patients who are critically ill and require immediate imaging and diagnosis. Moreover, imaging studies in a conventional film based emergency room tend to get misplaced or sometimes borrowed by one of the multiple consultants that might be involved in the care of a single patient. The effect of this is twofold; firstly, the study may never be returned for interpretation and secondly interpretation may be delayed. The PACS offers almost instantaneous access to all current and comparison imaging studies, hospital-wide.

One of the most common problems in the emergency room setting is the lack of access, due to time constraints or other factors, to previous imaging studies and reports. This results in many emergency room physicians not being able to review previous imaging studies and reports in conventional ER departments. The PACS provides access at all workstations to all of the previous imaging studies and reports that have been generated since the initial operation of the system. Prior studies from outside institutions of patients referred to our emergency room can be digitized into the PACS and made available for subsequent evaluation and comparison.

A relatively high percentage of examinations performed in the emergency room are portable radiographic studies that are obtained on patients who cannot easily be moved or positioned for optimal quality radiographs. Patients in the emergency room who may be immobilized, on life support, or uncooperative, pose technical challenges for radiology technologists. Computed radiography (CR), in conjunction with the use of a computer workstation, permits display of multiple window and level settings in order to optimally evaluate different parts of a single study. This has resulted in a decreased radiographic retake rate from 5% prior to PACS to 1% . This has been accomplished in conjunction with a perceived increase in the overall quality of radiographic studies in the ER by both radiologists and clinicians.

The availability of imaging studies hospital-wide has decreased the overall radiologic consultation rate. This impression was confirmed by interviewing the ER staff who state that while the consultation rate for radiographic images has decreased, the consultation rate for cross-sectional imaging studies has not changed.

Emergency Room staff judged the image quality for computed radiographic images to be generally superior to film for the ER setting. Window and level adjustments and magnification are the two most commonly used workstation tools. Workstations in an ER need to be easily accessible to the clinicians and are therefore not necessarily situated in a room where the lights can be dimmed. For this reason increased brightness of the monitors would help improve the image quality. Placing view boxes adjacent to a workstation would allow the ER physician to directly compare outside imaging studies with current studies on PACS. Outside studies are usually digitized during regular working hours only. Some ER physicians have expressed a preference that the workstation be located at eye level. This would allow viewing of images in the standing position which may be an advantage in a busy ER. Concerns have been expressed about powder from gloves used frequently by ER staff getting into the keyboard and mouse. Protective covering may be helpful.

In a survey of medical staff and ER physicians, one of the frequent comments was the discrepancy in the amount of time from when studies were available for review and when the reports were available in the hospital information system. Currently we do not use a digital dictation system. Therefore, reports are only available after they have been transcribed. This may be of no consequence in an outpatient setting where there is ample time between the patient's imaging study and the next clinic appointment. For ER and Critical Care patients however, availability of the radiologist's report is more crucial. Currently radiologists are annotating findings on examinations and calling the physician when appropriate. "Voice" annotation of an examination may allow the radiologist to provide a short report to the clinician before the full report could be available on the PACS. Voice recognition software would also provide rapid turnover of reports after dictation. On-line availability of images of normal variants would be helpful to both the ER physicians and the interpreting radiologists.

In conclusion, PACS has been well received by the ER staff at the Baltimore VA Medical Center. ER requirements for PACS are unique in some ways especially in the fast turnaround time required, requirements for rapid retrieval of old studies, and due to the fact that the patients pose difficulties technically in obtaining adequate quality studies. The PACS and CR offer particular advantages in the ER setting with regard to image availability and the ability to use the workstation to optimize image quality. Suggestions for improvement would include relocation of monitors and improved training for ER personnel. Voice or graphical annotation of abnormalities on images would further facilitate communication between ER clinicians and radiologists.

SESSION 10

Image Processing

Co-Chairs:

Hans Roehrig

Ronald B. Shilling

Application of B-spline Wavelets for High-Level, High-Quality Compression of Medical Image Data

D.F. Schomer, S.K. Thompson and J.D. Hazle
The University of Texas M.D. Anderson Cancer Center, Department of Diagnostic Radiology

Á.A. Elekes
Houston Advanced Research Center, Houston, Texas

J.C. Huffman
Silicon Graphics, Inc., Mountain View, California

L. Zhong and C.K. Chui
Texas A&M University, College Station, Texas

I. Introduction

As the trend towards an all digital radiology department continues, demand on the central image archive as well as local and wide area communication networks will increase. The capability for high quality image compression enables this evolution. We present a novel compression algorithm based on the minimally supported bi-cubic spline wavelet and its dual introduced by Chui and Wang [7] which has many advantages for the compression of medical images.

High-quality wavelet compression of medical images consists of three parts: (1) wavelet decomposition, (2) quantization, and (3) encoding (Figure 1). The development of an optimum coder/decoder for image compression requires integration of all of these components. The aim of signal representation and decomposition is to efficiently decorrelate the information content of the image. This is highly dependent on the selection of the wavelet basis function. The semi-orthogonal bi-cubic spline wavelet transform has a near-optimal time-frequency window and compact support.

Figure 1. Image Compression Overview

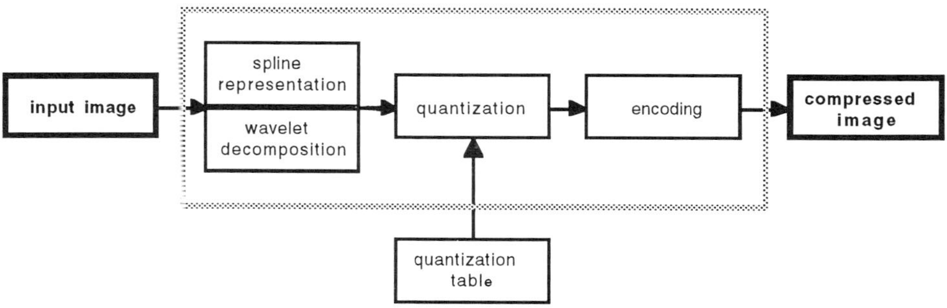

A software implementation of this algorithm was submitted to Working Group IV of the American College of Radiology-National Equipment Manufacturers Association (ACR/NEMA) to be considered as a component of the DICOM standard for lossy image compression. The proposed algorithm incorporates the following useful features:

- tractable computational complexity allowing efficient software implementation,
- block segmentation is allowed but not required,
- parallel implementation is simple,
- aliasing artifacts are reduced,
- relevant information can be localized and variable compression depth across the image is possible, and
- sequential, progressive, lossless and hierarchical encoding operations can be incorporated.

These advantages ensure that compression methods based on the spline-wavelet family generate minimal artifacts and better reconstructions than other wavelet compression methods [8]. The cubic-spline wavelets implemented in this algorithm are semi-orthognormal, symmetric, and compactly supported [3-6].

II. Wavelet Decomposition

Separable wavelets can be grouped into orthogonal and biorthogonal wavelets. Orthogonal wavelets are popular in image coding and are quite easy to implement. In compression applications, symmetric wavelets are preferred since they have linear phase or pseudo-linear phase properties. Their use prevents information loss through phase distortion in the associated finite impulse response filters (FIR). Symmetry in wavelets may be obtained only at the cost of giving up either compact support or orthogonality [2, 4]. Some of the most commonly used wavelets, such as the Daubechies and Coifman wavelets, are orthogonal wavelets and cannot be symmetric or antisymmetric. A new class of semi-orthogonal wavelets are used in this project. They have the unique advantage of providing symmetry while preserving both compact support and orthogonality.

II.1. Spline representation

The first step in the compression scheme is representation of the image data. Because the integral wavelet transform (IWT) is defined only for analog (continuous-time) signals, digital signals must first be mapped into the continuous-time domain in order for the IWT be meaningful. This is achieved through appropriate representation of the image. If the input signal is exactly represented, it is said to possesses the "perfect reconstruction" property (exact reproduction of the input signal if there is no processing of the transformed signal). Many popular compression schemes approximate the input signal with an infinite Fourier series rather than representing it exactly. These techniques are therefore subject to truncation error.

Splines are widely used in computer graphics and are easily adapted to medical imaging. The spline scaling functions for which this wavelet transform is defined exactly represent the input signal and therefore possess the "perfect reconstruction" property [4]. Spline-based wavelets are also attractive since processing may be performed in the spectral domain. Although most wavelet-based compression techniques allow for post-processing, none do so more naturally than those based on spline wavelets. Spline-based techniques are very well suited for edge-enhancement, feature recognition, and extraction and quantification.

II.2. Wavelet transformation

The wavelet transformation converts the spatial image into a "spectral image" with good energy compaction. Wavelet representations are determined by the choice of wavelet basis functions. Although wavelet theory was formalized only a decade ago they have proven to be an excellent transform for image compression [1, 2]. The Chui-Wang spline-wavelets on which this work is based can be formulated explicitly in the time (or spatial) domain [7]. Other wavelets must be computed either iteratively or by taking the inverse Fourier transform of certain infinite products.

We chose cubic spline wavelets because they are symmetric, semi-orthogonal and compactly supported [3, 4]. The Wavelet Research Laboratory at Texas A&M University has been working with these types of wavelets for several years. These wavelets are very well understood and are exploited in this implementation. The time-frequency window of these wavelets is near-optimal as dictated by the Uncertainty Principle; 0.8% away from the theoretical limit of 0.5 corresponding to the Gaussian function. The side-lobe/main-lobe ratio for the filter characteristics of a semi-orthogonal cubic spline wavelet is below -41 dB. By comparison, Daubechies wavelets (D_4) of the same order, produce a time-frequency window 292% away from theoretical limit of 0.5 and a side-lobe/main-lobe ratio of -21 dB. Further, the linear-phase property is guaranteed, since the cubic spline wavelets are even ordered and symmetric. These advantages assure that compression methods based on the spline-wavelet family generate minimal artifacts and better reconstructions than other wavelet compression methods [8].

III. Quantization

Compression is first accomplished by quantizing the coefficients in the decomposition subbands. The quantizer exploits the statistical characteristics of the coefficients in the subbands and the properties of the human visual system. In general, the higher frequencies are quantized more coarsely than the lower frequencies.

The quantized coefficients are compactly represented with binary codewords. Unlike blocked frequency-based compression methods such as JPEG, the output of the wavelet transform can be statistically modeled in the general case. This property allows the design of a quantizer which minimizes distortion for a target compression rate. Although a vector code book could be designed that would outperform a general uniform scalar quantizer, the computational overhead for designing the code book is prohibitive and a static code book performs poorly. The use of a scalar quantizer in conjunction with an entropy coder was considered a better solution.

IV. Lossless encoding

The purpose of encoding is to achieve compression by compactly representing the quantized wavelet coefficients by their statistical characteristics. We accomplish this with a tree-like algorithm in combination with an adaptive arithmetic coder. The lossless coder is based on ideas presented by Said and Pearlman [9]. Our tree parsing structure is similar to the one described in their paper, however, a different method for updating the list of insignificant sets was chosen and the method of storing the coefficients is different. The coder was also designed to take more care in determining the presence of descendants in sub-trees, leading to a more efficient algorithm. The arithmetic coder is a generic, adaptive coder with a binary tree seed-state. It has sufficient depth to cover all pertinent entries with a starting count of the one used for both zero and one states in all sub-states.

V. Discussion

Compression of images with a wavelet transform is accomplished in three general steps. The first step transforms the digital image into the spline-wavelet domain. This requires image representation with spline scaling functions to map the digital data into the contiguous-time domain so that the IWT is meaningful. At this point, no compression has been accomplished and the original image can be exactly regenerated due to the "perfect reconstruction" property. To compress the data-set, the coefficients defining the decomposition subbands are quantized, preserving those coefficients most relevant to image reconstruction. The final lossless encoding step further compresses the coefficient table but with no mathematical loss of information.

The computational complexity associated with our wavelet compressor is of the order O(n). This is significantly lower than the O(n log n) number of operations generally needed with DCT-based codecs. Enhanced versions of DCT based codecs such as Joint Photographic Experts Group (JPEG) or lapped orthogonal transform (LOT) based compressors may be even more demanding computationally. Medical images are generally non-stationary. That is, the statistical characteristics of the image vary between and over images. In order to encode images, the DCT and LOT-based compressors have to divide images into blocks or subimages which are stationary. Unfortunately, these techniques produce block artifacts. Wavelet-based compressors on the other hand do not have to subdivide images due to the compact nature of the basis functions.

The use of lowpass and bandpass filters in wavelet-based compression of images allows a parallel implementation of the codec in a natural way. Both of these operations can be simultaneously performed during the decomposition and reconstruction processes on every compression level.

By its very definition, wavelet decomposition is pyramidal. The decomposition is accomplished by critical downsampling the image. Due to the correlation between the image bitplanes and the spatial domain, the image may be reconstructed with different spatial resolutions and quality. Therefore, wavelet compression is ideally suited for hierarchical transmission and thumbnail browsing. Also, variable compression depth across an image can be implemented with ease. Important features can be extracted and retained at lower compression ratios, making intelligent archive architectures feasible.

In conclusion, a new algorithm has been developed specifically for medical image compression based on bi-cubic spline wavelets [4-6], optimized quantization and lossless encoding [9]. This algorithm was submitted to the ACR/NEMA Working Group IV to be considered as a lossy compression standard for the DICOM image format standard by our group in late 1995. This algorithm is based on semi-orthogonal spline wavelets with compact support. These wavelets have many remarkable mathematical characteristics which make them ideally suited for image compression [8]. These advantages guarantee that compression based upon semi-orthogonal spline wavelet families generate better reconstruction with minimal artifacts.

References

[1] I. Daubechies, Orthonormal bases of compactly supported wavelets, Comm. Pure and Appl. Math., 41, 909-996, 1988.

[2] I. Daubechies, Wavelets, CBMS-NSF Series in Appl. Math., SIAM Publ., Philadelphia, 1992.

[3] C. K. Chui and J. M. De Villiers(95 a) , Spline-wavelets with arbitrary knots on a bounded interval: Orthogonal decomposition and computational algorithms CAT Report # 362, Texas A&M University, 1995, submitted to Appl. & Comp. Harmonic Analysis.

[4] C. K. Chui, An Introduction to Wavelets, Academic Press, San Diego, 1992.

[5] C.K. Chui, Multivariate Splines, SIAM Publ., Philadelphia, 1988.

[6] C. K. Chui, Wavelets: A Mathematical Tool for Signal Analysis, SIAM Publ., Philadelphia, 1996, to appear.

[7] C. K. Chui and J.Z. Wang, Computational and algorithmic aspects of cardinal spline wavelets, CAT Report #235, Texas A&M University, 1990.

[8] J. Lu, R. Algazi and E. Estes A, comparative study of wavelet image coders Optical Eng. Visual Communic. and Image Proc. V, June, 1995.

[9] A. Said and W. A. Pearlman, A new fast and efficient image codec based on set partitioning in hierchical trees, IEEE Trans. Circuits and Sys. for Video Techn., 1993.

Interactive 3-Dimensional Registration of MR and ^{201}Thallium SPECT Brain Images

Richard Gorniak , Elissa Kramer, Marilyn Noz, Andrew Litt and Michael Gruber
NYU Medical Center
Edward Farrell
IBM Corporation

INTRODUCTION

In patients with brain tumors or uncharacterized mass lesions, thallium-201 (^{201}Tl) SPECT imaging of the brain offers unique information about lesion metabolism. Increased uptake of ^{201}Tl in a primary brain tumor can be used to differentiate high grade from low grade astrocytomas(1) or identify concentrations of high grade tumor cells within an otherwise low grade tumor. In treated patients, uptake on ^{201}Tl SPECT has been associated with poorer prognosis(2) . In glioma patients treated with radiation therapy, ^{201}Tl SPECT can be used to differentiate tumor recurrence from radiation necrosis (2). Finally, in the setting AIDS, ^{201}Tl SPECT has shown utility in differentiating primary CNS lymphoma from opportunistic infections(3). However, ^{201}Tl SPECT studies lack anatomic detail and suffer from poor spatial resolution. Even with state of the art collimation and triple-headed rotating gamma cameras, the full width half maximum of a SPECT study is 7-8 mm. Often there is little anatomic context in which to place the abnormal uptake because thallium does not accumulate significantly in normal brain structures.

In contrast, MRI produces high resolution anatomical images which can precisely identify the area of the brain affected and the surrounding structures. The spatial extent of abnormalities is well delineated. However, standard MRI is less effective in determining the metabolic activity of an abnormality. MRI cannot reliably differentiate primary CNS lymphoma from an opportunistic brain infection in AIDS patients (4) or high grade gliomas from low grade. In the treated patient with a history of primary brain tumor, MRI can neither definitively detect the areas of high grade transformation within a mass nor distinguish radiation necrosis from recurrence (5).

Through digital image registration, the complementary and unique information from each of these modalities can be combined, providing a composite image which integrates the metabolic with the anatomic information. The composite image localizes the abnormal metabolic activity within the anatomy of the patient's brain and in relation to any mass lesion. For example, areas of high grade tumor can be detected within a mixed astrocytoma and localized to a specific site within a complex mass depicted on MR. Similarly, metabolically active tumor may be identified within an area of necrosis or surrounding edema. This information could be invaluable in diagnosis, guiding biopsies, surgical planning and follow-up of treated patients.

Several methods have been described for registering radiologic image sets in two dimensions (6-9). Recently, with the greater availability of image workstations and more powerful computer processors, three dimensional approaches have been investigated(10-18) . In this paper we describe a method for registering corresponding image sets from ^{201}Tl SPECT and MRI in three dimensional space, using programs implemented with the IBM Visualization Data Explorer (DX) software. This method of registration, like the method described by Pietrzyk, et al.(16), relies on the innate faculties of the human visual system to interpret information. 2D and 3D images from both modalities are displayed simultaneously. The user then visually assesses mismatches between analogous structures apparent in both images and, by adjusting the translation and/or rotation of one image set, attempts to correctly match them.

METHODS

Patients

Twenty-four patients, 8 female and 16 male, aged 22-63 years, were referred to the Nuclear Medicine Department between April, 1994 and June, 1995 for evaluation of a known or suspected primary brain tumor(n=16) or for differentiation between AIDS-related opportunistic infection and lymphoma(n=8) (Table 1). Of the 16 primary brain tumor patients, 14 had previous surgical or biopsy confirmation of glial or neuronal tumors, 1 had suspected glioma, and 1 had progressive multifocal leukoencephalopathy. 12 of these patients had undergone previous therapy for their brain tumors. Of the 8 patients with AIDS and mass lesions on MRI, 2 patients had opportunistic infections, 1 a cerebral hemorrhage, and 5 lymphoma.

SPECT Imaging

^{201}Thallium SPECT studies were acquired at 20 minutes and approximately 2 hours after intravenous administration of 5 mCi of ^{201}thallium chloride. Using a triple-headed gamma camera (Triad, Trionix, Inc.) interfaced to a Sun SPARC 390 workstation (Sun Microsystems) and fitted with low energy, high sensitivity collimators, 4 degree projections of the head were acquired over a 360 degree interval into a 64 X 64 matrix for 70 seconds per view. A 20 % energy window was centered at the 80 keV photopeak of ^{201}thallium. The studies were reconstructed using a Butterworth filter with a 1.4 cyc/cm Nyquist frequency, a 0.6 cyc/cm high cut frequency and an alpha of 3.0. Attenuation correction using Chang's algorithm was performed.

MR Imaging

Patients were scanned on a 1.5T or 1.0T Clinical MR Scanner (Siemens Medical Systems, Iselin, NJ) with T1 and T2-weighted imaging. The T1-weighted study is an Magnetization Prepared Rapid Gradient Echo sequence (MP-RAGE). The MP-RAGE sequence utilizes a 3D short TR (TurboFlash) gradient-echo acquisition. MP-RAGE sequence parameters were TR /TE /TI /FlipAngle /Matrix /FOV /Scantime 12 /4 /300 /15 /180*256 /230/5:32. The advantages of the sequence are: heavy T1 contrast, relatively high signal/noise, post-processing capabilities, thin contiguous images, a short acquisition time and the presence of flow related enhancement. The MP-RAGE data set consists of 128 1.25 mm sagittal partitions that can be reconstructed in any plane because of isotropic voxel dimensions. For this study, 20 axial sections 5 mm thick with a 1.5 mm interslice gap were reconstructed.

Table 1: Patient Characteristics at Time of SPECT Scan

Num	Age	Sex	Diagnosis	Previous Therapy
1	35	f	glioblastoma multiforme	chem,rad
2	35	m	low-grade oligodendroglioma	none
3	48	m	anaplastic oligodendroglioma	resct,chemo
4	50	m	suspected glioma	none
5	44	m	non-Hodgkin'slymphoma	none
6	51	m	glioblastoma multiforme	resct,chemo,rad
7	22	m	astrocytoma grade II/III	rad
8	56	m	glioblastoma multiforme	resct,chemo,rad
9	37	f	astrocytoma grade I/III	none
10	39	m	grade II/IV astrocytoma	chemo,rad
11	41	m	non-Hodgkin'slymphoma	none
12	32	m	cytomegalovirus infection	none
13	61	f	focal encephalitis	none
14	55	f	non-Hodgkin's lymphoma	chemo
15	33	m	non-Hodgkin's lymphoma	resect
16	40	m	cerebral hemorrhage	none
17	55	m	glioblastoma multiforme	resct
18	39	m	ganglioglioneurocytoma	resct,rad
19	35	f	grade II/IV astrocytoma	resct
20	57	f	ganglioglioneurocytoma	resct
21	63	f	mixed astro/oligodendroglioma	resct,chemo
22	25	m	mixed astro/oligodendroglioma	resct,chemo
23	38	f	progressive multifocal leukoencephalopathy	none
24	56	m	non-Hodgkin'slymphoma	none

Previous Therapy:
none - follow up or anti- microbial/viral medication only
resct - resection
chemo - chemotherapy
rad - radiation therapy

Image Processing

The 3D registration program is implemented through IBM Visualization Data Explorer (DX), which provides an object-oriented, graphical programming interface. DX is based on the MIT X11 Window System and Open Software Foundation's Motif graphical user environment. DX uses a data-flow driven client-server execution model, and runs on UNIX workstations from most leading manufactures. Panel content, layout, and access were structured for convenient clinical use and ease of learning. Each image is fully annotated with variable names, display parameters, patient name, and scan date. The later data are automatically extracted from the image header. The HP9000/720 also served as the host machine running the DX executables.

Using Data Explorer's ExtractSurf And SPECTref

In the first step of the registration process, a 3D surface from the MR data set is extracted using the ExtractSurf program . Since the scalp is consistently visible in both the MR and the SPECT image sets, it is the anatomical structure on which the 3D surface is based. By entering a pixel value, the user identifies a surface that contains all points in the data set that have that value. This isosurface and a 2D MR image with a contour at the selected pixel value are displayed. Guided by these images, the user modifies the pixel value until the isosurface that best represents the scalp is selected. This results in the display of the surface representing the scalp plus any other surfaces that happen to form at this pixel value, such as portions of the brain or image noise external to the scalp. These areas are removed by "picking" or choosing the scalp surface with the mouse. All surfaces that are not continuous with the selected scalp surface are removed. This isosurface is then saved.

The SPECTref program is used to display and register the MR and SPECT images. First, the SPECT, MR, and MR surface data are loaded and then displayed, taking into account the voxel size of each image set. The display of images occurs in two windows, one referred to as the 2D display and the other as the 3D display. In the 2D display, a slice from each image set is shown with isovalue contours from the SPECT slice superimposed over the corresponding MR slice. These slices can be axial, coronal or sagittal sections at any location in the data sets. In the 3D display, the selected MR surface is shown. Using SPECTref, the SPECT isosurface best representing the scalp is interactively selected in much the same way the MR surface was selected. Once the SPECT surface is defined, both are displayed concurrently in the 3D display window. These images in the 3D display can be rotated, allowing the surfaces to be viewed from any angle.

To register the image sets, the SPECT data set is moved into the correct position with respect to the MR data by applying rigid body transformations. Using the registration control panel, the user can modify the six registration parameters, one translation and one rotation parameter for each of the three cardinal axes, which define the position of the SPECT data set in space. As the user adjusts the 3 translation and 3 rotation variables, both the 3D and 2D displays are updated, showing the effects of the newly chosen parameters. Using both the 2D and 3D images, the user attempts to match as closely as possible anatomical landmarks, such as the scalp and paranasal sinuses, depicted in both imaging modalities. Initially, the translation parameters are set so that the SPECT surface representing the scalp is roughly centered with the MR surface. Using an axial slice through the paranasal sinuses as a guide, the initial axial rotation is established. Next, the initial coronal and sagittal rotations are chosen by observing the difference in scalp contours between the SPECT and MR images as shown in the 3D and 2D displays. Once a rough estimate of the six parameters has been made, the registration is fine-tuned by examining a series of views of the 3D surfaces and 2D slices to determine how well the SPECT and MR images match globally and then modifying the registration parameters as necessary. Table 2 shows the 3D view and 2D section used at each step when modifying the listed registration parameters. Usually sections at a minimum 2 or 3 locations in the stated plane were examined at each

Step	*3-D Display*	*2-D Display*	*Translation*	*Rotation Axis*
1	Anterior	Coronal	Axial and Lateral	A-P
2	Left lateral	Sagittal	A-P and Axial	Lateral
3	Cephalad	Axial	Lateral and A-P	Axial
4	Posterior	Coronal	Axial and Lateral	A-P
5	Right lateral	Sagittal	A-P and Axial	Lateral
6	Caudal	Axial	Lateral and A-P	Axial

Table 2

step. This process of adjusting the registration parameters continues until the user is satisfied that the best registration has been achieved. Usually, one or two iterations of the fine-tuning process are required. The total time to process the images, depending on the image set and the load on the server, ranged from 20 to 60 minutes.

RESULTS

The utility of image registration using this method was evaluated qualitatively by comparing the location of lesion seen on the MR image with the location of increased thallium uptake. In 10 cases the area of increased thallium uptake corresponded to the entire lesion seen on the MR image (patients 6-15)(figure 1). In 5 cases the area of increased thallium uptake corresponded to a portion of the lesion seen on the MR image (patients 1-5)(figure 2). In 4 cases increased thallium uptake overlay an area at or near the border of the cavity left by surgical resection (patients 17-20)(figure 3). In 4 cases the area of the MR lesion was too close to the thallium activity in the scalp to be able to identify abnormal thallium uptake in the site (patients 21-24). In one case no increased thallium uptake was seen at the site of the MR lesion or in the remainder of the brain. This patient was found to have cerebral hemorrhage (patient 16).

DISCUSSION

Registration or fusion of images from multiple modalities offers the opportunity to combine very different kinds of information about an anatomic structure or a mass into one image. Until recently, most registration efforts have dealt with two dimensions at one time(6-9). Typically, transaxial slices from the same level are registered. Although the entire volume or slice set may be available, the ability to view these sets simultaneously as a three dimensional volume is usually lacking. Accurate matching requires that the anatomic planes of slice pairs be identical. Reproducible positioning for each type of image acquisition session may be used to obtain matched image sets, but in practice there is usually some variation in position between image data sets. For instance in our 2D algorithm(24, 25), the center-to-center match is better than the degree of overlap of like features (26). This is most likely due to differences between the anatomic planes of a slice-pair. Several three dimensional techniques have been developed to overcome this limitation(10-18).

Most registration algorithms rely to some extent on the matching of like features in pairs of image data sets. These features may be externally placed fiduciaries or intrinsic anatomic features. Fixed external references, like stereotactic frames or face masks, hold the patient's position constant between studies and provide external points of reference between the two images(27). External references must be used prospectively, decreasing their clinical convenience. Methods that utilize intrinsic features can be applied retrospectively since no special preparation is needed before acquiring images. The difficulty with these methods is the identification of the intrinsic features. The identification of these features may be automated, relying on image segmentation algorithms, or require various degrees of operator interaction. Image segmentation algorithms generally demand that well-defined features, usually based on pixel values, be present within the image data. While this often is possible in CT, MRI, or PET, the lower resolution, noisy images from ^{201}Tl SPECT lack sharply defined features which would lend themselves readily to image segmentation. Although semiautomated techniques of Tl SPECT-MR registration using Pelizzari's technique have been described(11,15),

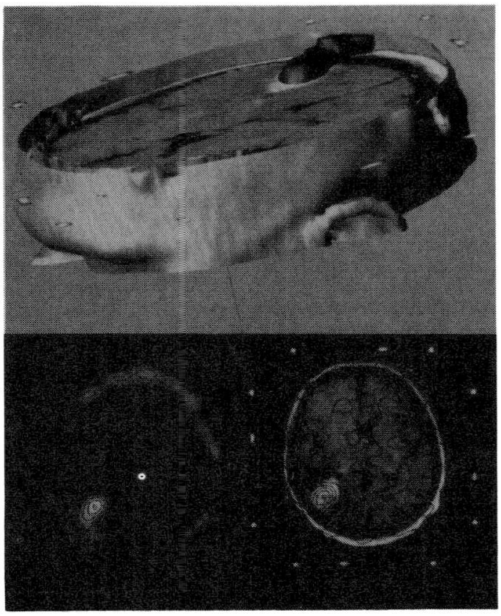

Figure 1

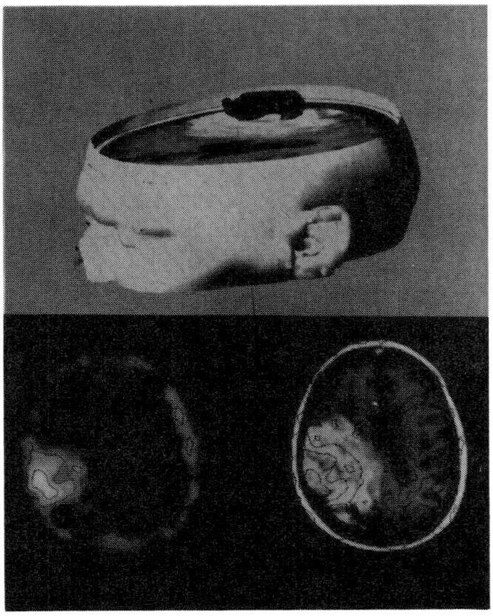

Figure 2

Figure 1 - Increased Tl-201 uptake corresponds to the entire tumor seen on the MR image (Pt. 6).

Figure 2 - Area of increased Tl-201 uptake corresponds to only a portion of the lesion seen on the MR image (Pt1).

Figure 3 - Increased Tl-201 uptake overlies an area near the border of the surgical cavity, representing residual tumor (Pt. 19).

top image - scalp surface extracted from MR(grey surface), axial MR slice, volume of increased Tl-201 uptake(black surface).

bottom image - left:axial SPECT image, right: axial MR slice with isovalue contours from the SPECT slice superimposed

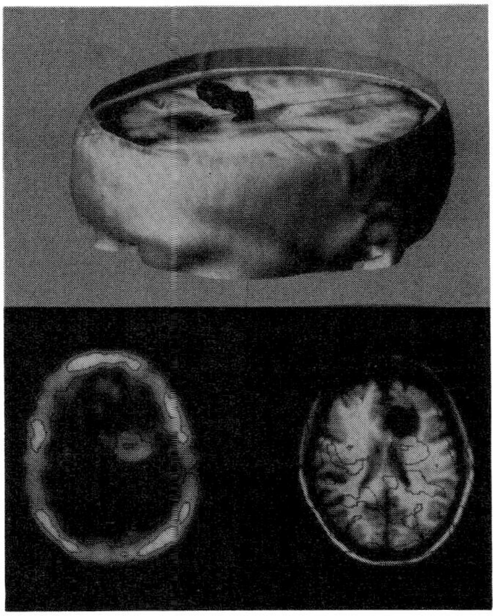

Figure 3

fully automated techniques have not been used because of the difficulty in segmenting ^{201}Tl SPECT. Even the scalp uptake is often patchy and irregular making it unsuited to image segmentation. In the work described here we have relied solely on operator-defined registration.

We feel that the human visual system is well suited for identifying structures on Tl SPECT images. Since registration methods rely on the identification of like structures, accurate determination of the like structures is key. While interactive techniques rely on the somewhat subjective perceptions of anatomy by the operator, they allow application of the user's ability to recognize and manipulate anatomical structures in a noisy image. For instance, a moderately experienced user can infer the "true" location of the scalp from the thallium uptake. Users need only limited knowledge to do this. The method described here has been used by medical students and technologists with success

The previously described interactive technique (16) utilizes multiple 2D slice sections in different planes to guide the registration process. The method described here adds 3D surface renderings to the display of information to assist the user in registration. 3D surfaces can help determine initial parameters when images are grossly misaligned and there is little or no overlap seen in the 2D slices. The 3D surface can also help the user in acquiring a global impression of the image sets .

The results presented here, while qualitative, show that it is possible to register ^{201}Tl SPECT and MR images of the brain retrospectively using this method. In this series of studies, this method was useful in demonstrating the presence of ^{201}Tl uptake in an MRI abnormality. Areas of recurrence in patients with tumor resections, small areas of high uptake within a larger mass lesion and patients with lesions with increased thallium uptake throughout the entire MRI lesion were demonstrated. The accuracy and inter- and intra-user reproducibility need to be addressed before this method can be applied to areas, such as biopsy and surgery planning. However, at present this method could be useful clinically. Once registered with an MR image set, areas of thallium uptake can be localized within that individual anatomy of the patient, enhancing our interpretation of both ^{201}Tl SPECT and MR and, as a consequence, improving our understanding of the clinical status of the brain tumor patient.

REFERENCES

1.Black KL, Hawking RA, Kim KT, et al. J Neurosurg 1989; 71(3):342-346.
2.Schwartz RB, Carvalho PA, Alexander E III, et al. AJNR 1991; 12(6):1187-1192.
3.Ruiz A, Ganz WI, Post MJ, et al. AJNR 1994; 15(10):1885-94.
4.Kupfer MC, Zee CS, Colletti PM, et al. Magn Reson Imaging 1990; 8:51-57.
5.Dooms GC, Hecht S, Brant-Zawadzki M, et al. Radiology 1986; 158:149-155.
6.Van den Elsen PA, Pol EJD,Viergever MA. IEEE Eng Med and Biol 1993; 40(3):26-39.
7.Mazziotta JC, Phelps ME, Meadors AK, et al. J Comput Assist Tomogr 1982; 11:948-954.
8.Hawkes DJ, Robinson L, Crossman JE, et al. Eur J Nucl Med 1991; 18:752-756.
9.Brown L. ACM Computing Surveys 1992; 24(4):325-376.
10.Alpert NM, Bradshaw JF, Kennedy D, Correia JA.J Nucl Med 1990;31:1717-1722.
11.Holman BL, Zimmerman RE, Johnson KA, et al.J Nucl Med 1991;32:1478-1484.
12.Kapouleas I, Alavi A, Alves WM, et al. Radiology 1991; 181:731-739.
13.Maguire GQ,Noz ME,Rusinek H, et al.IEEE Comput Graph Appl 1991;11:20-28.
14.Mangin JF, Frouin V, Bloch I, et al. J Cereb Blood Flow and Metab 1994; 14(5):749-762.

15.Pelizzari CA Chen GTY, Spelbring DR, Weichselbaum RR, Chen CT. J Comput Assist Tomogr 1989; 13(1):20-26.

16.Pietrzyk U, Herholz K,Heiss WD. J Comput Assist Tomogr 1990; 14(1):51-59.

17.Pietrzyk U, Herholz K,Fink G, et al. J Nucl Med 1994; 35:2011-2018.

18.Woods RP, Mazziotta JC,Cherry SR. J Comput Assist Tomogr 1993;17:536-546.

19.Noz ME, Maguire GQ. Computer Methods and Programs in Biomedicine 1988; 27(11):229-240.

20.Maguire GQ, Noz ME. . Medical Physics 1989; 16(5):818-823.

21.Baxter BS, Hitchner LE, Maguire GQ. In: AAPM Report No. 10. New York, NY: Am. Inst. of Phys., 1982: 10.

22.Reddy DP, Noz ME, M Maguire GQ, et al. In: H.U. Lemke K Inamura C.C. Jaffee, and M.W. Vannier ed. Computer Assisted Radiology - CAR '95. Berlin, West Germany: Springer-Verlag, 1995: 1339-1345.

23.Reddy DP, Maguire GQ, Noz ME, Kenny R. In: H.U. Lemke K Inamura C.C. Jaffee, and R Felix ed.Computer Assisted Radiology - CAR '93. Berlin, West Germany: Springer-Verlag, 1993: 253-258.

24.Kramer EL Noz ME. Nuclear Medicine and Biology. Int J Radiat Applic and Instrument Part B 1991; 18:27-42.

25.Birnbaum B Noz M,Chapnick J, Sanger J,et al. Radiology 1991;181:469-474.

26.Katyal S, Kramer EL, Noz ME, et al Cancer Res (Suppl) 1995; :5759s-5763s.

27.West J, Fitzpatrick J,. Wang M, et al. SPIE, Medical Imaging 1996; 2710:12pp.

Left Ventricular Kinematic Analysis and Cavity Measurements from the Trajectory of Geometrically 'True' Endocardial Edge on Planar ECG-Gated Myocardial Perfusion Scintigrams using Tc-99m-Tetrofosmin.

Dhan R. Jangid, Naresh Trehan
Departments of Nuclear Medicine and Cardio-thoracic Surgery,
Escorts Heart Institute and Research Center, New Delhi, INDIA.

I. INTRODUCTION

Initial attempts at left ventricular (LV-) geometric and kinematic analysis (G&K-A) from planar ECG-gated myocardial perfusion scintigrams (P-GMPS) has been discouraging because of erroneous assumption that the endocardial edge (EE) lies at inner border of P-GMPS. This 'inner' edge showed hyperkinetic motion with central collapse during closed-loop cine'-viewing of LV-systolic excursion. No serious attempt was made to localize the 'true' LVEE on the P-GMPS for calculating cord shortening fraction[1]. Also, no serious attention was given as to where exactly (in the geometric sense) the LVEE lies on perfusion scintigrams, while attempting regional wall motion analysis (RWMA)[2-4]. However, a geometric approach to the cinematic and numerical evaluation of cardiac functional parameters viz. LV-RWMA, LV-cavity size etc. would require exact localization of 'true' LVEE. We have formulated a theoretical model of P-GMPS by hybrid mathematical-computational method and found that the trajectory of geometrically true LVEE lies along circumferential count-rate maxima $[(C\phi,\max)_j]$ of the P-GMPS-sequence $[(Cx,\phi)_j]$. A computer algorithm was developed to 'image' the trajectory of LVEE from an actual multi-frame G-PMPS. This automatically generated image-sequence ($j=1,2,.........,N$) can be subjected to G&K-A for evaluation of LV- regional and global function.

II. PHYSICO-MATHEMATICAL FOUNDATION

Left ventricle (LV) is considered to be a thick walled hollow shell made up of proximal and distal halves with respect to detector of gamma camera (scintillation imaging system). The wall of the shell which represents the myocardium has internal (endocardial) and external (epicardial) radii, Ri and Ro, respectively and contains uniformly dispersed radioactivity.

Count rate ($Z(x)$) from myocardium in z-direction is given by,

$Z(x)=Zo(x)-Zi(x)$ where, $Zo(x) = \sqrt{Ro^2 - x^2}$ and $Zi(x) = \sqrt{Ri^2 - x^2}$; (Fig:1A)

Count-rate after photon attenuation from proximal half of the 'myocardial' shell (Φp) is given by,

$$Zp,a(x) = \int_{0}^{Z(x)} e^{-\mu z}\, dz = \frac{1}{\mu}[1 - e^{-\mu(Zo-Zi)}]$$

and, that from distal half of the 'myocardial' shell (Φd) is given by,

$$Zd,a(x) = Zp,a(x) \,.\, e^{-\mu(Zo+Zi)}$$

Linear cout rate profile (LCRP(x)) (Fig:1B) of a 1 mm thick concentric shaped (x,z)-slice of this 'myocardial' shell will then be given by,

$$Za(x) = Zp.a(x)+Zd,a(x) = \frac{1}{\mu}[1 - e^{-2\mu Zo} - (e^{\mu Zi} - e^{-\mu Zi}) \,.\, e^{-\mu Zo}]$$

which after considering myocardial systolic thickening (MST) correction factor (Fk) can be rewritten as,

$$Za,k(x) = (Fk/\mu).[1-e^{-2\mu Zo}-[2 \sinh(-\mu Zi)]\, e^{-\mu Zo}]$$

Where, $Fk = (R^3_{o,d}-R^3_{i,d})/(R^3_{o,k}-R^3_{i,d})$; $k = d, S_1, S_2, S_3, \ldots\ldots, ES$

$Fk = 1$, for end-diastolic (d=ED) frame.

Fig:1A. Right half of a concentric, ring-shaped 1-pixel thick slice of 'myocardial' shell

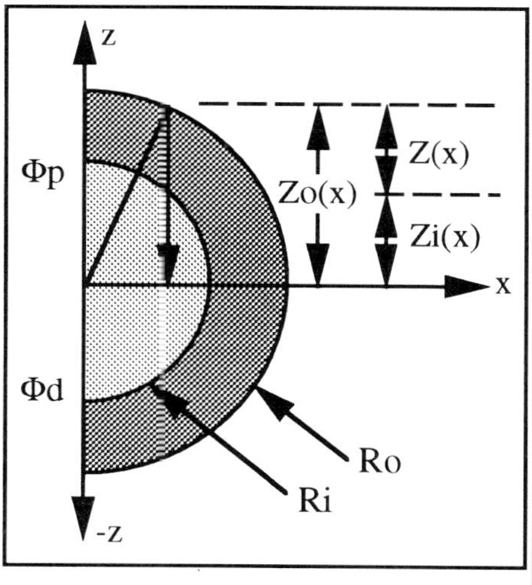

Fig:1B. Linear count-rate profile function (LCRP(x)=Za(x)) [——] and its first derivative [——].

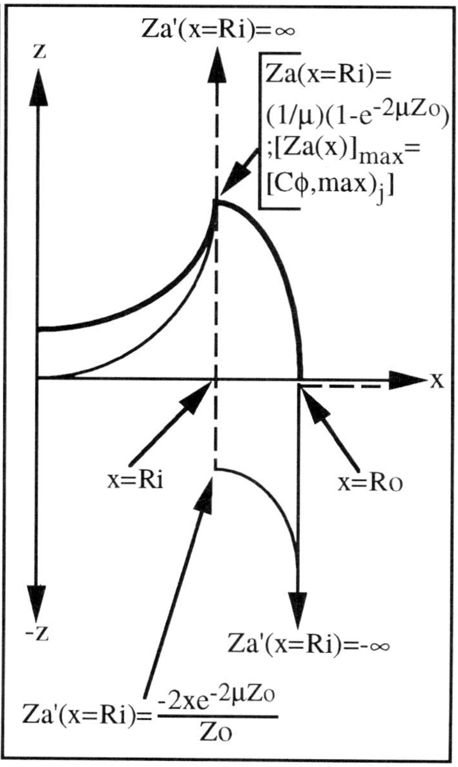

Since, there is the fixed radioactivity in the myocardium, MST would lead to decrease in the real myocardial count rate (MCR) per unit volume. However, apparent MCR from actual P-GMPS appears to increase during systole; this is because of finite spatial resolution

(S.D. of Gaussian line-spread-function; LSF(x)) of gamma camera-computer system), which can better resolve MCR spread over a larger area during systole. To take this in to consideration, Za,k(x) was convoluted with LSF(x) to obtain Ok(x) (i.e. Za,k(x) * LSF(x) = Ok(x)), the true "LCRP(x) of k-th frame of an actual P-GMPS"; Fig:3B.

Although the function Za,k(x) is piece-wise continuous, being singular (non-analytic) at Ri and Ro, yet it can still be found analytically that its maxima lies at Ri (i.e. LVEE) (Fig:1B). However, it could be convoluted with LSF(x) only numerically to obtain Ok(x). For the usual S.D. value (6 mm) of the LSF(x), the maxima of Ok(x) still lies at Ri only without significant centripetal/centrifugal drifting.

A preliminary radioactive cardiac phantom study by us did reveal that LVEE lies along the circumferential count-rate maxima $[(C\phi,\mathrm{max})_j]$ of a P-GMPS, thus providing experimental validation to the theoretically obtained position of geometrically true LV-endocardial edge[1].

III. PATIENTS AND METHODS

Patients: 9 normal individuals (<N>) and 13 patients with coronary artery disease (CAD; with ischaemia &/or infarction) were subjected to both myocardial perfusion scintigraphy as well as echocardiography for G&K-A.

Planar gated myocardial perfusion scintigraphy (P-GMPS) was performed in best-septal (BS) LAO-projection after injection of 15 mCi of Tc-99m-Tetrofosmin. Multi-frame perfusion scintigraphic study was obtained in the standard way assuring sufficient count density.This study was subjected to automated sequential image processing for obtaining 'true' LVEE (Fig:3A), using computer algorithm developed by us (Fig:2) .

Echocardiography (2D-ECHO) was performed in a projection matched view (in a plane orthogonal to direction of BS-LAO scintigraphy) to evaluate the corresponding LV- geometric and kinematic parameters.

IV. RESULTS AND DISCUSSION

Rigorous theoretical (hybrid mathematical-computational) modelling of LV-P-GMPS revealed that geometrically true LVEE $([C\phi,\mathrm{max}]_j)$ is defined by circumferential ('orthogonal') trajectory of radial count-rate maxima [(Cx,max)j] of the P-GMPS (Ok,(x)-sequence in (x,ϕ)-plane; see inset figure in Fig:2). Previous investigators possibly did not realize this fact and thus achieved lower correlation between P-GMPS and 2D-ECHO in measuring geometric parameters. Also, they faced kinematic uncertainties in regard to LV-RWMA carried out from standard P-GMPS[2-4].

Accurate G&K-A of LV has been made possible from the $(C\phi,\mathrm{max})_j$ (temporal profile of circumferential count rate maxima on multiframe scintigraphic study) on the $[\mathrm{Inv}(C'x,\phi)_j]$-sequence obtained by automated computerised image processing of actual P-GMPS (Fig:2, 3A & 3B).

Clinical results are depicted in Tables:1 & 2, and Fig:4. Measured geometric parameters by the two modalities were found to be essentially similiar with high/excellent correlation (Table:1 & 2). Also, excellent concordance especially within (±1) grade has been observed between P-GMPS and 2D-ECHO for RWMA (Fig:4).

Fig:2. Computer algorithm for generation of endocardial edge sequence

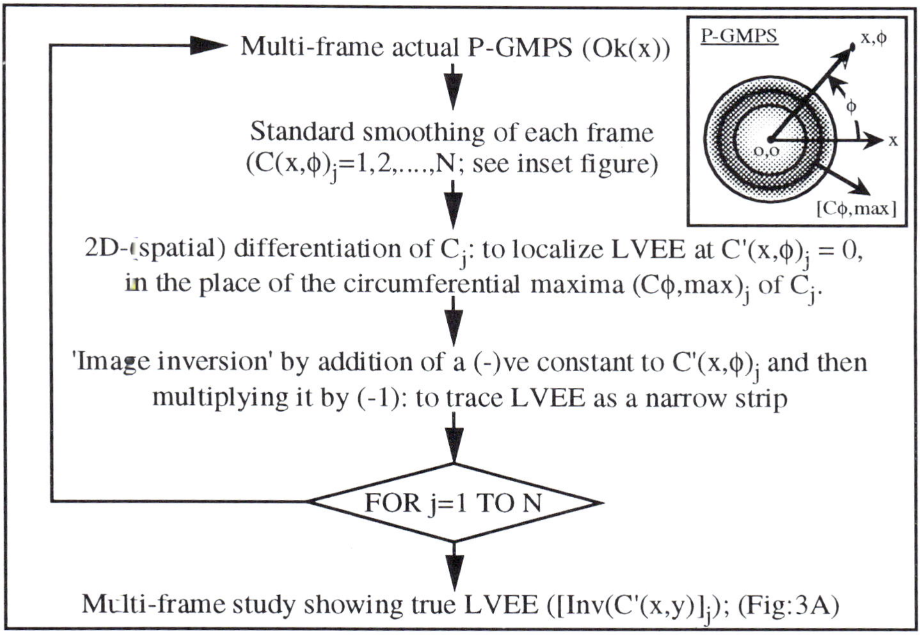

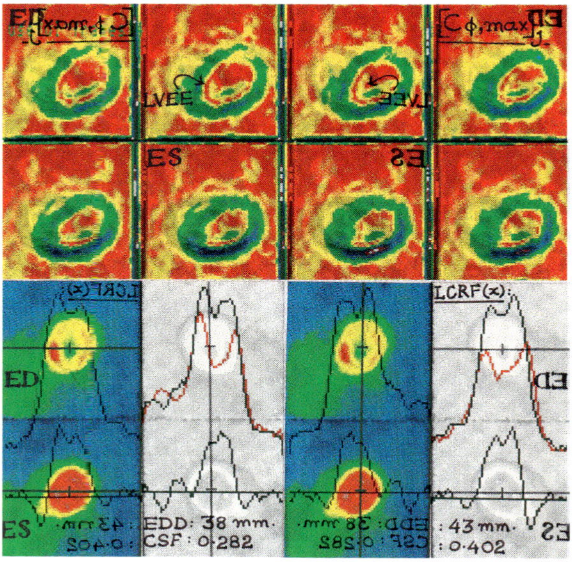

Fig:3A. Computer-generated multiframe endocardial edge (LVEE) sequence

Fig:3B. Orthogonal cord shortening fractions using true LVEE.

Table:1. Kinematic and geometric analysis for parameter evaluation using P-GMPS (in BS-LAO view) and 2D-ECHO (in geometrically matching section of four-chamber view)

	[Paired values for P-GMPS/2D-ECHO]					
	Kinematic analysis			Geometric analysis		
Pt.No.	AS	PL	AI	SAX-EDD	SAX-SF	LAO-ASF
Normal individuals (n=9)						
1.	0/0	0/0	0/0	46/45	0.348/0.356	0.48/0.50
2.	0/1	0/0	0/0	42/41	0.333/0.341	o.46/0.48
3.	0/0	0/0	1/0	39/41	0.282/0.293	0.42/0.46
4.	0/0	0/0	0/0	51/49	0.373/0.367	0.51/0.51
5.	0/0	0/0	0/0	50/51	0.320/0.314	0.46/0.44
6.	0/0	0/0	1/0	40/42	0.325/0.333	0.42/0.43
7.	0/0	0/0	0/0	43/41	0.395/0.390	0.52/0.53
8.	0/0	0/0	0/0	46/44	0.435/0.432	0.65/0.63
9.	0/0	0/0	0/0	47/45	0.426/0.422	0.62/0.63
Patients with coronary artery disease (n=13):						
1.	3/3	0/0	1/0	62/60	0.194/0.200	0.32/0.33
2.	2/2	0/0	0/0	55/52	0.255/0.250	0.41/0.39
3.	0/1	2/2	1/1	41/40	0.366/0.325	0.32/0.34
4.	4/3	1/1	0/0	64/63	0.141/0.159	0.24/0.22
5.	1/0	2/3	1/0	41/42	0.317/0.333	0.35/0.33
6.	4/3	0/0	1/2	66/62	0.136/0.145	0.28/0.26
7.	0/0	2/3	2/1	40/39	0.225/0.231	0.32/0.36
8.	0/0	1/1	3/3	51/50	0.275/0.280	0.40/0.38
9.	0/0	3/3	1/1	40/41	0.425/0.390	0.38/0.36
10.	0/1	3/3	0/0	46/48	0.391/0.396	0.40/0.41
11.	1/1	2/3	4/3	54/53	0.204/0.189	0.26/0.23
12.	0/0	2/2	0/0	39/40	0.410/0.400	0.38/0.35
13.	3/4	0/0	1/1	56/54	0.268/0.259	0.27/0.24

Myocardial segments in the matched projections:
AS = Anteroseptal; PL = Posterolateral; AI = Apicoinferior.
Grades of RWMA: 0 = Normal;1 = Hypokinesia-I (Mild-to-Moderate); 2 = Hypokinesia-II (Moderate-to Severe); 3 = Akinesia; 4 = Dyskinesia.

SAX-EDD (mm) = Short axis end-diastolic diameters
SAX-CSF = Short axis cord shortening fraction [(EDD-ESD)/EDD].
LAO-ASF = Area shortening fraction in LAO/4-Chamber view (using ellipses fitting on $(C\phi,max)_j$ of ED and ES frames).

V. CONCLUSION

Trajectory of geometrically 'true' LVEE lies along circumferential count rate maxima ($[C\phi,max]_j$) of an actual P-GMPS sequence and not at its subjective 'inner' border as assumed erroneously by previous investigators. G&K-A of true LVEE ($[Inv(C'(x,\phi)]_j$-sequence) derived computationally from P-GMPS has lead to excellent geometric correlation and kinematic concordance with 2D-ECHO.

Fig:4. Concordance of two imaging-modalities

2D-ECHO wall motion scores \ P-GMPS wall motion scores	0	1	2	3	4
0	36	6	0	0	0
1	3	5	1	0	0
2	0	1	2	2	0
3	0	0	2	4	2
4	0	0	0	1	1

Concordance rate:
Absolute = 48/66 = 72.7%
Within (±) 1 grade=100%

Table:2. Mean±S.D. and correlation (r) of parameters: P-GMPS/2D-ECHO.

Parameters	<N>	CAD
SAX-EDD	44.89+4.20/ 44.33+3.64; (r=0.911)	50.38+9.88/ 49.54+8.70; (r=0.991)
SAX-CSF	0.360+0.051/ 0.361+0.047; (r=0.993)	0.276+0.098/ 0.274+0.089; (r=0.986)
ASF	0.504+0.082/ 0.511+0.072; (r=0.970)	0.333+0.058/ 0.323+0.064; (r=0.934)

VI. REFERENCES

1. Najm YC, et al. The evaluation of ventricular fuction using gated myocardial imaging with Tc-99m MIBI. Eur Heart J 1989;10:142-148.

2. Tischler MD, et al. Validation of global and segmental left ventricular contractile fuction using gated planar technetium-99m sestamibi myocardial perfusion imaging. JACC 1994;23(1):141-145.

3. Verzijbergen J , et al. Combined assessment of technetium-99m SestaMIBI planar myocardial perfusion images at rest and during exercise with rest/ exercise left ventricular wall motion studies evaluated from gated myocardial perfusion studies. Am Heart J 1992;123:59-68.

4. Wackers FJTh, et al. Gated 99m-Tc-isonitrile myocardial perfusion imaging : disparity between endo- and epi- cardial wall motion. Circulation 1987;76(Suppl.IV):203-208.

5. Jangid DR. Trajectory of left ventricular true endocardial edge on E.C.G.-gated planar myocardial perfusion scintigraphy: geometric and kinematic implications in nuclear cardiac imaging. Proceedings of 1st Reg. Conf. of IEEE-Engg. in Med. & Biol. Soc., & 14th Conf. of Biomed. Engg. Soc. India 1995(Feb 15-18);pp 4.117-4.118

Inter and Intra-Observer Variability in the Perceived Direction of Motion with "3D" Cine Images: A Pitfall in Image Interpretation

Eliot L. Siegel and Zenon Protopapas
Department of Diagnostic Imaging, Baltimore VA Medical Center and Department of Radiology, University of Maryland Medical School, Baltimore, Maryland

Richard Weinstein, Thomas McLaurin and Eric Cameron
Department of Diagnostic Imaging, Baltimore VA Medical Center, Baltimore, Maryland

Bruce Reiner and Stephen Pomerantz
Department of Radiology, University of Maryland Medical School, Baltimore, Maryland

I. Introduction

During the past several years, there has been a trend toward an increase in the use of computer workstations for the primary interpretation of imaging studies. This is particularly true for Computed Tomography (CT), Magnetic Resonance Imaging (MRI) and Nuclear Medicine image interpretation. Although this use of soft-copy reading using computer workstations eliminates the artifacts and many of the limitations of film, the interpreting physician must now be aware of the potential pitfalls associated with the use of these workstation tools and the computer monitors.

Cine images can be particularly useful in the evaluation of bony structures in CT, MRI, and Nuclear Medicine and when viewing vascular structures in CT and MRI. Images can be obtained or reconstructed in multiple projections and displayed in rapid sequence resulting in a "three-dimensional" effect with the anatomic area of interest appearing to rotate 180 or 360 degrees.

This paper describes a potential pitfall in the interpretation of these "rotating" images in which it was discovered that the perceived direction of rotation (clockwise, counterclockwise, or oscillating) varies not only from observer to observer but changes over a short period of time for a single observer. Further, the perceived direction of rotation was found to be important in the "lateralization" of a pathologic process. Thus, the observed location (left vs. right) of a pathologic process depends upon the perceived direction of rotation of the cine image.

The purpose of this study was to determine the amount of inter and intra-observer variability in the perceived direction of motion of a "3-D cine" image and the effect of this phenomenon on lesion lateralization

II. Materials and Methods

One hundred subjects observed cine images obtained from a SPECT (Single Photon Emission Computed Tomography) nuclear bone scan which demonstrated an area of abnormal increased radiotracer uptake involving one side of the S1 vertebral body. The subjects were asked to describe the apparent motion of the pelvis as viewed on a computer workstation and whether it seemed to change during a 30 second observation period. They were also asked if they could mentally change the nature of the perceived motion and to determine the location (left vs. right) of the S1 abnormality.

III. Results

An equal number of subjects perceived the motion initially to be counter-clockwise in comparison to the number that perceived it to be clockwise with 10% reporting that it appeared to oscillate "back and forth" without completing a full revolution. During the first 30 seconds of observation, 75% of the subjects reported a spontaneous change in the apparent motion despite the fact that the cine display had, in fact, not changed. More than 90% of the subjects were subsequently able to change their perception of the direction of motion resulting in a change in the apparent side of the bone lesion.

IV. Discussion

Image interpretation of soft-copy and particularly cine images is subject to artifacts and pitfalls not encountered when images are interpreted using film. This study demonstrates that the apparent direction of motion of "three dimensional" reconstructed cine images can vary from subject to subject and can change unpredictably for a single observer over time. Although this phenomenon has been described in the perceptual psychology literature, we are not aware of any previous description in the imaging literature. Since the perceived direction of motion determines the apparent location of a pathologic process, this potential pitfall must be taken into account when interpreting these imaging studies using a computer workstation.

The Difference in Diagnostic Accuracy Between the Original Film and the Digitized Image of the Bone Scintigram

Shoji Terui, Takashi Terauchi and Hiroyuki Abe
Division of Nuclear Medicine, National Cancer Center Hospital, Tokyo, Japan

I. Introduction

Picture archiving and communication(PACS) has become a vital tool in radiology, but the images processed with an analogue type of gamma cameras have to be digitized for archiving. Picture archiving systems with film-digitizer have been developed in order to file these type of scintigrams. We have no experience in monitor reporting[1,2]. Here arises the question that monitor reporting to be able to rely on compared with the conventional film-screen system. Almost 6 months, we tried to compare in this paper the differential diagnostic accuracy between the original films(conventional film-screen system) and the digitized images on the monitor concerning the abnormal accumulations on the bone scintigram; the aim is our daily clinical reading.

II. Characteristics of the Hospital

The National Cancer Center Hospital in Tokyo is a cancer hospital and has 550 beds. The nuclear medicine department is independent from the other X-ray diagnostic division. The annual number of nuclear medicine examinations is around 3000 of whom approximately 80% are bone scanning.

III. Archiving and Display Architecture

Since 1992, our division of nuclear medicine has installed small local PACS(SIPACS ^{R}, Shimadzu Medical, Japan).

*Host CPU 32 bits with 4MB memory
*Local CPU 32 bits with 4MB memory
*System disk(600MB)
*Image display memory(32 MB, 2000x2000 matrix for 4 images)
*Diagnostic reporting console(a CRT size of 20 in., and a spatial resolution of up to 1000 lines)
*Film digitizer(LD-4500 R, Konica, Japan)

IV. Materials and Methods

From April 1992 to October 1992, 941 patients with clinically proofs of malignancies received bone scintigram. They were 371 males and 520 females(aged 11 - 85 years, with mean age, 56.6 years). The clinical diagnosis of these patients represented as following: 422 with breast cancer, 230 with lung cancer, 47 with prostate cancer, 41 with esophageal cancer, 25 with liver cancers and 176 with the other type of malignancies. Of these scintigraphy, 581 were the very first examination and 360 cases were the cases with the repeated one.

The examinations of Tc-99m bone scintigraphy were performed in the following way: a dose of 740MBq of Tc-99m HMDP was administered intravenously and the scintigraphic images were taken 2 - 3 hours later using 3 gamma cameras(Simens ZLC, Technicare sigma 410S, and Shimadzu LFOV). For the bone imaging, both the whole body and the spot images were taken in all patients. All these scintigrams were taken in 11 x 14 inches film. These films were digitized into 1024 x 1024 matrix in 12 bits with 0-3.5 range of optical density. The digitized image was displayed in 1024 x 1024 matrix in 8 bits on a 20 inch monitor. The monitor has a spatial resolution of up to 1000 lines. Whole body image was displayed in 512 x 1024 matrix and the spot images were in 512 x 512 matrix. Pixel value of the digitized image is fixed to linear and it's proportion to the reporting console is 1:1.

We compare the detection and the number of the abnormal accumulations on the bone scintigram between the monitor reporting and the conventional film-screen system in our daily clinical reading. Accumulations due to arthritis and the post surgical changes were excluded in this study.

The monitor reporting was scored initially by a radiologist and the result was compared with the result of the conventional film-screen system, a result arrived at by consensus of three experienced radiologists Drs.(S.T., T.T., H.A.). The window level was occasionally adjusted by a clinician-interpreter. In the process, we employ observer performance test with receiver operating characteristic(ROC).

V. Results

For the monitor reporting, 511(54.3%) of the 941 patients are registered in as having no abnormal accumulation and 514(54.6%) registered in as having abnormal accumulations. The coincidence was obtained in 846(89.9%) patients between the monitor reporting and the conventional film-screen system. However, 95(10.1%) patients were pointed out the mismatch.

ROC analysis showed that there were 81 false positives (16%), and 14 false negatives (3.2%). The sensitivity was 96.8%, but, the positive predictive value was 83.3%. Therefore, the diagnostic accuracy was 90%(Table 1). Of these 95 mismatched patients, 745 abnormal accumulations were pointed out on the monitor reporting. But, on the film-screen system, only 682 abnormal accumulations were confirmed. Comparing the film-screen system, 108 accumulations in the 45 patients were diagnosed as over-estimated and 66 accumulations in the 50 patients were missed on the monitor reporting. In these 50 missed cases, 17 abnormal accumulations of 14 patients were missed and these patients were diagnosed as normal appearance by the monitor reporting. The rest of the 36 patients were missed several accumulations in the multiple abnormal accumulations on the bone scintigram. Concerning about the 45 over-estimated patients, all of the 45 were diagnosed as having metastasis to the bone. But, 21 of these 45 patients could not pointed out any abnormal accumulation at all on the film-screen system, then the diagnosis have to change to normal appearance. The other 24 patients of the 45 were the patient with multiple abnormal accumulations and 56 of 282 accumulations(19.9%) were over-estimated on the monitor reporting.

Table 1. ROC Analysis of the Monitor Reporting

Number of tests		941
Case of correct test	True positive	420
	True negative	426
Case of test error	False positive	81
	False negative	14
Positive predictive value (%)		83.8%
Negative predictive value (%)		96.8%
Sensitivity (%)		96.8%
Specificity (%)		84.0%
Diagnostic accuracy (%)		89.9%

VI. Discussion

It is one of the key issue of filmless radiology to be able to rely on monitors for daily practical reporting in nuclear medicine[3]. The diagnostic accuracy of monitor that has to be at least equal to film based reporting.

There is no reports comparing the differential diagnostic accuracy between the film-screen system and the monitor reporting concerning the abnormal accumulations on the bone

scintigram. Our studies have shown that the monitor reporting have no diagnostic superiority over conventional film-screen system and show 10% mismatched diagnostic performance as optimal exposed conventional film-screen system. The reasons of this mismatch were considered the followings:(1) Our reporting room has not light-control system, so the interpreter sitting in front of the diagnostic console complain of early fatigue and eye strain, (2) the monitor of our installation was not a high luminance -it's only 50FL, (3) the difference of the density resolution between the monitor (8 bits-256 step) and the digitized image(12 bits-4096 step) resulted in loss of the contrast resolution through digitalization.
Actually, the interpreter adjusted window and brightness very occasionally. It confused the interpreter too much because there is no adequate scale on the digitized image for nuclear medicine. In questionable cases, the interpreter seems to be over-estimation about the accumulation.

Cancer patients were followed-up bone scintigrams for the evaluation of therapeutic effects consecutively. In our experience, the high rate of the false positive(16%) and the false negative(3.2%) results affect the patient's treatments and prognosis. The monitor reporting has decreased the diagnostic quality of bone scintigram in routine operation and it needs the increased amount of time necessary to perform this kind of work.
In conclusion, without film-screen check-up, the monitor reporting of the digitized images seems to be limited value in nuclear medicine. Here arise a problem to be solved in future.

References

1. Lyttkens K, Andersson B, Kehler M, Lindberg L. Bedside chest radiography using digital luminescence. A comparison between digital

radiographs reviewed on a personal computer and as hard copies. Acta Radiol 1992;33:427-430

2. Franken EA Jr, Smith WL, Berbaum KS, Kao SC, Sato Y. Comparison of a PACS workstation with conventional film for interpretation of neonatal examinations: a paired comparison study. Pediatr Radiol 1991;21:336-340
3. Fahey FH., Harkness BA., Gage HD., Eades CG., Williams RC. and Keyser JW Jr. Implementation and experience with a filmless positron emission tomography center. SCAR 94 Symposium for computer assisted radiology 1994;43-48

3D Reconstruction of Thoracic Vessels in Patients with Aortic Diseases from MRA Data

Beier J.
Virchow Klinikum Strahlem- und Poliklinik, Humboldt University Berlin
Diegold Th, Vogl Th and R. Felix
Virchow Klinikum, Strahlem- und Poliklinik, Humboldt University Berlin
Tröger J. and E. Fleck
German Heart Institute Berlin, Virchow Klinikum, Germany

1. Introduction

MR angiography has become an important modality in assessing aortic diseases like aneurysms, dissections and caliber changes. It represents a completely non-invasive examination without the need for contrast agent and without radiation. In the last years MRA has become an alternative and an addition to conventional angiography, CT angiography and ultrasound. Conventional diagnosis of 2D MRA images is limited to the assessment of vascular cross-sections, as presented in the slice images. Results are still far from satisfactory when it comes to visual inspection of two-dimensional images for answers to more complicated questions, such as the configuration of a stenosis or the shape of a bifurcation or the course of a given vascular system. Hence, three-dimensional representation of vessels is very helpful. By providing the surgeon with high-quality three-dimensional reconstructions of the present status of the aortic anatomy, the surgery can be planned and optimum techniques can be selected.

2. Segmentation and 3D Reconstruction

High-resolution magnetic resonance angiography (MRA) examinations were performed using the following acquisition parameters: slice thickness 3.0 - 6.0 mm, no gap, field of view 350 - 450 mm, calibration 0.65 - 0.90 mm/pixel, TR: 29 ms, TE: 7 ms, matrix 256 x 512, 1 acquisition, Magnetom SP 63, 1.5 Tesla (Siemens, Erlangen, Germany). The generated images were transferred for further processing to external workstations (SUN Sparc 20, SGI Indy) via a housewide network (Ethernet).

The first processing step at the external workstation is the segmentation of relevant structures in the MRA slices, e.g. the true and the false lumen of a dissection, aneurysms, plaques and calcifications. For segmentation of the image data, different manual and automatic procedures were implemented:

- manual drawing of contours using the mouse,
- manual demarcation of Bezier and cubic spline base points,
- automatic region growing: seed point, two thresholds, minimal region area,
- automatic cost matrix contour tracing.

The contours can easily be manipulated (move, add, delete base point, region editor) or by morphological functions (erosion, dilation). The resulting contours are assigned to specific objects („aorta", „lumen", „plaque", etc). The contours are stored in a database and can be retrieved for further processing at a later time.

Fig. 1 demonstrates the program for image segmentation. Several menus help the user to create and manipulate objects and contours. The resulting contours of all or individual objects are displayed in the image. A pictorial image browser helps to navigate through the image stack. These functions allow the comfortable and fast processing of the image data even with a large number of MRA slices.

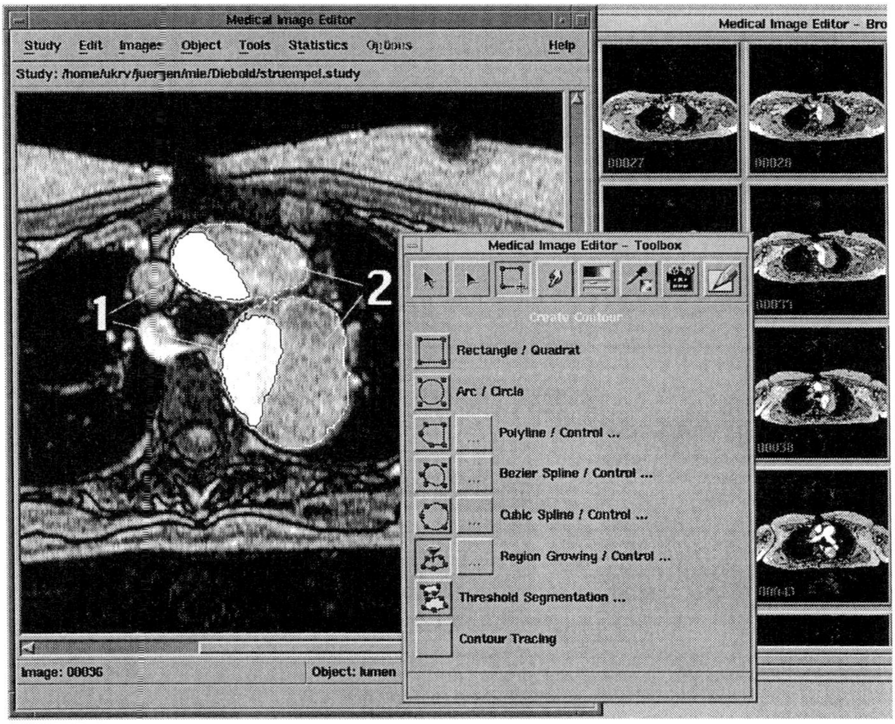

Fig. 1: Image segmentation of MRA images
(1: remaining flow within the aorta, 2: aortic dissection)

3. Visualization

After completion of the contour detection, the images are 3D reconstructed by two methods: 1. maximum intensity projection (MIP) and 2. shaded surface display.

We have implemented software for the visualization of volumetric image data in MIP and volume rendering mode. This software is based on the IAP

software (ISG Technologies, Mississauga, Canada) and allows the display from orthogonal (axial, coronal, sagittal) and further arbitrary projections.
Due to the high signal intensity of the blood vessels in the MRA images, it is generally sufficient to calculate the MIP images from unsegmented MRA data. In cases with mutiple overlays it was helpful to use segmented images instead to obtain a more suuficient result.

Fig. 2 shows the coronal MIP image of a MRA examination (55 slices, 0.88 mm/pixel, 2.7 mm slice thickness, no gap) of a patient with an extented dissection in the aortic arch (Marfan syndrom). Due to the projection in this MIP image, the vessels overlay and are hard to distinct from each other. The non-perfused (false) lumen of the aorta cannot be seen at all in this image.

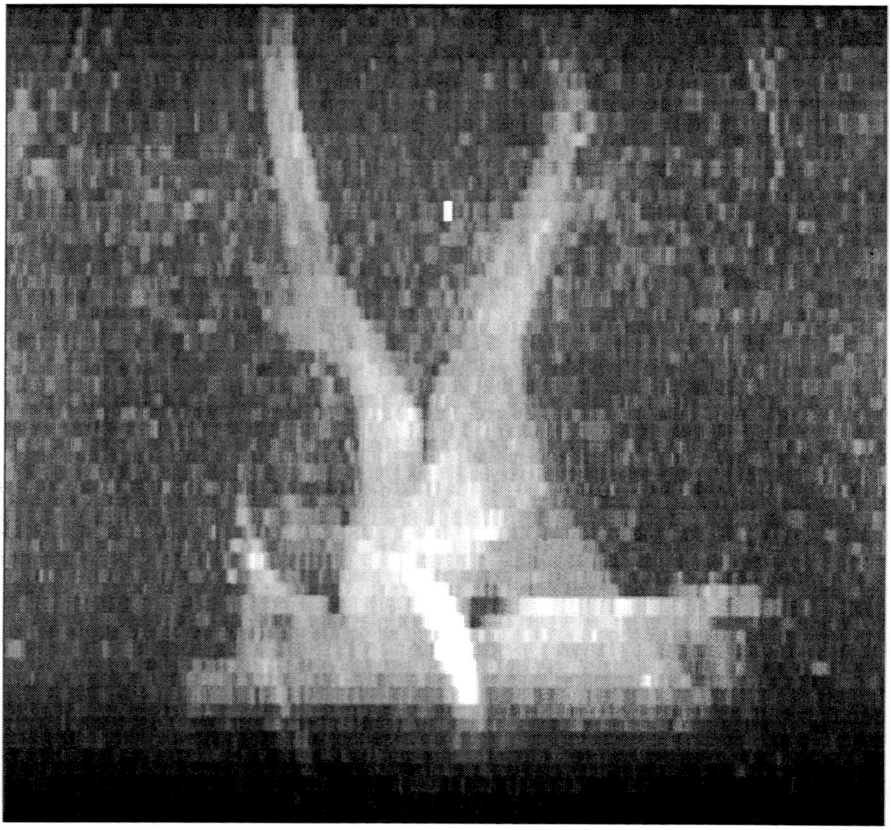

Fig. 2: Maximum intensity projection image of the aortic arch (dissection caused by Marfan syndrom)

In addition to the MIP technique, all 2D contours of an object are triangulated to form a three-dimensional surface. The result of this triangulation process is transferred into the AVS software (Advanced Visual Systems, Inc. [3]). The resulting 3D data can be displayed and manipulated interactively with AVS: arbitrary rotations, translations and scalings can be performed. Objects can be moved separately, thus allowing the assessment to be free from superimpositions by other structures. Each object has properties of its own, like color, intensity, hue, reflection, texture, opacity, etc. With one or more light sources perspective effects and shadow casts are to be generated. This 3D scene can be animated and the original MRI data can be integrated, too. We have developed special AVS modules for the reading of ACR-NEMA/DICOM images and calculated triangulated surfaces. The integration of original MRA data in the 3D scene is possible by different methods:

- The display of a bounding box and a coordinate system emphasizes the perspective of the observers eye. The spacing information is read automatically from the ACR-NEMA files, thus, the axes are labelled in absolute values (mm).
- One or more cut planes through the MRA volume allow the display of slice data together with the other three-dimensional objects. The orientation of the cut planes is arbitrary and does not has to be orthogonal. Brightness and contrast are adjusted by sliders. When using oblique cuts, an interpolation for the reformatting can be switched on, thus, avoiding hard steps between adjacent slices.
- From the data cube of the entire examination a second cube is cut away. The MRA data is mapped on the walls of the remainder. The wall positions are adjusted interactively.
- The original MRA data can be mapped directly on the surfaces of segmented 3D objects.

A composite visualization of 3D objects of different type in one common 3D space was used to display the stent and surrounding structures: objects triangulated from contours, isosurfaces from thresholding, volume rendering, and original MRA data (cut planes, data cubes). Furthermore, this 3D scene can be animated by the AVS animator. The user just defines two (or more) states of the 3D scene and a sequence of images is computed with a specified number of steps in between. This can be the rotation of the entire scene, a zooming, or a change of the opacity of individual objects.

Fig. 3 shows the reconstructed object surfaces of this patient. The perfused lumina are displayed with a solid color, the aneurysm due to the Marfan syndrom is displayed with transparency. Compared to the corresponding MIP image, this kind of representation is independent from object superimpostions and the individual vessel can clearly be distincted from each other. Furthermore, signal inhomogeneties within the stack of MRA images (see Fig. 2) have no impact on the visualization of the vessels.

4. Planning and Control

The 3D reconstructions help the physician to show the position, shape, and extent of a lesion (aneurysm, dissection, stenosis) and its spatial relation to surrounding structures. The indication and feasibility of a possible intervention is assessed and supported using this knowledge. Quantitative parameters are obtained by distance measurements in the 2D slices and within the 3D space by indicating surface points.

In a study together with the cardiologists and cardiosurgeons, we created 3D reconstructions of the thoracic aorta in 10 patients with different aortic diseases (aneurysms, coarctations, Marfan syndroms). Questions of surgical interest are: location of the neck of the aneurysm, its size and extent, caliber differences, dissection type, and stenoses or dilatations of surrounding vessels. The three-dimensional reconstructions we provided help in answering these questions and in planning surgical interventions.

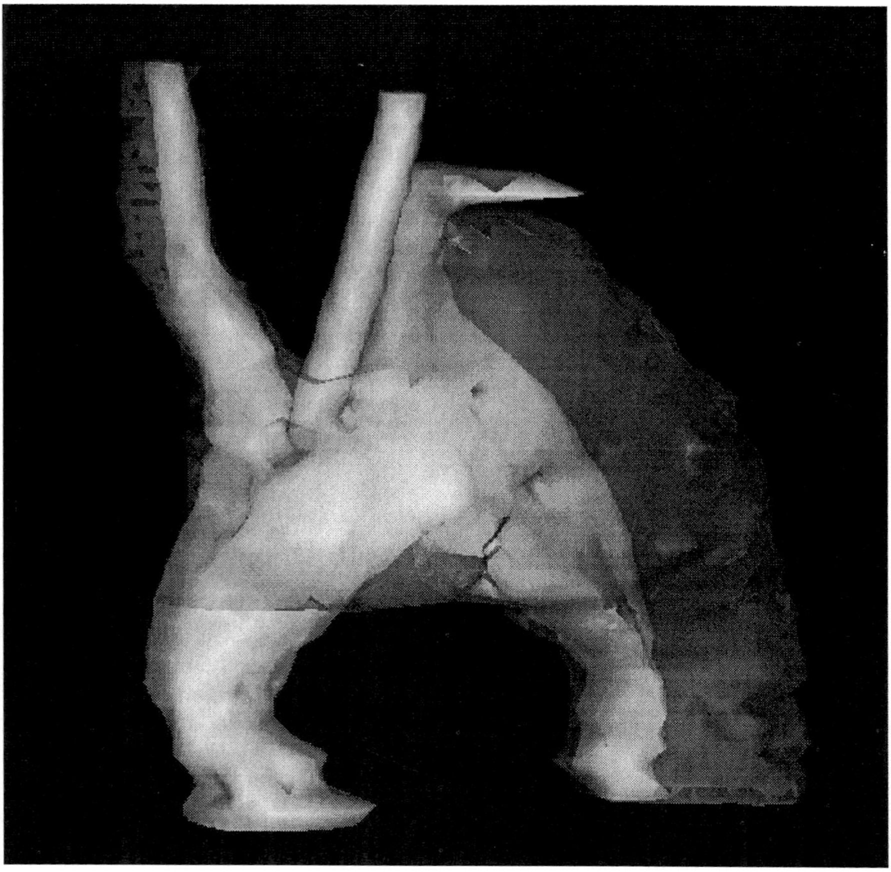

Fig. 3: Surface representation of the aortic arch
(free lumen (opaque), dissection (transparent))

5. Conclusions

The three-dimensional surface reconstructions of the aortic vessels based on the MRA examinations allow a better assessment of the vessel geometry and exact measurements compared to the maximum intensity projection technique.

Furthermore, MRA represents a three-dimensional, high resolution modality. As a non-invasive examination, it only requires the intravenous injection of contrast agent. Thus, MRA has become a comparative and competitive modality to conventional angiography and spiral CT angiography in the diagnosis of aortic vessels.

By providing the physician with high-quality 3D reconstructions of the aortic region the surgery can be planned and long term follow-ups can be controlled.

References

[1] AVS Manuals: AVS User´s Guide, AVS Developers´s Guide, AVS Module Reference, AVS Animator, Advanced Visual Systems Inc., 300 Fifth Avenue, Waltham, MA02154, USA, 1994

[2] Beier J, Siekmann R, Müller F, Stalke J, Biamino G, Fleck E, Felix R Three-Dimensional Reconstruction of Implanted Aortic Stents using Computed Tomography, Comp. in Card 1995, pp. 549 - 552

[3] Beier J, Siekmann R, Müller F, Stalke J, Biamino G, Fleck E, Felix R: Planning and Control of Aortic Stent Implantation using 3D Reconstructions based on Computed Tomography, CAR 96, in press

[4] Rubin GD, Walker PJ, Dake MD, Napel S, Miller DC: Three-dimensional spiral computed tomographic angiography : an alternative imaging modality for the abdominal aorta and ist branches, J Vasc Surg, 1993, 18(4), pp. 656 - 664

3-D Reconstruction of Upper Airway MR Images in Healthy and Anesthetized Volunteers

O. Esch, M.D., R. Garza, M.S. II, M. Mathru, M.D., R. Patterson, Ph.D., D. Brunder, Ph.D., G. Hillmann, Ph.D., M.W. Willcott, Ph.D. and E. vanSonnenberg, M.D.

Departments of Radiology, Anesthesia, Orthopedics, and the Office of Academic Computing, University of Texas Medical Branch, Galveston, Texas

I. INTRODUCTION:

During anesthesia, hypotonia of the pharynx causes associated structures such as the tongue, uvula, and epiglottis to relax and thus obstruct the airway. It is the traditional view that the hypotonia of the tongue is responsible to a large extent for such obstruction. Since the underlying mechanisms that lead to airway obstruction during anesthesia are similar to those leading to sleep apnea, we have shown that anesthesia-induced pharyngeal narrowing could be counteracted by applying nasal continuous positive airway pressure (CPAP).[1] Nasal CPAP restores patency to the pharyngeal airway by creating a positive transmural pressure that functions as pneumatic splint. In this study, we quantified the volume of the upper-airway in three

different states: awake, during anesthesia, and during anesthesia with continuous positive airway pressure . The volume of air between the tip of the uvula and the tip of the epiglottis in each state is the determining factor. We investigated the volume change from collapse or expansion of the upper airway during different states with the anesthetic agent Propofol which is widely used to induce intravenous general anesthesia. Its properties can include relaxation of the upper airway muscles, and airway obstruction. We approached this task by measuring degree of collapse from two angles: a traditional approach with two radiologists blinded to the study manually measuring predefined distances from 2D sagittal MR images, and a computer aided system using a locally developed semi-automated boundary tracer. Data from each approach were used to correlate the degree of upper-airway volume changes during the different states of anesthesia to determine the degree of airway obstruction and the effectiveness of CPAP to relieve obstruction.

II. MATERIAL AND METHODS:

MR acquisition

In 5 healthy volunteers (aged 27-34 yr.), sagittal and axial T1-weighted images (slice thickness 3 mm or less, TR 500 msec, TE 25 msec) were obtained on a 1.5TE magnet using an anterior surface neck coil (General Electric). Images were obtained during the awake state, propofol sedation, and propofol plus 10 cm H20 nasal CPAP application. Propofol was administered in 50 mg increments every 30 sec to a maximum of 300 mg, or until the eyelash reflex could not be evoked

Manual calculation

Two radiologists blinded to the state of anesthesia independently measured the following minimum anteroposterior distances: pharynx to dorsum of the tongue (Diam T); pharynx to epiglottis tip (Diam E); pharynx to soft palate (Diam SP). Airway volume was calculated using Diam E and mean axial radii at each level, assuming this space as a truncated cone. Statistical analysis was performed using a two-tailed Student t-test.

Computer-aided calculation

Images were obtained in a proprietary format and consisted of 3 mm thick contiguous slices in an axial plane with a field of view of 20 and a matrix of 256 X 128 pixels. After file transfer and conversion to flat file format, images were reconstructed in a three dimensional model using a suite of locally developed medical image analysis software packages on a SunSparc 10 and Kubuta Pacific Titan 3000 workstation. On the Sparc platform, three different programs were used to contour image boundaries, calculate the volume, and create the graphics file necessary to visualize the 3D reconstructions respectively. The expertise of a blinded radiologist using the Wrist program manually corrected the soft tissue structures' outline in the digitized flat file images. The contour information resulting from the boundary points of each soft tissue structure was saved to a data file (.dat) consisting of x, y and z coordinates. After processing all slices, the coordinates for each structure were collected and grouped by the do_stats program for calculating volume of each structural object and other statistical characteristics. The algorithm for volume calculation involved stacking the outlines along the z axis at the corresponding interval and interpolating the space between each pair of slices. The interpolation defined the space between each continuos slice as a conic frustum. The resulting frusta's volumes were then added and the airway volume estimated.

Computer-aided visualization

After statistically analyzing the data sets and calculating the geometric parameters, correctness of the boundaries was demonstrated. Visualization of the location of each soft tissue component (object) was performed, and spatial relationship among each other confirmed by conversion of the contour data file (.dat) consisting of x, y and z coordinates into a graphics file (.tri). The do_avs program made this a simple procedure using an algorithm that involved covering the boundary data set obtained from the slices with triangular tiles. The program used the contour points as vertices for the bases and apices for the generated trianglular tiles. The resulting graphics file (.tri) was remotely acquired via network by the Kubuta workstation. This workstation housed the commercial available Evans and Sutherland AVS system. The graphic file (.tri) were then converted to AVS geometry by a locally developed AVS input module. The resulting 3D models viewed by the standard geometry viewer were colored, shaded, rotated, and enlarged for inspection from all conceivable angles. This process was repeated for each patient and state.

III. RESULTS:

Manual calculation

	mean Diam T (mm)	mean Diam E (mm)	mean Diam SP (mm)	mean Volume (mm3)
Awake	11.63	10.63	6.57	4200.6
Sedation	7.88	7.00	2.71 #	2437.6
Sedation CPAP	12.88*	9.63	8.43*	5847. 1*

* Significant compared to sedation (p=0.0136)
# Significant compared to awake state (p=0.0025)

Minimum anteroposterior diameter of the pharynx at the level of the soft palate decreased from 6.6 ± 2.2 mm (SD) in the awake state to 2.7 ± 1.5 mm ($P < 0.05$) during propofol anesthesia and increased to 8.43 ± 2.5 mm ($P < 0.05$) after nasal CPAP application. Anteroposterior diameter of the pharynx at the level of the dorsum of the tongue increased from 7.9 ± 3-5 mm during propofol anesthesia to 12.9 ± 3.6 mm ($P < 0.05$) after nasal CPAP. Pharyngeal volume (from the tip of the epiglottis to the tip of the soft palate, assuming this space to be a truncated cone) significantly increased from 2,437 ± 1,008 mm3 during propofol anesthesia to 5,847 ± 2,827 mm3 ($P < 0.05$) after nasal CPAP application.

Computer-aided calculation

	mean Volume (mm3)
Awake	2360.66
Sedation	1393.94
Sedation CPAP	3186.26 *

* Significant compared to sedation (p=0.0406)

Pharyngeal volume (from the tip of the epiglottis to the tip of the uvula) significantly increased from 1393.94 ± 1670.70 mm3 during propofol anesthesia to 3186.26 ± 1959.32 mm3 ($P < 0.05$) after nasal CPAP application.

IV. CONCLUSION:

The volume calculations and the spatial relationships visualized from the 3D model indicate that the airway narrowing during sedation occurs at the level of the soft palate and not at the level of the tongue; obstruction was relieved by the application of nasal CPAP. Image reconstruction of the upper airway resulted in significantly improved understanding of complex spatial changes during anesthesia and more accurate measurements. This was particularly important since these findings differ from the traditional view that airway obstruction during anesthesia is caused by hypotonia of the tongue and movement towards the posterior pharyngeal wall. The manual volume calculations were less accurate than the computerized, but this did not influence the statistical significance of relative upper airway changes. The computerized process was complex and time consuming but did offer advantages: unique and superior to the manual approach was the use of a visualization tool to illustrate anatomical changes and thus complementing both manual and computerized measurements. Visualization of complex image objects and their relationship proved to be a useful tool for the radiologists involved, but was absolutely essential for the non-radiologists to better understand the mechanisms of upper airway obstruction.

V. REFERENCES

1. Mathru M, Esch O, Lang J, Herbert M, Chaljub G, Goodacre B, vanSonnenberg E: Magnetic Resonance Imaging of the Upper Airway. Anesthesiology 84, No. 2: 001-007, Feb 1996.

2. Tagare H, Elder K, Stoner D, R Patterson, Nicodemus C, Viegas S, Hillman G: Location and Geometric Description of Carpal Bones in CT Images. Annals of Biomedical Engineering 21: 715-726, 1993.

Automated Total Lung Capacity Measurement from Computed Radiography Chest Images

Siu K. Yu, Lianne Tan, Karen Finlay, Craig Coblentz and Claude Nahmias

Department of Radiology, Chedoke-McMaster Hospitals and McMaster University Hamilton, Ontario, Canada

I. INTRODUCTION

Total lung capacity (TLC) measurements are useful in the management of lung disease. A radiographic method is desirable as chest radiographs are easily obtainable. Barnhard et al[1] developed a radiographic method using two views of the chest. The method models the chest as a stack of elliptical cylindroids, and considers the contribution of non-gas containing structures in the estimation of the TLC. The value and accuracy of this radiographic TLC determination have been previously confirmed[4-5]. However, the time involved in performing the method on film has, in part, limited its use. With the ability to manipulate digital images acquired by computed radiography, we developed a fast and easy-to-use automated technique for determining TLC based on Barnhard's multiple ellipsoid method. The automated technique and its results are presented in this paper.

II. METHODS AND MATERIALS

36 standard posterior-anterior (PA) and left lateral computed radiographs of the chest at maximum inspiration were obtained at a target distance of 6 feet. The radiographs were taken with the patient erect; and the arms of the patient were raised for the lateral exposure. The magnification factors for each view were obtained directly by taping a reference object of known size to the sides of the chest (axillary line for the PA view, anterior midline for the lateral view) as suggested by Bush et al[2].

The radiographic images were directly acquired using a Fuji AC-1 computed radiography system and transferred to a Sun Sparcstation IPX for TLC measurement using the automated technique. Based on Barnhard's method, the total thoracic volume was estimated by the volume of five elliptical cylindroids from which the non-gas containing portion, occupied by the diaphragm, heart, pulmonary tissue and pulmonary blood, was subtracted to give the estimation of TLC. User-interaction is limited to identifying 5 anatomical locations on each view. The volumes of pulmonary tissue and pulmonary blood were estimated using the method suggested by McGaff et al[6].

Image Segmentation

The digital radiographs with a grey-scale of 1024 are stored in pixel matrices of 2048x2048. In order to speed up the segmentation process, the matrix size of both views is resampled to 638x638. This matrix size was chosen because it is the maximum allowable for displaying both chest views on the same screen using our display programs. A 9x9 median filter is applied to both images since it preserves edge information while removing noise[3]. In order to enhance the contrast between the lungs and the other tissues, the pixel values of the images are altered so that pixels with values higher than an upper threshold value are set to a predefined maximum value; pixels with values lower than a lower threshold value are set to a predefined minimum value; and pixels with values bounded by the upper and lower thresholds are rescaled linearly.

PA View

With both PA and lateral images displayed on the same screen, the user is prompted to identify five points on the PA view. The locations of the points are : a lung apex (PA1), both costophrenic angles (PA2 & PA5), and both cardiophrenic angles (PA3 & PA4), as shown in Figure 1a. The user is given an option to either use an average magnification factor (derived from 20 patient cases), or to select two more points for measuring the size of the reference object for calculating the magnification factor. The user is also required to enter the weight of the patient in order to estimate the pulmonary tissue and pulmonary blood volumes.

The PA view is thresholded to obtain a binary image which indicates the rough location of the boundaries of the lungs. The two lungs are first identified as being separated by the maximum pixel value in each row of the mediastinal region of the image. Each lung is then divided vertically into two regions, separated by the minimum pixel value for each row of the image within that lung region. The threshold value for each row in each region is calculated as:

$$T_{ij} = min_{ij} + g_{ij}(max_{ij}-min_{ij})/2 \qquad (1.1)$$

where T_{ij} is the local threshold value for row i and region j; min_{ij} and max_{ij} are respectively the minimum pixel value and maximum pixel value for row i and region j; and g_{ij} is a normalizing factor tailored to each region j.

Since the lungs are bounded by the rib cage, all possible edges of the ribs within each lung are located by tracking the maximum gradient. A Sobel filter[3] is passed through the original image to obtain a gradient image. The searching algorithm is applied at every 5th row of the gradient image, from the apex down to the level of the costophrenic angle, with starting points lying on the estimated lung region boundaries obtained from the binary image. If a search extends beyond the lung apex or beyond the costophrenic angles, or tracks a rib curvature back to the estimated lung region boundary obtained from the binary image, then that particular search is terminated. This search algorithm is applied to both the costal and the mediastinal boundaries. When all of the search paths are exhausted, the inside edges of the ribs are identified, and the costal and mediastinal contours of each lung, as well as the cardiac notch, are outlined as shown in Figure 2a. Assuming the cardiac notch is located below the 3rd ellipsoid and above the specified points PA3 and PA4 in the left and right heart borders respectively, the long diameter of the heart is estimated as the longest possible line joining the left heart border with point PA4 of the right heart border; and the second diameter of the heart is found by constructing lines extending perpendicularly from the long diameter to the furthest points of the left and right heart borders. The diaphragmmatic contours of each lung are outlined by searching along the maximum gradient starting from one costophrenic angle to its nearest cardiophrenic angle.

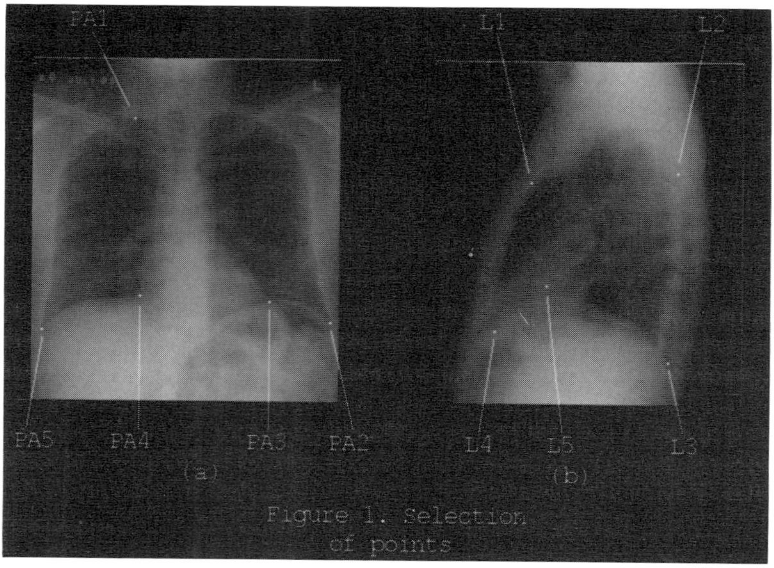

Figure 1. Selection of points

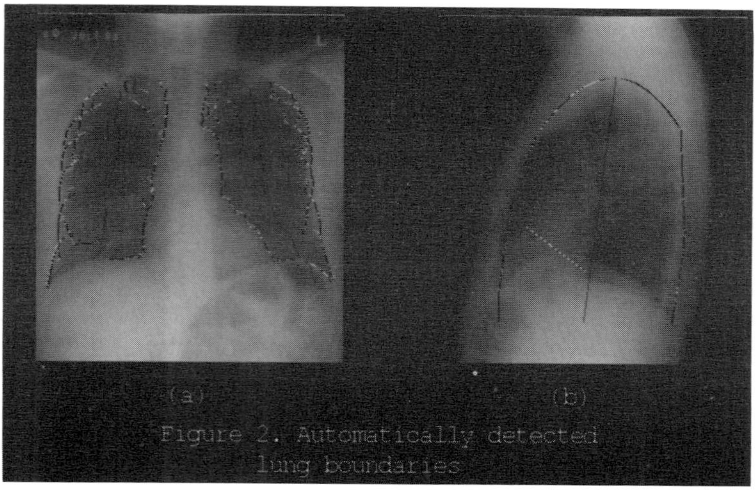

Figure 2. Automatically detected lung boundaries

Lateral view

Similar to the segmentation procedure of the PA view, the user is required to identify five points on the lateral view. The first two points (L1 and L2 in Figure 1b) are required to identify the apical region in which the lung boundary becomes difficult to identify. Points L3 and L4 identify the posterior and anterior costophrenic angles. The last specified point (L5) should be the center of the heart. Again, the user is given an option to either use an average magnification factor, or to select two additional points for measuring the size of the reference object for calculating the magnification factor.

The postero-inferior lung margin (i.e. between points L2 and L3 in Figure 1b) is assumed to follow approximately the contour of the body. Thus, the body contour is first outlined by thresholding the image, and then a copy of this contour is moved anteriorly, based on the distances between L2 and L3 and the body contour, to estimate the posterior lung margin. A central axis which roughly divides the lung into two equal sections is formed by joining the mid-point between points L1 and L2, and the mid-point between points L3 and L4. This line is extended to the height of the lung apex as specified on the PA view. The anterior lung margin is then estimated by flipping the posterior lung contour about this central axis. The anterior lung contour is then adjusted to align itself with points L1 and L4.

The anterosuperior lung margin is estimated by fitting a parabolic function to point L1 and the top of the central axis. Similarly, the posterosuperior lung margin is outlined by fitting a parabolic function to point L2 and the top of the central axis. The estimated lung contour and the calculated central axis are shown in Figure 2b.

The long diameter of the heart is assumed to be at a 60 degree angle from the central axis. The edges of the heart are estimated by starting at point L5 and searching along the long diameter until one of the following conditions is met : (a) the gradient is smaller than a predefined value, (b) the line is crossing the estimated anterior lung contour, or (c) the line is passing from the 4th to the 5th ellipsoid.

Manual correction

Once the contours of the lungs are outlined in both PA and lateral views, the required measurements are automatically performed and superimposed on the displayed images The total thoracic volume, the volumes of the heart and the diaphragm, and the resulting TLC are automatically calculated and displayed (Figure 3). The operator can view or save the on-screen results and perform any manual correction if required. If, for example, the automatic segmentation has incorrectly identified a lung boundary point, manual correction simply involves two mouse clicks: identifying the point and selecting its correct location. All of the measurements are automatically updated.

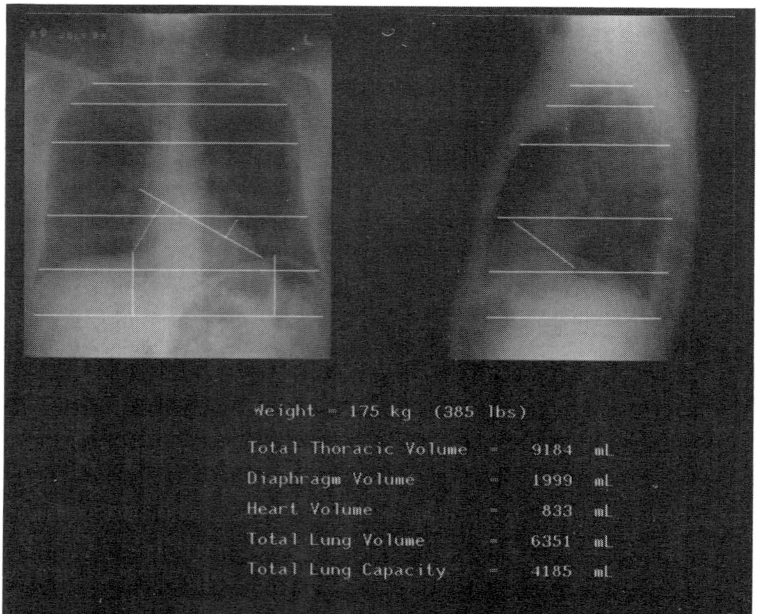

Figure 3. Results of automated TLC determination

III. RESULTS

TLC values obtained by this automated technique ranged from 2745-8082mL (mean = 5344mL) for 36 patients, ranging in age from 9 to 78 years (mean = 51years). The initial image pre-processing part of the automated technique, which is performed separately without any user interaction, requires 4 minutes on a Sun Sparcstation IPX. The time then required by a trained user to select the points is less than 10 seconds, and the actual lung segmentation and TLC computation requires 9 seconds.

On the PA view, the edge tracking routine would sometimes stop at the high intensity clavicles, identifying them as the edges of the thorax. A quick manual adjustment of the endpoint corrects this error. In a few cases, significant differences in inspiration between the PA and the lateral exposures caused an underestimation of the thoracic volume, since the automated method assumes identical inspiration in both views and extrapolates the sectioning lines from the PA to the lateral view. Often, minor adjustments to the endpoints of the sectioning lines were made, according to the judgment of the operator, to refine the accuracy of the segmentation. Of 19 cases for which TLC was recorded before and after manual correction, R=0.90, with a mean relative error of 14.3%.

In a parallel study for twenty of the cases, the gold standard TLC values were taken to be those measured on film by a radiologist familiar with the Barnhard method. The differences between automated TLC and manual TLC values ranged from 10-646mL, with a mean difference of 221mL, and mean relative error of 4.1%. Correlation between the two methods was high, with R=0.98.

IV. DISCUSSION

Compared to the manual film-tracing procedure, which, with practice, still requires 20 minutes of a radiologist's time per case, the automated technique with an easy-to-use graphical interface significantly reduces the actual amount of radiologist involvement to less than 20 seconds. Alternately, point selection can be performed by technologists trained to identify the 10 anatomical landmarks required by the program. The radiologist is then involved only in assessing the accuracy of the automated lung segmentation and in making quick manual corrections on-screen when necessary.

The need for manual correction must be assessed on a case by case basis, depending on the pathologic state of the lungs or the presence of high intensity objects within the pleural outline. Manual correction is easy and can be done within seconds.

With an automated technique, the limitation to a 5 elliptical cylindroid model of the thorax can be removed. Increasing the number of sections is expected to improve the accuracy of the automated boundary detection without significantly increasing the computation time.

V. CONCLUSION

The automated technique presented here for determining TLC based on the multiple ellipsoid model provides a fast and accurate way of obtaining TLC from digital chest radiographs. As this method can easily be extended to more than 5 sections, there is potential for increased accuracy in the TLC measurement. As well, the speed and ease of use of the computer program makes it feasible for routine clinical use.

REFERENCES

1. Barnhard HJ, Pierce JA, Joyce JW, and Bates JM: Roentgenographic determination of total lung capacity: a new method evaluated in health, emphysema and congestive heart failure. Am. J. Med. 28:51-60, 1960.
2. Bush A, Denison DM: Use of different magnification factors to calculate radiological lung volumes. *Thorax* 41:158-159, 1986.
3. Gonzalez RC, Wintz P: *Digital Image Processing.* Reading, MA, Addison-Wesley 191-195, 1987.
4. Greene R: Radiographic measurement of thoracic gas volume. *Radiol Clin North Am* 1:63-71, 1971.
5. Lloyd HM, String ST, and Dubois AB: Radiographic and plethysmographic determination of total lung capacity. *Radiology* 86:7-14.
6. McGaff CJ, Roveti GC, Glassman E, Milnor WR: The Pulmonary blood volume in Rheumatic heart disease and its alternation by isoproterenol. *Circulation* 27:77-84, 1963.

Gamma Knife Planning: A Time-Critical PACS Data Sink

M. Wiltgen, G. Gell, R. Pitzler and A. Kainz
Department for Medical Informatics, Statistics and Documentation
K.H. Feichtinger
Department of Radio Oncology
G. Papaefthymiou
Department for Neurosurgery, University of Graz, Austria

1 Introduction

PACS (Picture Archiving and Communication System) has been developed to manage and handle the images in a radiological department[1-3]. In a PACS the image acquisition modalities, the archive and the digital viewing stations are interconnected in a network. PACS means digital processing, archiving, transfer and display of image data. Beside advantages like reduced costs for archive space, fast image transfer and handling, PACS eliminates local dependencies by providing immediate access to the images also from peripheral (non radiological) departments.

At the Department of Radiology of the University of Graz a PACS[4-5] has been running as part of the daily routine since 1989.

2 PACS configuration and routine operation

To date the PACS incorporates four CT-scanners (Siemens), two MRI-scanners (Philips), one DSA (Siemens), one Ultrafast-CT (Siemens) and one DLR (Agfa) as modalities. In addition, two radiotherapy planning systems, 8 reporting („MagicView") and several viewing („PV") consoles are included. Two archive units (ISA) with a total of three jukeboxes for optical disks (320 GB online) and another archive (52 GB online) mainly used for DLR images serve as longtime archives. The network hardware is based on FDDI and Ethernet. The PACS (fig.1) is a heterogeneous system and partially consists of a Siemens SIENET PACS with several components supplied by IMAGE DEVICES (located in the pediatric radiology) and on the other hand, of some components of an older Siemens PACS version. The modules are based on SUN SPARCstations and VAX systems. The PACS is connected with a Radiological Information System (RIS) so that the management of the image archives is done by the RIS using patient data to select and retrieve the images. The RIS has been developed in-house and is used routinely since the late 1970s.

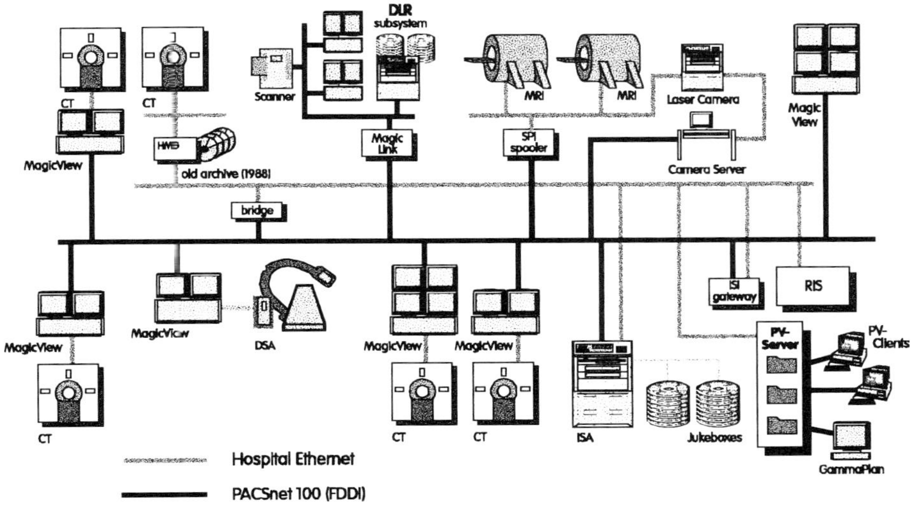

Fig. 1 PACS configuration

All the images produced from CT, MRI, Ultrafast CT, DSA and DLR are routinely stored in the optical archives. The PACS is used for different tasks including: archiving, retrieval of previous examinations, reporting of selected examinations on the digital reporting consoles and image distribution to selected places within the hospital.

3 Image transfer to the planning workstation

As an additional feature to the tasks performed by the PACS, selected MRI examinations required for the planning of LEKSELL GAMMA KNIFE treatments can be sent directly from the MRI scanner to a planning workstation. The image transfer is initiated at the console of the MRI scanner by the radiographer. The images are transferred to and temporarily stored on a server (PV_SERVER, fig.1); the user at the planning station can access the images via an NFS (Network File System) mount.

4 Gamma Knife

The LEKSELL GAMMA KNIFE (fig.2) is an instrument which allows irradiation of intracranial lesions with high precision. The irradiation unit contains 201 Co-60 sources, arranged in a sector of a hemispherical surface. The radiation beam of each single source first passes a special collimating system (a stationary collimator system and an interchangeable final collimator system located in the so called collimator helmet) and then through the center point of the hemisphere. This means that all radiation beams intersect in this central region and deliver a dose-rate of 3.7 Gy/min (time of loading[6]). Outside the central area the dose-rate decreases very rapidly. The spherical geometry of the treatment unit gives an nearly spherical radiation volume with a diameter of approx. 4, 8, 14 and 18 mm (depending on the collimator helmet)[7].

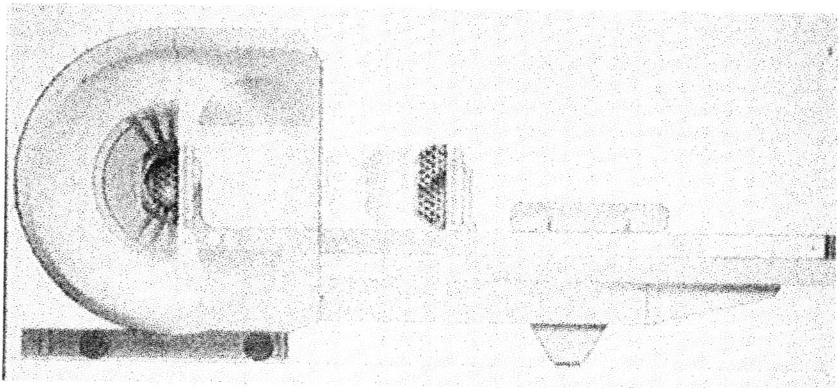

Fig.2: Schematic view of the Leksell Gamma Knife with radiation unit and collimator helmet

The main principle of Gamma Knife treatment is to bring the intracranial lesion in the area of beam intersection, i.e. the center of the collimator helmet. Depending on the size and the shape of the lesion several positions with different collimator helmets can get necessary. The dose applied to the tumor indicates the treatment time for each position.

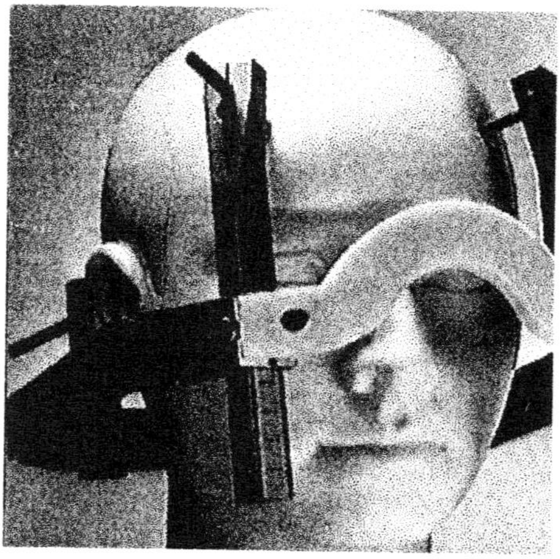

Fig.3: Skull with attached Stereotactic Frame

5 Gamma Planning

Before the treatment planning diagnostics (MRI, CT or angiography) the Stereotactic Frame has to be screwed to the patients skull (with four pins, local anesthesia) (fig.3). This frame provides the coordinate system to determine the cartesian position of the lesion and it allows the fixation of the patients head within the collimator helmet. The

LEKSELL GAMMA PLAN (LGP) is a treatment planning software implemented on a HP workstation that works on digital images (MRI, CT or angiographic).

6 Benefits of Gamma Planning in a PACS Environment

Gamma Knife irradiation and treatment planning are highly dependent on the quality of the planning images because the whole planning procedure is solely picture based. In contrast to common diagnostic images it is not sufficient to know that there is a tumor in the brainstem region. The success of the treatment depends highly on the quality of tumor localization and therefore it is essential to get its exact Cartesian coordinates.

Without being connected to a PACS it is necessary to re-scan hardcopies in order to get digital images, thus inevitably losing a lot of contrast and brightness and reducing the quality of the digitized image.

The duration of the whole treatment procedure should be as short as possible to reduce emotional and physical stress for the patient. This applies not only to the treatment of old or narcotized patients. The ability of directly importing images from the net significantly shortens the planning phase preceding the treatment, as PACS supplies the LGP with flawless quality images in acceptable short time.

There is no need to scan the skull in all directions, because with the LGP software sagittal or coronal reconstructions based on axial images can be performed. Those reconstructions are even more accurate than directly taken sagittal or coronal images, because the axial distortion is the smallest.

Furthermore PACS reduces the ongoing costs because no hardcopies need to be processed. The daily patient throughput also is improved as the quick image access frequently - depending on the complexity of the individual cases - permits the treatment of a second patient during the same day shift.

In individual cases (e.g. appearance of multiple metastases) PACS offers convenient possibilities to immediately discuss alternative or additional treatments with radio oncologists - even in different sites.

7 Epilogue

Summing up, the following advantages of supplying radiological images in digital form can be enumerated:

- Reduced emotional and physical stress for the patient due to the significantly shortened planning phase preceding the treatment.

- No loss of information concerning the localization of structures essential to the successful planning of the irradiation.

- Reduced ongoing costs because no more hardcopies are needed and the utilization of the treatment device (Gamma Knife) is improved.

- Convenient possibilities to discuss alternative treatments with radio oncologists - even in different sites.

Conclusively the network provided images are considered an important improvement for a successful and efficient Gamma Knife treatment.

8 References

1. Akisada M., Okaniwa H., Tsuneyoshi H. and Okabe T.
Some Consideration on Hospital-wide PACS from the Experience in Tokyo Hitachi hospital
In Computer Assisted Radiology, Proceedings of the International Symposium CAR91 (Eds: Lemke H. U., Inamura K., Jaffe C. C., Felix) Springer, Berlin, Heidelberg, New York, (1993) 15-19

2. Meyer-Ebrecht D.
Picture Archiving and Communication Systems (PACS) for medical application.
International Journal of Bio-Medical Computing 35 (1994) 91-124

3. Mosser H., Urban M., Pärtan G. and Hruby W.
Clinical Routine Operation of a Filmless Radiology Department: 20 months Experience
In:. Boehme J., Rowberg A., Wolfman N. (eds)
Computer Applications to Assist Radiology
Proceeding Book of the SCAR 94 Symposium for Computer Assisted Radiology
Winston-Salem, North Carolina, June 12-15, 1994, 30-38

4. Wiltgen M., Gell G., Kainz A. Pitzler R, Ebner F., Kern R., Fazekas F., Kapeller P. and Stollberger R.
Quantitative Evaluation of Reporting from Monitor in Comparision to Hardcopy
In Computer Assisted Radiology, Proceedings of the International Symposium CAR95 (Eds: Lemke H. U., Inamura K., Jaffe C. C., Vannier M.W.) Springer, Berlin, Heidelberg, New York, (1995) 570-574

5. Wiltgen M., Gell G., Pitzler R. and Kainz A.
An Integrated PACS-RIS: Experiences and Developments
In:. Boehme J., Rowberg A., Wolfman N. (eds)
Computer Applications to Assist Radiology
Proceeding Book of the SCAR 94 Symposium for Computer Assisted Radiology
Winston-Salem, North Carolina, June 12-15, 1994, 213-218

6. Obenaus B., Kindl P., Feichtinger K.H., Stücklschweiger G.
Measurement of dose rate in the Leksell Gamma Unit with a semiconductor diode. Z. f Med. Phys. 4: 46-49.

7. Kindl P., Obenaus B., Feichtinger K.H., Stücklschweiger G.
High resolution measurement of dose distribution in the Leksell Gamma Knife. Z.f. Med. Phys. 4: 215-219.

FOCUS SESSION

The Visible Human Project™ of the National Library of Medicine

Michael J. Ackerman, Ph.D.
Office of High Performance Computing and Communications, National Library of Medicine, Bethesda, Maryland

The Visible Human Project™ has its roots in an observation made in 1987, that the medical school community needed a better way to teach anatomy. A "digital cadaver", in the public domain, would allow every medical school to share in its development and benefit from its existence. This idea was supported by an earlier 1986 long-range planning effort of the National Library of Medicine (NLM). It foresaw a coming era where NLM's bibliographic and factual database services would be complemented by libraries of digital images, distributed over high speed computer networks and by high capacity physical media. Not surprisingly, it saw an increasing role for electronically represented images in clinical medicine and biomedical research. It encouraged the NLM to consider building and disseminating medical image libraries much the same way it acquires, indexes, and provides access to the biomedical literature. As a result of the deliberations of consultants in medical education, the long-range plan recommended that the NLM should "...thoroughly and systematically investigate the technical requirements for and feasibility of instituting a biomedical images library."

Early in 1989, under the direction of the NLM Board of Regents, an ad hoc planning panel was convened to explore in-depth the proper role for the NLM in the rapidly changing field of electronic imaging. After much deliberation, the NLM Planning Panel on Electronic Image Libraries made the recommendation that NLM should undertake a first project, to build a digital image library of volumetric data representing a complete, normal adult male and female.

The initial aim of the Visible Human Project™ was the acquisition of transverse Computerized Tomography (CT), Magnetic Resonance (MR) and cryosection images of a representative male and female cadaver. The corresponding transverse sections in each of the three modalities were to be registered with one another. A contract for acquisition of these pixel-based data was awarded in August 1991 to the University of Colorado at Denver. Victor M. Spitzer, Ph.D. and David G. Whitlock, M.D., Ph.D. are the principal investigators.

It took almost two years to find an appropriate male cadaver and two and a half years to find an appropriate female cadaver. The male data set consists of MR, CT and anatomical images. Axial 12-bit, 256 x 256, MR images of the head and neck and longitudinal sections of the rest of the body were obtained at 4 mm intervals. The CT data consists of axial 12-bit, 512 x 512, CT scans of the entire body taken at 1 mm intervals. The axial anatomical images are 2048 pixels by 1216 pixels where each pixel is defined by 24 bits of color, about 7.5 megabytes. The anatomical cross-sections are also at 1 mm intervals and coincide with the CT axial images. There are 1871 cross-sections for each mode, CT and anatomy. The complete male data set is 15 gigabytes in size.

The female data set consists of similar MR and CT scan data. However the axial anatomical images were captured at 0.33 mm intervals in order to match the pixel spacing in the horizontal plane thus enabling developers to work with cubic voxels. Every third axial anatomical image coincides with an axial CT image. There are 5189 axial anatomical images and 1829 axial CT images. The complete female data set is 39 gigabytes in size.

The Visible Human Project™ data sets are designed to serve as a common reference point for the study of human anatomy, as a set of common public domain data for testing medical imaging algorithms, and as a test bed and model for the construction of image libraries that can be accessed through networks. The data sets are being applied to a wide range of educational, diagnostic, treatment planning, virtual reality, artistic, mathematical and industrial uses by over 500 licensees in 26 countries.

The data sets are having their greatest effect on health care and health education. They are used as a normal reference and as an aid in the diagnostic process. Programs under development will be used to educate patients about the need for and purpose of surgery and other medical procedures as well as to permit physicians to plan surgery and radiation therapy. The images from the Visible Human data sets are used in several prototype virtual reality surgical simulators. Educational materials that make use of the Visible Human data sets are beginning to be used by students from kindergarten to practicing health care professionals.

NLM has begun a second phase of the Visible Human Project™, turning the data sets into a true interactive data base. The digital image library under development by NLM from the Visible Human data sets may be the first truly "digital" library in that the library's contents were never intended to be in any format other than digital.

The larger, long-term goal of the Visible Human Project™ is to produce a system of knowledge structures, which will transparently link visual knowledge forms to symbolic knowledge formats. Methods still need to be developed to link image data to symbolic text-based data which is comprised of names, hierarchies, principles and theories. Although experiments are being done using generalizable linkage methods, like the use of hypermedia where words can be used to find pictures, and pictures can be used as an index into relevant text, standards do not currently exist for such linkages. Basic research is also needed in the description and representation of structures, and the connection of structural-anatomical to functional-physiological knowledge. The goal is to make the print library and the image library a single, unified resource for health information.

Image Guided Frameless Stereotactic Cranial Surgery

Kevin O. Lillehei, M.D.
Associate Professor Surgery, Division of Neurosurgery, University of Colorado Health Sciences Center, Denver, Colorado

The application of computer technology to the field of medicine has forever changed the way in which we practice. Its impact has been most apparent in the disciplines of Neurology and Neurosurgery. With the development of Computerized Tomographic (CT) scanning in the 1970's, and then Magnetic Resonance Imaging (MRI) and Positron Emission Tomography (PET) in the 1980"s, our ability to intricately image the brain has improved dramatically. Along with this ability to better visualize the brain, however, has arisen a need to more effectively treat lesions so identified, particularly those lesions which are deep seated or in eloquent areas of the brain. To address this need, Neurosurgeons again turned to computer technology, applying it to the field of stereotactic neurosurgery. Initially this gave rise to the fixed head frame coordinate systems such as the Brown-Robert-Wells (BRW) system, which proved to be very convenient for biopsing lesions but cumbersome for use in open craniotomies. Nevertheless, the availability of this technology had a major impact on the practice of neurosurgery in the 1980's. As more precise guidance systems were needed for open craniotomies, these systems evolved, combining the accuracy and ease of CT and MRI imaging, with computer based three dimensional imaging, and new frameless coordinate systems. This has given rise to image guided frameless stereotactic identified pre-operatively within the brain, is outlined on a three-dimensional computer reconstruction and then projected stereotactically through the lens of an operating microscope, over the surface of the brain by use of a "heads-up" display. This in turn, precisely outlines for the surgeon the extent of the lesion within the brain and also allows the identification of areas of "risk", for the surgeon to stay away from. With the coupling of the three dimensional computerized imaging to a robotically controlled microscope, not only is the image precisely located in space, but the program will then allow the surgeon to plan an approach to the lesion on the 3-D reconstruction, which will be followed in real-time space by the microscope. Examples of this system is use will be presented in the treatment of primary and metastatic tumors of the brain.

Posters and Demonstrations

Developments of CT System Using Singular Value Decomposition Method

Masahiro Daibo, Tomeo Minamihaba, Tatsuo Hasegawa, Takami Kumagai and Mitsuru Fujisawa
Iwate Industrial Research Institute, 3-35-2, Iiokashinden, Morioka, Iwate, Japan
Norio Tayama
Iwate University, 4-3-5,Ueda, Morioka, Iwate, Japan

1 INTRODUCTION

The aim of this work is to develop a very fast CT system with low cost for the industrial fields. It is desirable to visualize inside of running object very fast such as heart or coronary artery. There are same request in the industrial fields in order to improve reliability of the machine parts or electric devices. If it is carried out to check defect inside for all of the parts very fast without increasing costs, unexpected failure will be decreased. If the CT achieve test without many projection and massive calculation, the reconstruction time will be shorten, then a wide variety of application will be possible. A few projection will contribute to not only shorten time for projection data acquisition but also simplify rotation device. The fast CT may produce on different kind of fabrication, such as a manufacturing test under the processing in real time.

This paper reports a new CT system that can reconstruct a CT image from a few directions of projection based on singular value decomposition method. This CT system does not require a large amount of calculation after acquisition of projection data. Computing time at reconstruction decreases because the projection model is defined and a constant matrix is calculated before practical X-ray projection. The CT image is obtained by one operation of matrix multiplication with the constant matrix.

2 METHODS

Figure 1 illustrates our newly developed CT algorithm. A calculation space that sampling function is placed on each grid is prepared. A high spacial frequency of the calculation space is eliminated using sampling theorem. Then, Angeles and intervals at which the projection lines intersect with the calculation space are modeled. Note that the model needs to correspond to actual geometry of X-ray projection. The distance of the projection line and sampling function on the grids assumed to be a variable, and we calculate influence coefficient by line integration along the projection line. The influence coefficient represents what rate the density at each sampling point has influenced from the projection line.

The linear equation to which the influence coefficient, the pixel density, and the projection value is made. The linear equation of each projection line is set up corresponding to paths of penetrating X-ray beams. And next, the simultaneous equations and the least squares errors are solved by using the SVD (Singular Value Decomposition) method. We obtain the pseudo-inverse matrix C+ by the cutting singular method. The matrix C+ is stored as the constant matrix in the memory. Finally, the matrix C+ and the measured projection vector are multiplied, and the product is a reconstructed CT image.

In addition, to shorten time for reconstruction, we use filtering process. We set a threshold and extract dominant components of the matrix C+ that the absolute value is not near zero. The rest of components are a small fraction for the reconstructed image, because the density of the reconstruction image is calculated by accumulation a row vector of the matrix C+ multiplied by the scalar of projection data.

3 RESULT

As object to be check inside, we used electrolysis condenser. The projection dates have been acquired by a micro focus X-ray TV (TOSHIBA tosmicron 6125R) with a rotation device. Fig. 2 shows the reconstructed image by our new method. In this case, we used condition that the number of directions of projection was 8 (each 22.5 degree) , the total number of the sampling point was 64 × 64=4096. We assume that the good endpoint of rank for cutting singular value decomposition is about 500, because value of the rank begin to decrease around 500 in this case. The threshold of filter have been chosen 0.001. In the result, the size of filtered pseudo-inverse matrix is reduced to 1/20. The net reconstruction time, exclude file I/O, is 66ms with a work station (SPECrate_fp92=4645), which means that it will be possible to reconstruct 15 frames per second. If acquisition time for projection data is reduced enough, this method will achieve real time CT.

4 CONCLUSION

An experimental demonstration of the CT using newly developed SVD method with filter processing has been presented. This technique will potentially result in the development a real time CT to observe a dynamic phenomenon with low cost for either industry or medical purpose.

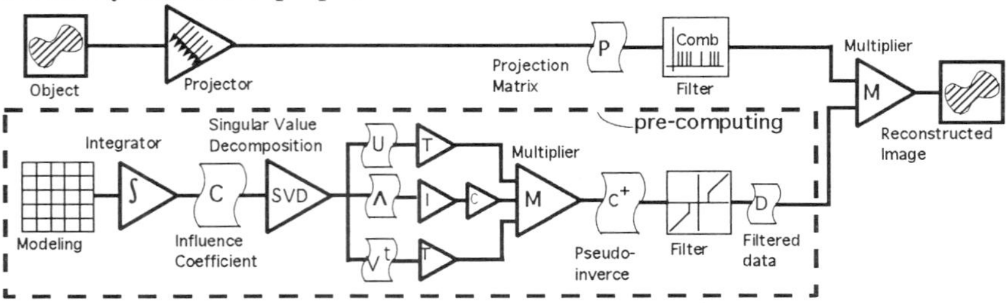

Fig. 1 Newly developed CT algorithm.

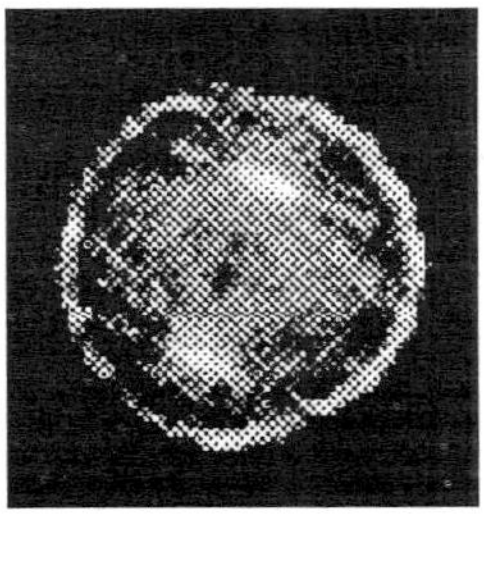

Fig. 2 Reconstructed cross section of electolysis condenser by new method, with only 8 derections of projection, 64 × 64 sampling point.

References

1. N. Tayama et al., Fast Visualization for 3D Smooth Density Distribution From a Few Projections, ASV'94, G16, pp.681-686 (1994).
2. A. Albert, Regression and the Moore-Penrose Pseudoinverse, Academic Press (1972).

A Filmless Radiology Learning File for the Internet

Chakri Inampudi, M.D., T.L. Kamplain and J.K. Smith, M.D., Ph.D.
University of Alabama at Birmingham

Purpose: Construct and demonstrate the utility of a computerized, filmless radiology learning file accessible over the world wide web (Web). The Web is an internet service that allows access to computer documents including text format styles and images and can provide hypertextual linkages to other documents anywhere on the internet.

Methods: Our teaching file runs on a Macintosh PowerPC using WebSTAR server software. The images to be used in the teaching file are transferred from CT, MRI, and Ultrasound machines over the local hospital network or digitized from 35mm slides using a slide scanner. Raw images are windowed, leveled, reduced, and cropped and then converted to Compuserve GIF format. The image manipulations are semiautomated using simple macros to speed case construction. Text documents used in the teaching file are created in the standard HyperText Markup Language (HTML) format using a text editor. HTML is an Internet standard which allows platform independent remote display and linkage of text and image documents. Templates and simple macros are used to rapidly build the cases in a standard format with history and images presented on the first page, followed by images, findings, diagnosis and discussion on the next page.

Each page contains links to the teaching file case list and the next case to make case review quicker.
Results: The learning file currently contains over 200 cases and is used regularly by our residents. It has been accessed by radiologists as far away as Australia. The "Home Page" of our teaching file provides the user with a menu containing categories to choose from, or the cases may be viewed as unknowns. Each of our completed cases contains a brief medical history, several images, findings, a diagnosis, a discussion, and appropriate references. The Web server also provides information about our residency training and fellowship programs and our faculty, as well as links to UAB Web servers and other relevant sites.

We have incorporated user suggestions to attempt to optimize usability and speed of case presentation, two of the most often cited reasons for not using electronic learning files. Decreasing image size greatly speeds case retrieval and images are routinely reduced to the minimum size that will still demonstrate the findings. Links directly to the next numerical case in a category greatly reduce the number of intermediate documents that must be retrieved thus dramatically increasing rate at which the cases may be reviewed as unknowns.

Conclusions: A filmless, on-line radiology learning file can be constructed with minimal computer hardware and software investment and has wider accessibility than traditional film based learning files. Improvements in speed of case presentation have resulted in increased resident usage. Visit our home page at: *http://www.rad.uab.edu.*

Automated Evaluation of Portal Images Using an Artificial Neural Network

Stephen M. Humphries and Francis D. Newman

Departments of Radiology and Radiation Oncology, University of Colorado Health Sciences Cer
Denver, Colorado

Harold J. Cline

Department of Radiation Oncology, Lutheran Medical Center, Wheat Ridge, Colorado

I. INTRODUCTION

Portal imaging is used in radiotherapy to verify patient positioning under the exact conditions of treatment. Acquired using the therapy accelerator, portal images show the orientation of anatomical landmarks relative to field borders. Weekly portal images are compared with an ideal set up image taken at the start of a patient's treatment course in order to assure that the correct anatomy consistently falls within the treatment beam. The emergence of electronic portal imaging devices makes it possible to acquire and process these images digitally. As more complicated treatment techniques for radiation dose escalation are pursued, accuracy and efficiency in portal imaging will be vital to assure proper patient positioning. This work shows the utility of an artificial neural network (ANN) approach to automating the portal image evaluation process.

II. METHODS AND MATERIALS

Using MATLAB (the MathWorks, Inc.) run on a desktop PC, simulation of a counterpropagation neural network has been performed. The network is trained with transformations of the set up image intended to mimic portal images that show translation and rotation of anatomic landmarks relative to field borders. The counterpropagation network (CPN) is a three layer competitive network that combines ANN structures known as instars and outstars[1]. The instar and outstar layers complement each other in that the instars function to classify inputs into groups based on training and the outstars give the desired response corresponding to each classification group. When an input image is introduced to the CPN the instars that represent the two training images that most closely resemble the input, based on a Euclidean or some other metric, are activated. Each instar gives a fractional output such that an interpolation is performed between the trained outputs for the first and second place training images. For example, assume a network has been trained with nine images rotated between -20° and 20° in 5° increments. Introducing an input showing a rotation of -8° will cause the instars corresponding training images rotated to -10° and -5° respectively to be activated.

An interpolation between the trained responses associated with the winning training images gives the result at the outstar layer.

III. RESULTS

As one might expect, accuracy increases with more extensive training. Exhaustive training would give near perfect results, however this is very impractical. Using the training scheme described above accuracies of $\pm 0.5°$ have been achieved in a network designed to evaluate rotation. Comparable results have been seen in networks to evaluate translation. At this point, combinations of translation and rotation have not been evaluated. However, these results suggest that similar levels of accuracy could be seen with training to include such combinations.

A new image similarity measure suggested by Cios and Shin [2] has been employed to determine winning instars on the competitive layer of the CPN. It is worthwhile to note that use of this similarity measure significantly improves the network's ability to interpolate compared to a CPN using a Euclidean metric.

IV. CONCLUSIONS

Further work to improve results while keeping training to a reasonable level is ongoing. The results presented here are seen as very promising and prove that artificial neural networks are appropriate for portal image evaluation.

REFERENCES

1. Hecht-Nielsen R: Applications of counterpropagation networks. Neural Networks 1(1) 131-139, 1988.

2. Cios KJ, Shin I: Image recognition neural network: IRNN. Neurocomputing 7(2) 159-185, 1995.

Application of a PC-based Multiparameter Full-Color Composite Display Technique in Musculoskeletal MR Imaging

Todd R. Hazelton, M.D.
Department of Radiology, University of South Florida College of Medicine, Tampa, Florida
H. Keith Brown, Ph.D.
Department of Physical Therapy, North Georgia College, Dahlonega, Georgia

INTRODUCTION

Advances in computer graphics hardware now allow full-color (24-bit) digital image processing applications to be readily performed on lower cost personal computer (PC) workstations. A PC-based method for generating full-color composites from multiparameter magnetic resonance (MR) image sets has been described.[1] Using this technique, a 486 PC with 24-bit graphics display capabilities was utilized to create color composite images from gray scale MR image sets of selected musculoskeletal cases.

METHODS

MR imaging was performed on a 1.5-tesla General Electric Signa Advantage imager (GE Medical Systems Group, Milwaukee, WI). Acquired image sets included both spin echo and fast spin echo T1-, proton density, and T2-weighted images, as well as STIR images. The selected image sets were transferred to a high performance PC with a 486 microprocessor. Specific color masks were applied to the gray scale images using custom image processing software. In a process analogous to NASA's Landsat system for generating composites from multispectral remote sensing data, spatially aligned, color masked image sets were then combined into a single image using the red-green-blue (RGB) color model.

FEATURED CASES

1. MR imaging of the knee demonstrating synovial hypertrophy and chondromalacia in a 9 year old male with hemophilia A and a history of frequent episodes of hemarthrosis.
2. MR imaging of the knee in a 12 year old male with osteochondritis dissecans.
3. MR imaging of the hips showing avascular necrosis of the femoral heads in an 18 year old female with a history of Hodgkin's disease and bilateral hip pain.
4. MR imaging of the femur in a 14 year old male with osteosarcoma.
5. MR imaging of the knee in a 15 year old which shows post-traumatic disruption of the anterior cruciate ligament and a large joint effusion.

SUMMARY

With this simple tissue segmentation algorithm, pathologic processes of the musculoskeletal system can be displayed within the context of near-natural appearing full-color MR images which summarize differential T1 and T2 information.

---

[1]Brown HK, *et al.* PC-based multiparameter full-color display for tissue segmentation in MRI of adnexal masses. ***J Comput Assist Tomogr*** 1993;17:993-1005

Nuclear Medicine Goes Filmless: Experience with a MiniPACS

M.J. Chamberlain, K.Y. Gulenchyn, R.B. Jammal and B.T.A. McKee
Division of Nuclear Medicine, Department of Radiological Science, Ottawa Civic Hospital and Department or Radiology, University of Ottawa, Ottawa, Ontario, Canada

I. INTRODUCTION

A heterogenous collection of five gamma cameras were linked through a network of Sun workstations operating Hermes software (Nuclear Diagnostics) using an Interfile header to give unified display, analysis, reporting and archiving. In the initial year of filmless operation, we have processed about 16,000 studies. On the basis of the advantages realized in this first year, we are now increasing the size of our on-line image database to 18 Gbytes, and adding more display/processing/review workstations (fig. 1).

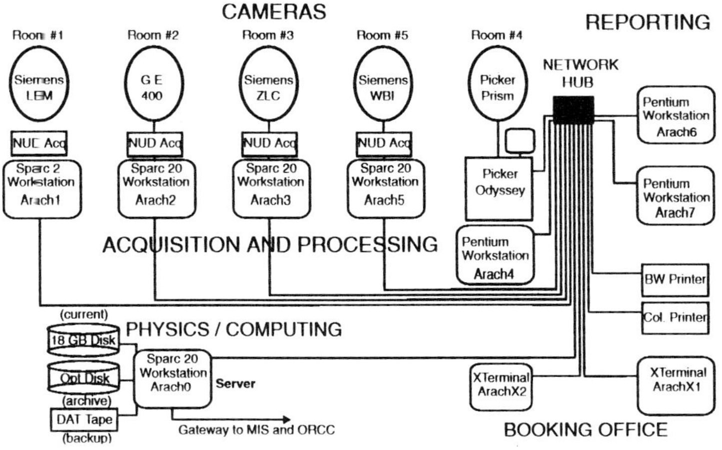

Fig. 1. Network configuration of Nuclear Medicine cameras and workstations, O.C.H.

II. BENEFITS

The anticipated benefits of the separation of the proprietary acquisition function from the processing, display and archiving functions have all been realised (Table 1).

Table 1. Anticipated benefits

1. Enhancement of diagnostic interpretation.
2. Avoids film processing, repeat scans due to incorrect exposures, misplaced films.
3. Separation of acquisition and processing for future purchases.
4. Common processing software for all acquisition protocols.
5. Utilization of imaging cameras not tied to processing capabilities.
6. Image archive uses non-proprietary file header.

Perhaps more interesting were some benefits that we had not fully anticipated, listed in Table 2.

Table 2. Additional benefits

1. Better service to referring physicians and patients through paper copies.
2. Better service to physicians visiting the department through quicker access to images.
3. Benefits of image database - teaching, research, etc.
4. Computer-based quality control.
5. Opportunities for display and processing of multi-modality images.

The use of laser printers to provide cheap paper output of the images has proved popular, empowering patients and referring physicians. Physicians, who bypass a trip to the film library and have quick access to their patients' data, are encouraged to visit the department, creating opportunities for teaching and consultation. Real-time remote consultation has been demonstrated using a workstation in the adjacent Cancer Clinic. There are many benefits for teaching and research from the digital image archive, and these benefits can be leveraged by sharing instructional material between teaching hospitals. The availability of digital images for camera quality-control independent of manufacturer is an advantage which we are only beginning to utilize. We have also imported images from CT, MRI and PET. Although we have the software capability to display and manipulate these multi-modality images, issues of access and header compatibility will slow utilization.

III. OTHER EFFECTS

On switching to a filmless workplace, we have seen the workload shift in ways not fully anticipated, with an uneven distribution of benefit and detriment. (Table 3).

Table 3. Additional workload

1. Clerical staff retrieves images from digital archive, but still maintains the film archive.
2. User training and preparation of user documentation.
3. More physician time spent reporting.

As the digital archive grows, the retrieval of archived studies for comparison with current studies and for printing becomes more time consuming. We are reducing this impact by increasing the size of our "current" image directory to hold images for one year, increasing to 4 years when compression is available. As technologists and interns train and rotate, there are novice users requiring training. Attention to training and user documentation has smoothed acceptance of the system. The additional reporting time used by the physicians is a consequence of the extra image manipulation available, and is accepted because it does lead to an enhancement of the diagnostic interpretation.

Because the imaging software is used by technologists and physicians in an environment subject to distractions and interruptions, it should be consistent and easy to operate. An operation which takes a few extra seconds becomes an irritation when repeated a hundred times a day.

Despite our best planning, some of the points discussed above were not obvious until the system was in use for some time. Flexibility on the part of the users and the vendor is helpful.

IV. CONCLUSIONS

We have implemented a Nuclear Medicine MiniPACS and operated it for over a year. It has met its goals, and has provided additional benefits, such as paper copies, which were not all anticipated. At the same time, changing workloads have required some flexibility. It has been well received by staff in the department and by referring physicians.

Data Base and Management System for Clinical Positron Emission Tomography (PET) Study

Hinako Toyama, Yuko Amou, Kenji Ishii, Keiichi Oda and Michio Senda
Positron Medical Center, Tokyo Metropolitan Institute of Gerontology, Tokyo, Japan

I. INTRODUCTION

Since nuclear medicine provides a good environment for the evaluation of picture archiving and communication system (PACS) because of the relatively small amount of digital data, its system and clinical application has been reported by many authors.[1,2,3,4)] However, no PACS is commercially available because the principles of system are different in the institute. We have developed a human friendly database and data management system for a clinical use on a positron emission tomography (PET) study. This system is based on a general purpose data base "GBASE" (Ricoh Co.Ltd. JAPAN) which works on a UNIX work station.

II. SYSTEM CONFIGURATION

A block diagram of hardware for our database system is shown in Fig. 1. PET images and the associated data are transformed to a Dr_View format and stored into a juke box. The address of the data and information of the patient, the study and the data are registered into the database at the same time. In a data processing and display unit, we use "Dr_View" (Asahikasei Joho System Co. Ltd. JAPAN) system. The data base consists of a tree structure of records (PATIENT, STUDY, SCAN and DATA) and several table records (INSTITUTE, RESEARCHER, DISEASE, STUDY_NAME, STUDY_PARADIGM, etc.). The management system consists of three parts : registration, retrieve and update. In this system, new record(s) of PATIENT and/or STUDY is/are created when the data file is registered for the first time and the basic information of the patient and the positron emission tomographic (PET) study is read from the header of the data file and are stored automatically. This system has a user friendly interface to retrieve and update the data quickly and easily by using work sheets explicitly and implicitly. This data base works on the network system and is retrieved from any work station.

III. CLINICAL APPLICATIONS

We applied this system to 800 patients and 1000 studies in our PET center during 5 years. We connected this data base to the data processing system "Dr_View" and reporting system[4)]. We can search for the data files to be processed either from study paradigm, study date,

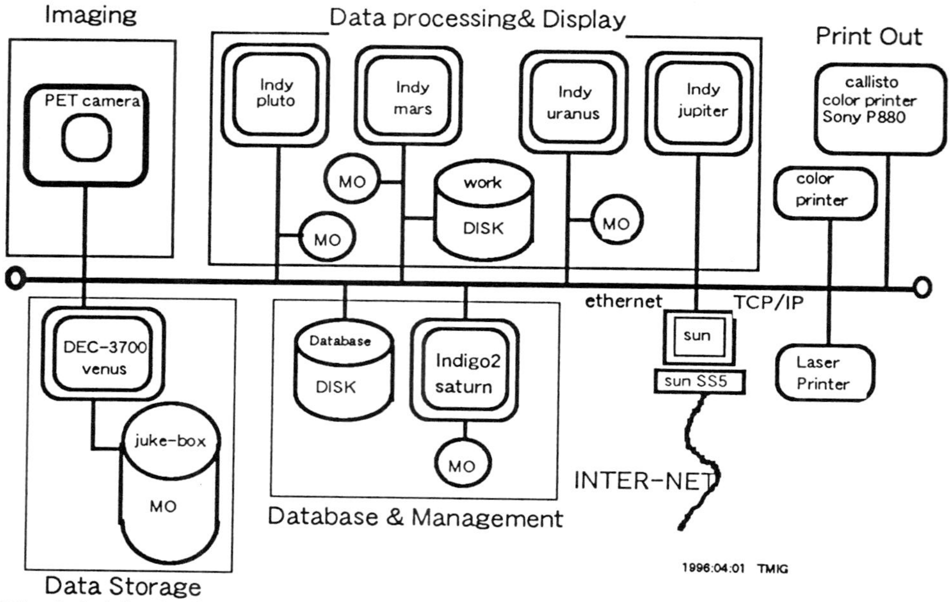

Fig.1 A block diagram of our database and computer system. This system consists of an imaging unit, a data sorage, data processing and display unit, a database and management unit and print out devices.

radiopharmaceutical or basic patient information and transfer them into the data processing tool automatically. A statistical analysis was performed on patients, PET studies and the relational data such as clinical diagnosis, age, gender.

IV. DISCUSSION

In this system, we can easily upgrade the hardware and the software of the database system and the data processing and display unit, independently. The good connectivity between both systems was considered. Since the data management system is written in C language and uses a MOTIF for screen management, it is easy to be transfered into other UNIX work station with a few modifiction.

References

1. Juni JE. NucNet:A singel-vender clinical picture archiving ans communication system - Description and reflections. Seminars in Nucl Med XX:193-204,1990

2. Brown PH, Krishnamurthy GT. Design and operation of a nuclear medicine picture archiving and communication system. Seminars in Nucl Med XX:205-224,1990

3. Line BR. Nuclear medicine information management system. Seminars in Nucl Med XX: 242-269,1990

4. Jamzad M, Ishii K, Toyama H and Senda M. A human friendly reporting and database system for brain PET analysis. Annals Nucl Med 10: 99-104, 1996

Universal System for Mass Medical and Radiological Monitoring

E.K. Kirilenko
Scientific Technical Centre "Viria Ltd", Kiev, Ukraine

In our previous paper we have described the automated spectrometric systems (MRC module) for the fast and accurate determination of gamma-radiating isotopes count of human body. It has been designed in order to control regularly the radioactive contamination of people living in territories that were polluted because of Chernobyl disaster. Our general aim is to put into operation a number of such identical modules in different districts of Ukraine and to network them. This large scale network gives the possibility to accumulate the data of the population's radiological check-up in order to detect the most dangerous areas for living and to plan a number of steps to provide the people's safety and to save the health of generation. The introduction into databases the results of population's medical observations allows to study changing in the human health under the continued effect of the small radiation doses.

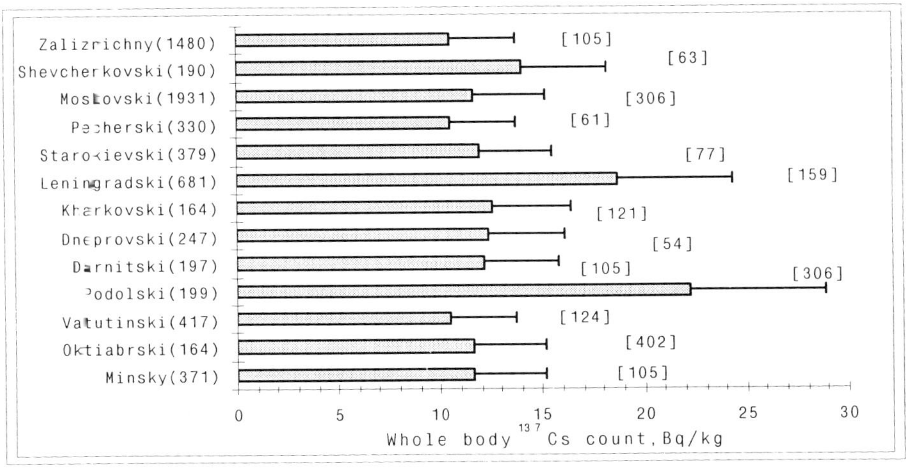

Fig1. Average whole body ^{137}Cs count per kg weight for 6700 persons living in 13 districts of Kiev is plotted against their place of residence. The number of the examined persons is in round brackets and the extreme ^{137}Cs values are shown in square brackets.

Now the source of such network exists in Ukraine. There are 30 MRC modules that operate in Kiev and other towns. In this paper we present the results of statistical processing of overall database received from 5 MRC modules.

We also have investigated the distribution of the internal radioactive contamination among the district residents . For example in Podolsky district 27% of people had less than 10 Bq/kg contamination, 32% of people had (10-20) Bq/kg and 28% of people had (20-30) Bq/kg . 13% of residents had the level of contamination higher than 30 Bq/kg but only 1 person had the extreme level 306 Bq/kg.

In the paper we also describe an operation of the updated MRC module that includes the apparatus for the spectral analysis of heart-beat. The connection of this device to the MRC module allows to evaluate a human stress level, a state of his vegetative nervous system, a working capacity, an adaptation reserves concurrently with the radiological measurement and to create a total database of patient's medical and radiological observations . The duration of the measuring is 5 minutes. The results of such concurrent check up of group of workers are shown in Fig.2. and Fig.3. The presented data show one of the possibilities of MRC module application in combination with the different medical devices.

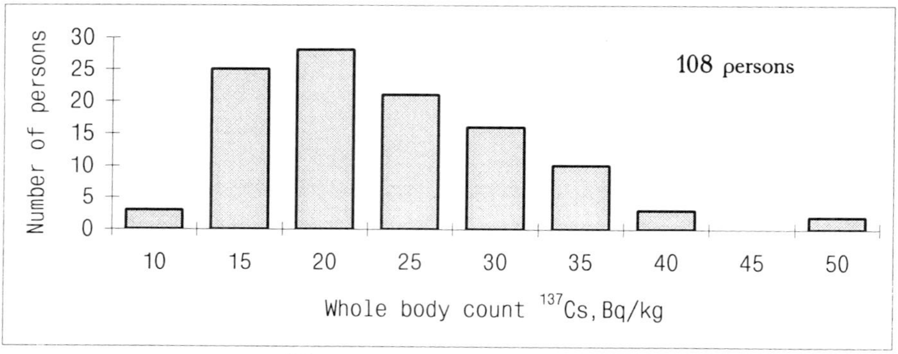

Fig.2. The distribution of ^{137}Cs whole body count among the persons.

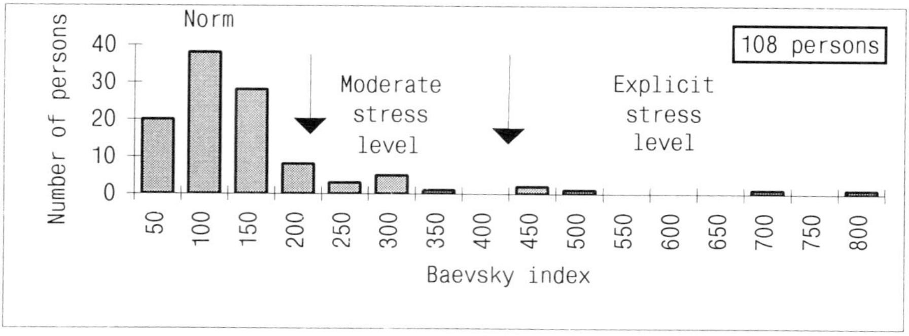

Fig.3. The results of the stress level analysis based on the Baevsky index evaluation .

Project BRAHMS: PACS Implementation at Brigham and Women's Hospital

William B. Hanlon, Ethan F. Fener and Scott D. Davis
Department of Radiology, Harvard Medical School, Brigham and Women's Hospital, Boston, Massachusetts

Jeffrey W. Downs
IDX Corporation, Burlington, Vermont

ABSTRACT

Project BRAHMS is a clinical imaging system that has been implemented at Brigham and Women's Hospital (BWH) for use by referring physicians. The purpose of the system is to provide customers of BWH radiological services with fast, local area, on-line access to digital radiological images and diagnostic reports, for consultation and review. The system provides an alternative to film.

Differentiating features of the BRAHMS system include: full integration with the Radiology Information System (RIS), decoupling of the database search engine from the display software (to allow the integration of third-party image viewers), and focus on the clinician, not the radiologist, as the target user. BRAHMS can be best conceptualized as a PACS for referring physicians.

Phase I of the project which is now complete includes: acquisition of CT and MR digital image data, validation and indexing of data in the RIS, storage on-line of images for thirty days, and deployment of eleven viewing stations (Unix workstations) in selected departments and clinics. The first sites to receive BRAHMS workstations were Neurology, Hematology/Oncology, Neurosurgery, and Thoracic Surgery. Seven of the viewing stations are located on campus, connected via Ethernet LAN; two stations are located at a neighboring institution via an extension of the LAN across the street; and another two viewing stations are located off campus connected via T-1 communication links. A variety of image-viewing options are available, from easy-to-use fast browsers, to sophisticated data fusion and teleconferencing applications.

The BRAHMS system has been very well received by the clinicians, as evidenced by focus group sessions, personal interviews, testimonials, unsolicited comments, and usage statistics. The BRAHMS system averages about 300 accesses per week and usage is increasing. Enhancements requested by users include; additional modalities on-line (NM, US, CR, angiography), and a long-term archive for review of historical exams. These enhancements are planned for Phase II, pending administrative approval and funding. Additional Phase II features will include adoption of DICOM file format and messaging where appropriate, and development of a platform-independent version of the image browser.

Development of this PACS has proceeded in partnership between BWH and IDX Corporation (Burlington VT) since 1993. The system is marketed by IDX as "IDXview", and has received 510K clearance from the FDA.

A New Rapid Technique to Digitize Filmed Images – A Comparison of a High Resolution Digital Camera to Other Established Digitization Methods

Michael F. Dowe, Jr., Michael P. McDermott, Andrew D. Vennos, Michael J. Marks, Michael A. Grimm, and Eliot L. Siegel

University of Maryland Medical Systems, Department of Diagnostic Imaging, Baltimore, Maryland

A high resolution digital camera was used to digitize CT, MRI, ultrasound and conventional radiographic films. An interactive computer based comparison of the digital camera with established methods for digitizing filmed images is presented. This new digital camera technique is compared to laser-based dedicated film scanning, desktop flatbed scanning, desktop 35mm slide scanning, PhotoCD digitization of 35mm film, and video frame grabbing. Important differences including product cost, resulting pixel depth and resolution, file size, and typical scan times of the varying methods are evaluated. Sample images from each method will be displayed to enable direct comparison.

In recent years there has been a steady increase in the use of digital images in Radiology for diagnostic examinations as well as in teleradiology and PACS. During this same period the rapid growth in personal computer multimedia capabilities as well as increased access to the internet has created additional applications for digital imaging in the creation of teaching files, multimedia exhibits and in publishing. Digital images offer several advantages over conventional methods in the creation of teaching files. The images are high resolution and high quality with better preservation of gray-scale than copy film. The images can be fine-tuned once acquired using commercially available software to optimize visualization of findings. Digital images offer long-term stable convenient storage, which can be accessed rapidly and which can be easily shared over the internet. Unlike conventional copy film, there is no loss of quality if the image is distributed and copied multiple times.

Archived digital images are easily exportable to several hard copy formats. They may be exported to dye sublimation printers which produce images that are virtually indistinguishable from photographs and which may be annotated at the computer rather than directly onto the photograph. The same images can be printed to slides and transparencies for lectures, can be incorporated into multimedia programs for the production of computer-based teaching files, and can be used in exhibits, posters and publications.

We find the new high resolution digital cameras to be superior to other commercially available methods for digitizing filmed images to be used in the production of teaching files, multimedia exhibits, etc. for a number of reasons. The digital camera is versatile and may be used for all photographic jobs (including documents for optical character recognition). It is fully function and portable and can completely replace a conventional camera. When using the digital camera there is no need for hardcopy intermediate (eg. slides / negatives must be produced for slide scanning). Digital cameras also offer rapid image acquisition time, it is possible to apply the full pixel matrix to any size original by changing lenses and when physically connected to computer, allows real-time adjustment of photographic technique. The major disadvantage is expense, however prices are now and will likely continue to decrease and resolution / dollar will increase over time making this a reasonable investment for any department or practice with a strong commitment to digital archiving, teaching files, and / or multimedia exhibits.

The recent introduction of several high resolution digital cameras offers a promising, cost effective method for rapid, high volume, high resolution digitization of filmed images.

Improvements to Backprojection for Lowering Experimental Error

G. Kashman
Long Beach VA Medical Center, Long Beach, California and
University of California-Irvine, Irvine, California

O. Nalcioglu
University of California-Irvine, Irvine, California

N. Milne and K. Lyons
Long Beach VA Medical Center, Long Beach, California

I. INTRODUCTION AND PURPOSE

In any medical imaging modality, it is desirable to identify the largest sources of experimental error before attempting to improve images. Removing a small error while a much larger one is present could be ineffective. Further, there is no way to determine in advance whether a single error or multiple errors of similar size are blocking progress. In the current state of development in SPECT imaging, the two errors which are commonly believed to cause the greatest part of the remaining image degradation are directional scatter and collimator blur. After some attention to geometrical arrangements, it can be decided that collimator blur is described by linear systems theory and can be removed by simple deconvolution. It does not appear to be as easy to remove the directional scatter. In this paper, we are primarily interested in removing directional scatter but to prevent difficulties in recognizing the errors, the distant dependent collimator blur was removed also. Both additions to the algorithm improved images of the Jaszczak phantom.

II. DECONVOLUTION OF THE COLLIMATOR

Collimator error is well known to be depth dependent. Therefore, the point spread function should be expected to be spatial variant. Since a given pixel in the image is influenced by many views at many distances away, it was decided that the spatially variant point spread function should be applied to the views themselves. In order to do this, each view was replicated repeatedly to form a two dimensional array, see fig. 1. Each replicated copy of the view is a different distance from the collimator and can be deconvolved for the point spread function for that distance from the collimator. Backprojection can be done by rotating this array to a proper angle and adding it to the backprojection sum. The point spread function to be used is known, at least approximately, and can be found in Vol. I of Barrett and Swindell[1].

III. ANALYSIS OF DIRECTIONAL COMPTON SCATTER ERROR

At the beginning of the study of directional scatter, an experiment was done to demonstrate the appearance of the error. Two long strips of masking tape were stretched down the length of the bed track on an ADAC two headed camera. The tapes were elevated above the floor at a height near the center of the camera's field of view. The bed, which is removable, was not present. A source of TcO4 was connected to one tape while a standard 2 cm saline bottle of the type used to dilute injections was connected to the other tape to serve as a scatterer. An image was obtained both with the ADAC computer and with a backprojection program written for this project. A sinogram was produced, and raw views were examined. It was noticed in the raw views that blurring of the source could only occur in the raw views during the time that the source was behind the scatterer but not otherwise. In the great majority of the views, a non-blurred image of the primary source was available to the backprojector. This makes intuitive sense and is also consistent with the known angular behavior of Compton scatter. Data tables for Compton scatter[1] indicate that scatter is smaller at 180 degrees (complete reflection) than at 0 degrees (complete transmission), and is smallest for 90 degree angles, which would lead to the observed behavior. A more serious difficulty was the fact that the scatterer fed inconsistent information to the backprojector. This can be seen in the sinogram from the single source - single scatterer experiment, fig. 2. Here the source is seen forming a proper sine wave but the scatterer only forms a short segment of a sine wave intersected by the source sine wave. In terms of the backprojection algorithm, the scatterer appears to be a blinking source which is only illuminated for a short time during the scan. Since backprojection cannot deal with changing sources, erroneous rays which stretched completely across the image were generated in a small number of consecutive views. These rays would actually form an image of the scatterer if the scatterer was seen in all views but in actuality form a streak across the image. This phenomenon occurs in C/T brain scans where it sometimes causes streaks between the clinoid bones. It is referred to as Houndsfield artifact. The Houndsfield artifact was associated with Compton scatter in a paper by Glover[2] in 1982.

From the preceding analysis of the raw views and sinogram, it was decided that the directional Compton scatter errors would be minimized if rays were more directly associated with their primary and scattered sources and not written for long distances across the backprojector. This can partly be done by the use of a theorem due to Edholm[3] where data from the back half of the image can be removed from the sinogram. This is often referred to as the energy-distance theorem or the frequency distance theorem. In this theorem, the back half is specified with respect to moving coordinates which are connected to the detector head of the camera. The method described in the theorem works by taking the 2-D Fourier transform of the sinogram and zeroing the second and fourth quadrants. After zeroing, the inverse 2-D Fourier tranform is applied to produce the corrected sinogram. By taking a narrower angle than the 90 degrees for a full quadrant, sections of the image can be selected which are smaller than one half. Currently, our program only divides the image in halves. This prevents activity in the rear of the image from scattering off voxels in the front, but does not prevent activity in the front of the image from scattering off other pixels which are also in the front of the image. In the future, we wish to expand the program to divide the image into smaller sections, but eventually a choice will have to be made between the amount of computer time available and the number of sections into which the image is divided. Up to the present time, we have not had good results utilizing the back half of the data to produce the back half of the image. Instead it appears the image is optimized by using only the front half of the sinogram data in the front half of the backprojector to produce the front of the image. In terms of directional scatter this would mean that it is better not to view sources behind the scatter at all.

IV. RESULTS

First, a control image of a Jaszczak phantom was produced using a standard filtered backprojection method. The algorithm included Nowak's method[4] in which views are collected for a full 360 degrees but they are only written half way across the backprojector array. The rear of the backprojector is filled by the view which differs in angle by 180 degrees. This idea was originally based on each view being most accurate for points nearest the view, but it also has value as a directional scatter removal method. The algorithm also included a Butterworth filter. Scan parameters were 128x128 pixels, 128 stops, 45 sec/stop, VXUR collimator. Images were taken on an ADAC dual head Genisys camera. Images are shown in fig. 3a for 25 pixel thick slices and in fig. 3b for 5 pixel thick slices. The 5 pixel thickness is equivalent to what is possible near the high end of patient exposure levels. The thicker slice can only be used in quality control situations. Next, Edholm's method of removing the back of the image from the sinogram was included and also, collimator deconvolution. These images are shown in fig. 3c for 25 pixels and fig. 3d for 5 pixels. The general improvement in resolution which is seen especially toward the center was due to the inclusion of the collimator deconvolution while the improvement in visualizing the coating of Tc on the top of the air bubble was due to Edholm's correction. It was surprising that collimator deconvolution improvements could be made even with a VXUR collimator because this collimator is a great improvement over collimators made in earlier years. What was not revealed in making this image was whether or not the algorithm is removing artifacts which are directly related to directional scatter. A run was made on the data containing the small isolated scatterer and source, and the image of the scatterer was removed by the algorithm of Edholm's theorem, but this is not conclusive proof that directional scatter in complex images will behave the same way. There also did not appear to be much interaction between the collimator blur and the directional scatter, which was feared in the beginning

V. CONCLUSION

Detailed analysis of the directional scatter problem in SPECT showed it to have features which were entirely SPECT related besides those that affect ordinary static images. Because SPECT in many ways has higher overall image quality than static imaging, it sometimes handles directional scatter better and sometimes worse. Those times when SPECT is better are reminiscent of the human eye's ability to recognize a rotating object behind a frosted glass better than a fixed object in the same circumstances. SPECT even allows some kind of a look behind the glass. Unfortunately, SPECT also malfunctions in these cases and makes streaks across the image. Using this analysis of the artifacts, improvements were made to a standard backprojection method which although lengthening reconstruction time, showed improvements in the image. It was further learned that even with very good collimators, collimator deconvolution improves the image.

VI. BIBLIOGRAPHY

1) Barrett, H. H., and Swindell, W., Radiological Imaging, Vol. 1, Academic Press, 1981.

2) Glover, G., "Compton Scatter Effects in CT Reconstructions," Med. Phys., pg. 860, Vol. 9, No. 6, Nov/Dec 1982.

3) Xia, W., Lewitt, R. M., Edholm, P. R., "Fourier Correction for Spatially Variant Collimator Blurring in SPECT," IEEE T-MI, Mar. 1995.

4) Hellman, R. S., Nowak, D., Collier, B. D., Isitman, A., Eisner, R., "Evaluation of Distance-Weighted SPECT Reconstruction for Skeletal Scintigraphy," Radiology, pg. 473, Vol. 159, No. 2, May 1986.

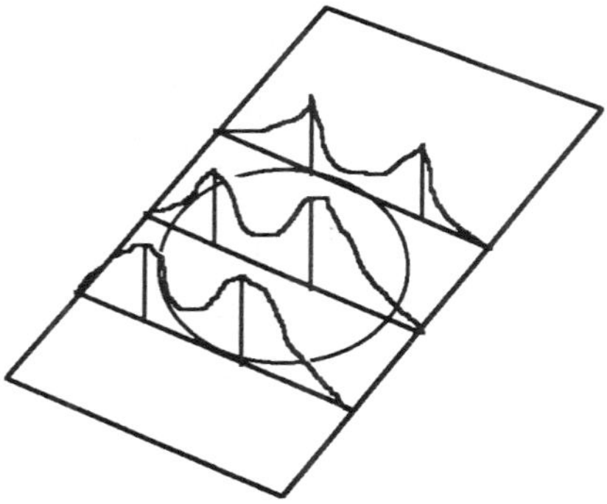

Fig. 1: Showing the layout of the collimator deconvolution algorithm

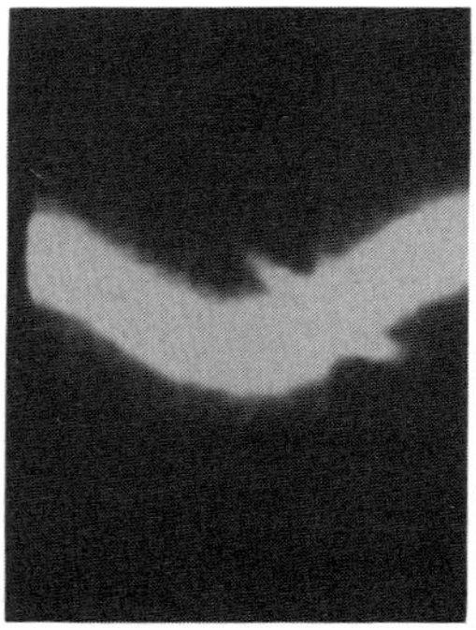

Fig. 2: Sinogram from single source - single detector experiment.

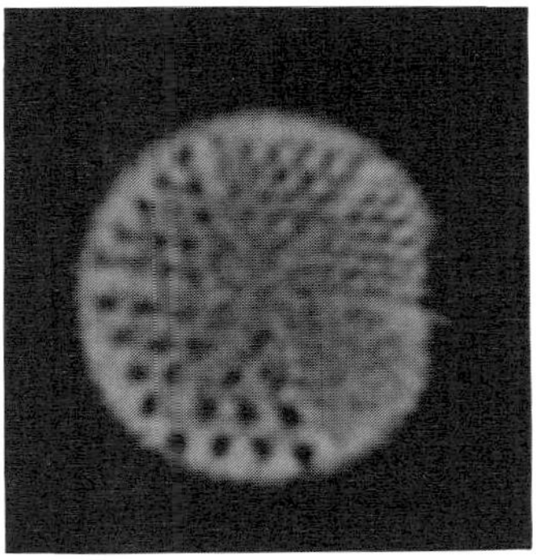

Fig. 3a: Control Jaszczak phantom image, 25 pixels thick.

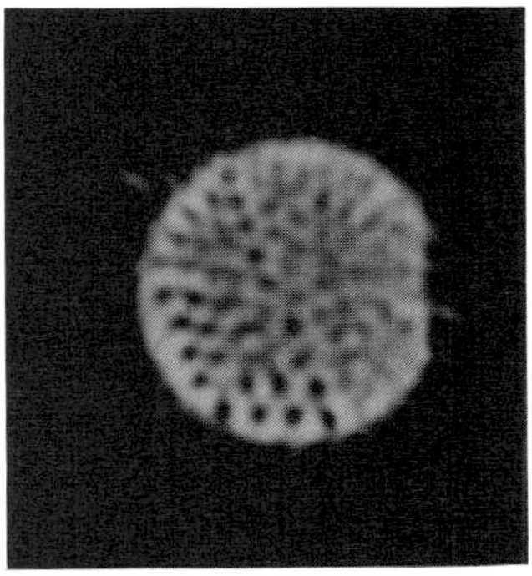

Fig. 3b: Control Jaszczak phantom image, 5 pixels thick.

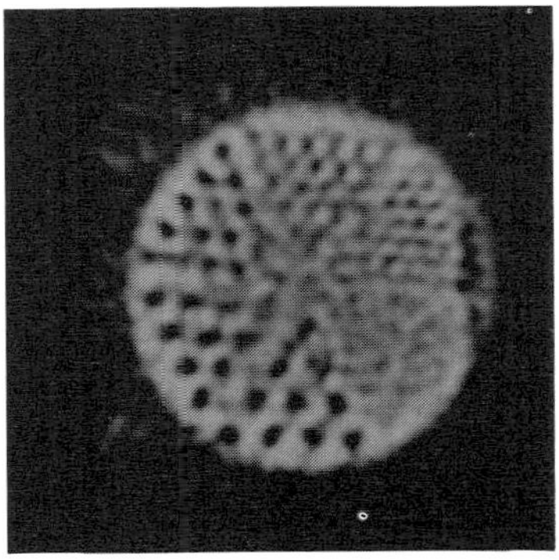

Fig. 3c: Improved Jaszczak phantom image, 25 pixels thick.

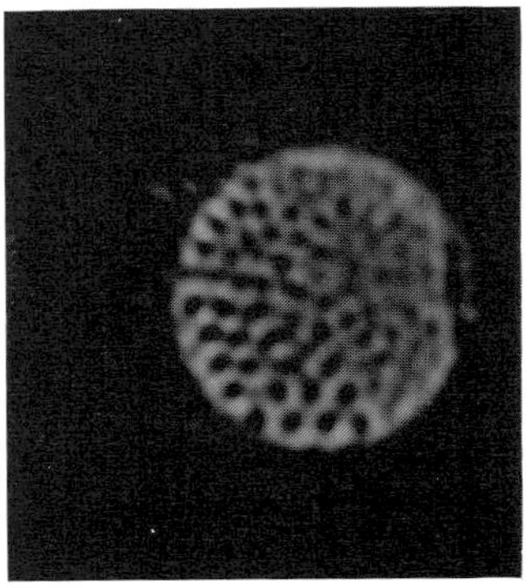

Fig. 3d: Improved Jaszczak phantom image, 5 pixels thick.

Author Index

AUTHOR INDEX